PSYCHOPATHOLOGY AND PSYCHIATRY

PSYCHOPATHOLOGY AND PSYCHIATRY

IVAN P. PAVLOV

WITH A NEW INTRODUCTION BY
GEORGE WINDHOLZ

TRANSACTION PUBLISHERS
NEW BRUNSWICK (U.S.A.) AND LONDON (U.K.)

New material this edition copyright © 1994 by Transaction Publishers, New Brunswick, New Jersey 08903. Originally published by Foreign Languages Publishing House, Moscow, U.S.S.R.

All rights reserved under International and Pan-American Copyright Conventions. No part of this book may be reproduced or transmitted in any form or by any means, electronic or mechanical, including photocopy, recording, or any information storage and retrieval system, without prior permission in writing from the publisher. All inquiries should be addressed to Transaction Publishers, Rutgers—The State University, New Brunswick, New Jersey 08903.

Library of Congress Catalog Number: 93-5454
ISBN: 1-56000-707-9
Printed in the United States of America

Library of Congress Cataloging-in-Publication Data

Pavlov, Ivan Petrovich, 1849-1936.
  [Psikhopatoligiia i psikhiatriia, English]
  Psychopathology and psychiatry/Ivan P. Pavlov; with a new introduction by George Windholz.
     p. cm.
  Translated from the Russian by D. Myshne and S. Belsky.
  Originally published: Moscow: Foreign Languages Pub. House, 1961?
  Includes bibliographical references and indexes.
  ISBN 1-56000-707-9
  1. Neuropsychiatry. 2. Neuropsychology. I. Title.
  [DNLM: 1. Mental Disorders—collected works. 2. Nervous System—collected works. WM 7 P338p 1993a]
RC341.P3313 1993
616.89—dc20a
DNLM/DLC
for Library of Congress   93-5454
                                                              CIP

CONTENTS

INTRODUCTION TO THE TRANSACTION EDITION 1

Psychopathology and Psychiatry

Experimental Psychology and Psychopathology in Animals . . 13
On Sleep 31
On Inhibition and Sleep 34
Conditions for Active and Resting States of the Cerebral Hemispheres 44
Some Facts About the Physiology of Sleep 53
Psychiatry as an Auxiliary to the Physiology of the Cerebral Hemispheres 60
Concerning the So-Called Hypnotism in Animals 70
Relations Between Excitation and Inhibition, Delimitation Between Excitation and Inhibition, Experimental Neuroses in Dogs 72
Normal and Pathological States of the Cerebral Hemispheres 87
Inhibitory Type of Nervous System in Dogs 100
Internal Inhibition and Sleep Are Essentially the Same Physicochemical Process 109
Transitional Phases Between the Animal's Waking and Complete Sleep (Hypnotic Phases) 126
Different Types of Nervous System. Pathological States of the Cerebral Hemispheres as a Result of Functional Influences Exerted on Them 147
Pathological States of the Cerebral Hemispheres as a Result of Functional Influences Exerted on Them 167
Application to Man of Experimental Data Obtained on Animals 187
Physiological Teaching on Types of Nervous System or Temperaments 208
Some Problems of the Physiology of the Cerebral Hemispheres 220

An Attempt of a Physiologist to Digress into the Domain of
   Psychiatry 225
Physiology of the Hypnotic State of the Dog 232
On Neuroses in Man and Animals 247
Experimental Neuroses 251
Essay on the Physiological Concept of the Symptomatology
   of Hysteria 255
Physiology of Higher Nervous Activity 282
Example of an Experimentally Produced Neurosis and Its Cure
   in a Weak Type of Nervous System 298
Feelings of Possession (Les Sentiments d'Emprise) and the
   Ultraparadoxical Phase 303
Attempt at a Physiological Interpretation of Compulsive
   Neurosis and Paranoia 309
General Types of Animal and Human Higher Nervous Activity 325
Experimental Pathology of the Higher Nervous Activity . . 355
The Conditioned Reflex 378
Types of Higher Nervous Activity, Their Relationship to Neu-
   roses and Psychoses and the Physiological Mechanism of
   Neurotic and Psychotic Symptoms 387
The Problem of Sleep 393

NOTES (Compiled by Prof. L. Rokhlin) 413
NAME INDEX 439
SUBJECT INDEX 441

INTRODUCTION TO THE TRANSACTION EDITION

Ivan Petrovich Pavlov's theory of higher nervous activity is concerned with organisms high on the phylogenetic scale, such as dogs, apes, and humans, and their adaptation to changing external environments. The theory encompasses normal as well as abnormal activities. In the 1920s, Pavlov and his disciples—Pavlovians—used laboratory experimentation to study the etiology and therapy of neuroses. In addition to laboratory experiments, Pavlov devoted much time and effort in the 1930s to the systematic study of psychopathology in the clinical setting. However, it is very possible that Pavlov's interest in psychopathology came much earlier; it might have appeared in his youthful years in Ryazan, Russia.

Pavlov's interest might have stemmed from his concern for the condition of his mother, Varvara Pavlova. After the birth of her third child, she developed a "nervous disorder"; she suffered terrible headaches that extended over parts of her head, a skin disorder that led to a partial loss of hair, and she would withdraw for days into a locked room. Pavlov's disciple, P. K. Anokhin suggested that Varvara's condition had been organic, but this was only a guess on his part because he never examined her.

Years later Pavlov took psychiatry courses at the University of St. Petersburg, where the examiner, I. P. Merzheevskiy attested in 1879 that Pavlov passed a course in nervous and psychiatric disorders. In 1930, Pavlov recalled that he had once studied psychiatry at the university but had forgotten what he had learned. This is not surprising because after receiving the M.D. degree in 1883, Pavlov's scholarly achievements were first in circulatory and later in digestive physiology. Nevertheless, Pavlov was still interested in psycho-pathology. In 1901, he began the systematic study of the conditioned reflex phenomena, and in 1903 he delivered at the International Medical Congress in Madrid a programmatic speech titled "Experimental Psychology and Psychopathology in Animals."

In 1918, Pavlov ventured from the laboratory to the psychiatric section at the Udelninskaya Hospital in Petrograd, where the psychiatrist V. P. Golovina demonstrated to Pavlov two catatonic patients. Pavlov interpreted the condition of the two patients in terms of his theory of higher nervous activity which was based on laboratory experiments with dogs as subjects. Pavlov proposed that neural inhibition spread over those parts of the patients' cerebral cortex that controlled motor movements. In the 1920s, Pavlov serendipitously encountered abnormal behavior in laboratory dogs and in the 1930s he and his disciples began to systematically study abnormal psychology and psychiatry. To this end, they devoted considerable effort and time.

The Pavlovians used two fundamental approaches in their study of neuroses and psychoses: the conditioned salivary reflex method with dogs as subjects and the observation of neurotic and psychotic behavior in humans.

The first method was based on the laboratory discovery of conditioned reflexes. In 1898, Pavlov's student S. G. Wolfson found that salivary secretion in dogs depended upon the nature of foods; moist foods evoked a lower rate of salivary flow than dry foods. Wolfson also noticed, serendipitously, that his dogs salivated when these foods were presented at a distance. Salivation to food presented at a distance was an anomaly; according to the classical, Cartesian conceptualization, a reflexive action occurred only when environmental stimuli impinged directly on the sensory receptors of the reflex. During the 1910s, Pavlov explained that salivation to food objects presented at a distance occurs because it was mediated by the cerebral cortex.

Thus, Pavlov, who at that time was working on the process of digestion, became interested in the function of cerebral hemispheres, mainly that of the cortex. But the method he used to study the function of the cortex differed from contemporary methods. Since the latter part of the nineteenth century, the method frequently used in the study of the function of the cortex was extirpation. Pavlov, however, rejected extirpation as too crude to determine the intricate function of the cortex. Assuming that salivary flow was a precise indicator of cortical function in the organism's interaction with the external environment, Pavlov rejected extirpation in favor of the conditioned salivary reflex. That is, for the Pavlovians, the conditioned salivary reflex was primarily of methodological importance. Other conditioned reflexes, such as the alimentary and orienting, were considered as having far greater adaptive properties but were poor indicators of cortical activity.

During the first decade of the twentieth century, Pavlov and his students discovered the fundamental principles of the function of the cortex. The following paradigmatic experiment shows acquisition of the conditioned reflex. When any indifferent stimulus was followed by swallowing food (unconditioned stimulus or UCS) which evoked salivation (unconditioned response or UCR) then, after several pairings, the indifferent stimulus became an effective evocator (conditioned stimulus or CS) of salivary flow (conditioned response or CR). The conditioned reflex was established between the CS and the UCS because both occurred simultaneously. Once the CS was repeatedly presented, but not reinforced with the UCS, the CR slowly extinguished. But, once the conditioned reflex was established, stimuli similar to the original CS evoked similar CRs, that is, became generalized. When two CS were presented, each evoking a CR, and when the first of these was reinforced, whereas the second was not, the presentation of the first CS evoked a CR, but the presentation of the second CS did not evoke a CR, that is, differentiation.

Pavlov was mainly interested in the function of the cortex in the organisms' adaptation to the external environment. The conditioned reflex findings were explained in terms of hypothetical physiological process. Two distinct processes, excitation and inhibition, either irradiated or concentrated over the cortical regions. Thus, in the experiment on the acquisition of the conditioned reflex, an indifferent stimulus impinged, as a locus of excitation, on the cortex, then the excitation irradiated over the cortex merging with irradiation stemming from the UCS that formed its own locus of excitation in the cortex. This physiological connection was, on the psychological level, expressed as an association between the CS and the UCS. Failure to reinforce the established CS with UCS resulted, on the cortical level, in the generation of inhibition that irradiated from its locus over the cortex, and which resulted in the disestablishment of the connections previously made between the loci of excitation of the CS and UCS. On the psychological level, there occurred a disassociation between the CS and the UCS, resulting in the extinction of the conditioned reflex. Thus, Pavlov conceptualized the organism's complex interaction with the environment as one which was mediated by an intricate interplay of excitation and inhibition which irradiated and concentrated in the cortex.

The higher organism's motivation to act in the environment emerged in the subcortical regions of the cerebral hemispheres in the form of complex unconditioned reflexes, or instinct. But, survival of higher animals through activities generated by instincts alone was unlikely because such activities were too rigid. Such instinctual activities were insufficient to react to the continuously changing environment. However, the organism's survival was greatly enhanced by the more flexible conditioned reflexes. That is, the struggle for existence, which led to the survival of an individual for some longer period of time, was enhanced by proper acquisitions and extinctions, as well by generalizations and differentiations, of conditioned reflexes.

However, in a changing environment, a previously established acquisition or extinction of conditioned reflexes could become dysfunctional. This meant that the adaptation of the organism to the external environment could be inappropriate. Serendipitous events in Pavlov's laboratory provided evidence for conditions leading to the organism's failure to adapt successfully to the environment.

In 1914, the ophthalmologist N. R. Shenger-Krestovnikova attempted to determine the threshold of visual differentiation in dogs. She conditioned each animal to respond to a circle of light projected on a screen in a dark room, but not to respond to an ellipse. Then she projected a series of figures with changed proportions of the horizontal and vertical diameters. The dogs salivated to most proportions, save to that of 9 to 8 for horizontal to vertical diameters. The dogs whined, yelped, and were very excited. Pavlov, who was familiar with Josef Breuer's and Sigmund Freud's case of Anna O., realized that the dogs' unusual behavior resulted from a conflict between excitation and inhibition and referred to this phenomenon as "experimental neurosis."

In 1924, Pavlov's Leningrad laboratory was inundated during a flood. When some time later the laboratory dogs that had been rescued with great difficulty were used again in experiments, their previously conditioned reflexes disappeared. Instead, the dogs did not eat and showed much fear. It took the Pavlovians considerable effort to recondition the dog. Pavlov concluded that there was a similarity between the dogs's reaction and traumatized human behavior.

Therefore, in the 1920s, Pavlov was certain that the dogs' inability to adapt flexibly to the changing external environment was the result of conflicts and traumatic experiences. Soon Pavlov would link these discoveries to actual human cases of neuroses and psychoses. To that end, Pavlov, under the guidance of psychiatrists, studied the abnormal behavior of hospitalized patients in mental institutions.

Almost every second Wednesday afternoon, Pavlov and a group of psychiatrists, among whom the most prominent were B. N. Birman and A. G. Ivanov-Smolenskiy, met in seminars now known as "Clinical Wednesdays." The seminars took place in either the nervous or psychiatric clinics attached to Leningrad hospitals. Human neuroses were studied in the Nervous Clinic at the Neuro-Psychiatric Hospital, whereas psychoses were considered in the Psychiatric Clinic at the Balinskiy Psychiatric Hospital. As a rule, the seminars followed this course. The psychiatrists introduced cases with the objective of allowing Pavlov to familiarize himself with the widest range of abnormal disorders. After the introduction of a case, which consisted of the description of the patient's anamnesis, the patient was brought into the room. Usually, Pavlov asked the patient to describe his condition. Surprisingly, Pavlov did not use the conditioned reflex method with the patients, but occasionally hypnosis was used! After the patient left, Pavlov asked the psychiatrists to elaborate on the characteristics of the diagnosed disorder and to express their views on the case at hand. Pavlov, then, explained the etiology and recommended a therapy of the disorder from the perspective of the theory of the higher nervous activity. In this way Pavlov linked theory, derived from laboratory experiments on animals, with actual disorders found in humans derived through observing neurotic or psychotic patients.

Pavlov's explanation of abnormal disorders in humans took into consideration the interaction between the organism's innate aspects and environmental conditions. Three related processes were considered to be responsible for abnormal human behavior: the temperaments, the second signal system, and the impact of the environment. The temperaments, according to Pavlov, were the innate characteristics of higher organisms. Pavlov reached the conclusion that there were differences in temperaments after observing the behavior of dogs in the laboratory where some were cowardly while others were bold. By the 1930s, Pavlov concluded that temperaments were primarily the result of three properties of the nervous processes: the strength, equilibrium, and mobility of excitation and inhibition. The strength of the nervous processes referred to the extent to which the organism was able to withstand taxing environmental conditions. The equilibrium of the nervous process pertained to the relation between excitation and inhibition. In the cases of equilibrium, no processes predominated over the other, whereas disequilibrium manifests itself either in overexcitement or undue restraint. The organism's mobility, or speed in reacting to the changing environmental conditions, was important to survival because life or death depends upon a judicious reaction to the environment.

It could be expected that a combination of these three characteristics would produce many types of temperament, but in reality only four have been observed. In 1935, Pavlov described these four types of temperament. The weak type was most susceptible to behave abnormally; its lack of powerful excitatory and inhibitory nervous processes made it unable to deal with, or withstand the pressure of taxing environmental conditions. The strong type did not easily succumb to difficult environmental conditions and, therefore, was not prone to behave abnormally. This was certainly true if the strong reactions of excitation and inhibition were in equilibrium and responded rapidly to changing environmental conditions. However, the strong type was prone to abnormal behavior if its excitatory and inhibitory processes were in equilibrium, but its reaction to the environment was sluggish.

The strong type was also prone to abnormal behavior if its excitatory processes were much stronger than the inhibitory processes. In this case the dog became very excited but its actions were not inhibited in environmental situations that demanded such restraint.

This typology of temperaments pertained to dogs, but Pavlov did not consider the activity of dogs and humans to be on the same plane. The main difference between humans and other higher animals was in the second signal system. The second signal system was the unique humans characteristic of language.

The basic reaction of higher organisms to the environment was reflexive. But reflexes could be conditioned when a previously indifferent stimulus became associated with the stimulus which, originally, triggered the reflex. In this case, the conditioned stimulus became a signal to the organism, signifying a characteristic of the environment. For instance, the location of food became a signal indicating where this food was to be found and a certain movement of a predator became a signal to the prey to escape. Conditioned stimuli constituted the first signal system. However, human beings, unlike the other higher animals, used and responded to language. Therefore, language constituted the second signal system, a symbolic activity ranging from single words to complex sentences.

The relations of the first and second signal systems characterized human personality types. Individuals with the first signal system predominating over the second signal system, were prone to respond to environmental stimuli and were denoted by Pavlov as *artistic*. Individuals with the second signal system predominating over the first signal system were denoted by Pavlov as *thinking*. Individuals with equally strong first and the second signal system, were rarely found. Leonardo da Vinci belonged to the latter because he was a great artist as well a profound thinker. However, individuals in which both systems were weak, were found quite often.

The relative dominance in artistic and thinking characteristics was related to specific neuroses. Thus, the weak, predominantly artistic type was prone to hysteria, which manifested itself in temporary paralyses and convulsions, as well as in emotional outbursts and fantasies. The weak, predominantly intellectual type tended toward psychasthenia, which manifested itself in lack of realism, in an inappropriate understanding of the environment, and in obsessions and phobias. Weakness of both the artistic and intellectual processes was associated with neurasthenia, which manifested itself in general exhaustion. However, nowhere did this typology imply that the artistic type was hysterical or that the thinking type was psychasthenic per se. Neuroses were the consequences of the individual's nervous system inability to withstand a taxing environment.

Among the psychoses, schizophrenia interested Pavlov most. Thus, in the Psychiatric Clinic, Pavlov saw from 1931 to 1936, forty-five schizophrenic patients. Pavlov considered schizophrenia to be the result of an overwhelming neural excitation in the brains of individuals with a weak nervous system. He devoted considerable time to finding a cure for schizophrenia, finally recommending the prolonged sleep therapy to reduce neural excitation. This therapy was initiated in the 1920s by the Swiss psychiatrist J. Klaesi. Pavlov was unaware that this therapy was of limited effectiveness and dangerous to patients' lives because this became known shortly before Pavlov's death.

The articles and excerpts included in this volume constitute a selection of Pavlov's works in psychopathology and areas related to psychopathology spanning more than three decades. Not all selections pertain directly to psychopathology, such, for instance, as Pavlov's conceptualization of sleep. The inclusion of such topics is, however, important to the understanding of Pavlov's concept of inhibition as it contributes to the understanding of the organism's self-regulating activity and schizophrenia.

Pavlov's last twenty-five years of life were traumatized by social and political events in Russia. Pavlov considered himself a Russian patriot and a liberal and could not reconcile himself with the policies of the Soviet rulers. Pavlov's initial reaction to the Soviet regime was to emigrate, but Lenin rejected this request by maintaining that Pavlov's contribution to the construction of the communist society was invaluable. Pavlov remained in the Soviet Union, but did not remain silent. Pavlov maintained that the Soviet regime was based on lies and lawlessness. In 1923, Pavlov openly attacked Nikolai Bukharin, at that time one of the most important of Russia's Bolshevik rulers, by pointing out that his, Bukharin's, conceptualization of Marxist theory was internally inconsistent. Pavlov's plea for freedom of inquiry was met by Bukharin with derision.

Pavlov's theory of higher nervous activity could be now considered to be mainly of historical value. As such, it could be placed side by side with its contemporary, Sigmund Freud's psychoanalysis. Post-Pavlovian psychologists and psychiatrists may argue, perhaps with some justification, that inference of neural processes from experimental findings obtained with the conditioned reflexes method has less validity than the direct neurophysiological investigation of the structure and function of the brain. Nevertheless, the theory of higher nervous activity guided the work of Pavlov and his disciples. Laboratory findings such as the concepts of "experimental neurosis" are considered important contributions to the understanding of conflicts and neuroses. It is, therefore, possible that the most important contribution of Pavlov and his disciples to modern psychology consists of the formulation of a well-developed theory that, if subjected to systematic experimental testing, may explain many vexing problems in abnormal psychology and psychiatry.

George Windholz

PSYCHOPATHOLOGY
and
PSYCHIATRY

EXPERIMENTAL PSYCHOLOGY AND PSYCHOPATHOLOGY IN ANIMALS[1]

Regarding the language of facts as most eloquent, I shall take the liberty of proceeding directly to the experimental material, which gives me the right to speak on the subject of my present communication.

To begin with, this is the history of the transition of the physiologist from research into purely physiological problems to the sphere of phenomena usually called psychical. Although this transition took place suddenly, it occurred in a perfectly natural way, and what seems to me most important in this respect, without changing the, so to speak, methodological front.

In studying over a period of years the normal working of the digestive glands, and analysing the constant conditions of this work, I came upon conditions of a psychical character, which, incidentally, had been observed by others before me. There were no grounds for neglecting these conditions, since they participated constantly and prominently in the normal physiological process. I was obliged to investigate them if I wanted to make a really thorough study of my subject. But how? All that follows in my exposition supplies the answer to this question.

From all our material I shall select only the experiments with the salivary glands—organs which apparently play a very insignificant physiological role; however, I am convinced that they will become classical objects for the new type of research about which I shall have the honour of telling you today; part of this research has already been carried out and part is in the planning stage.

In observing the normal working of the salivary glands one cannot but be amazed by the high degree of their adaptability.

Give the animal dry, hard food substances and there will be an abundant salivary secretion—give it liquid food and the secretion will be much smaller.

It is obvious that for the chemical testing of the food, for mixing it and converting it into a lump to be swallowed, water is required—and the salivary glands supply it. From the mucous salivary glands there flows for every kind of food, saliva rich in mucin—a lubricating saliva, which facilitates the smooth passage of the food into the stomach. All highly irritant substances, such as acids, salts, etc., also produce a salivary secretion which varies in accordance with the strength of their stimulating action; clearly, as we know from everyday experience, the purpose of this secretion is to neutralise or dilute the substances and to cleanse the mouth. In this case the mucous glands secrete fluid saliva containing little mucin. For what would be the purpose of the mucin here? If pure insoluble quartz pebbles are placed in the mouth of a dog it will move them around, try to chew them, and finally, it will drop them. There is either no secretion of saliva at all, or at most two or three drops flow out. Again, what purpose would the saliva serve here? The pebbles are easily ejected by the animal and nothing remains in the mouth. But if sand is placed in the dog's mouth, i.e., the same pebbles but in pulverised form, there will be an abundant flow of saliva. It is clear that without saliva, without fluid in the oral cavity, the sand could neither be ejected, nor forwarded to the stomach.

Here we have exact and constant facts—facts which seem to imply intelligence. But the entire mechanism of this intelligence is absolutely plain. On the one hand, physiology has long known about the centrifugal nerves of the salivary glands, which now chiefly cause water to enter into the saliva, and now accumulate in the saliva special organic substances. On the other hand, the internal lining of the oral cavity consists of separate areas which act as receptors of different special stimuli—mechanical, chemical, thermal. Moreover, these stimuli may be further subdivided, the chemical, for example, into salts, acids, etc. There are grounds for assuming that the same thing is true of the mechanical stimuli. It is in the areas acting as receptors of special stimuli that the specific centripetal nerves have their origin.

Thus, the reactions of adaptation are based on a simple reflex originated by definite external conditions acting only on certain kinds of centripetal nerve endings; from here the excitation passes along a definite nervous path to the centre, and thence, also along a definite path, to the salivary gland, evoking its specific function.

In other words, this is a specific external agent evoking a specific reaction in living matter. At the same time we have here a typical example of what we call "adaptation" or "fitness". Let us dwell for a moment on these facts and terms, since they play, obviously, an important role in modern physiological thought. What, exactly, is the fact of adaptation? It is, as we have just seen, simply the exact co-ordination of the elements making up a complex system and of the entire complex with the surrounding world.

But the same thing can be observed in any inanimate object. Take, for example, a complex chemical object. This object exists thanks to equilibration between its separate atoms and groups, between the object as a whole and the surroundings.

In exactly the same way the immense complexity of the higher and lower organisms exists as a whole so long as all its constituents are delicately and strictly co-ordinated and equilibrated both with one another and with the external conditions.

The analysis of the equilibration of this system is the prime task and aim of physiological investigation as purely objective investigation. There can hardly be two opinions on this point. Unfortunately, so far we have no purely scientific term to denote this fundamental property of the organism, its external and internal equilibrium. Many people hold that the terms now in use—fitness and adaptation (despite their natural-scientific, Darwinist analysis) —bear the stamp of subjectivism, which leads to misunderstanding in two opposite directions. The rigid adherents of the physico-mechanical theory of life see in these words an anti-scientific tendency—a retreat from pure objectivism to speculation and teleology. On the other hand, philosophically inclined biologists see in every fact relating to adaptation and fitness proof of the existence of a special vital force, or, as it is now more and more often called, spiritual force (vitalism, apparently, gives way to animism), which defines its own goal, chooses its means, adapts itself, etc.

And so, in the afore-mentioned physiological experiments with the salivary glands we, in our investigation, remain strictly within the bounds of natural science. We shall now pass to another sphere of phenomena which, it would seem, belong to quite a different category.

All the foregoing objects, which, after being placed in the mouth, influenced the salivary glands in different and at the same time definite ways, exert on these glands exactly the same action, at least qualitatively, when placed at a certain distance from the dog. Dry food produces much saliva—moist food only a little. A thick, lubricating saliva flows from the mucous glands to the food substances. Various inedible irritants also produce secretion from all the glands, including the mucous glands. But it is fluid and contains but a small amount of mucin. Pebbles, when shown to the animal, have no effect on the glands, while sand evokes profuse salivation. These facts were partly obtained and partly systematised in my laboratory by Dr.

S. G. Wolfson. The dog sees, hears, and smells all these substances, pays attention to them, rushes to them if edible or agreeable, but turns away from them and resists their introduction into the mouth when disagreeable. Everybody would say that this is a psychical reaction, psychical stimulation of the animal's salivary glands.

How should the physiologist regard these facts? How can he establish them? How to analyse them? What are they compared with physiological facts? What are their common features and in what way are they distinguished from one another?

Must we, for the purpose of getting to know the new phenomena, penetrate into the inner state of the animal, visualise its feelings and desires in our own way?

It seems to me that for the naturalist there is only one answer to the last question—an emphatic "No". Where is there even the slightest indisputable criterion that our conjectures are correct, that we can, for the sake of a better understanding of the matter, compare the inner state of even such a highly developed animal as the dog with our own? Further: Is not the eternal sorrow of life the fact that in most cases human beings do not understand each other and cannot enter into the inner state of the other? And then, where is the knowledge, where is the power of knowledge that might enable us correctly to comprehend the state of another human being? At first, in our psychical experiments with the salivary glands (for the time being we shall use the term "psychical"), we conscientiously endeavoured to explain our results by imagining the subjective state of the animal. But nothing came of this except sterile controversy and individual views that could not be reconciled. And so we could do nothing but conduct the research on a purely objective basis; our first and especially important task was completely to abandon the very natural tendency to transfer our own subjective state to the mechanism of the reaction of the animal undergoing the experiment and to concentrate instead on studying the correlation between the external phenomena and the reaction of the organism, i.e., the activity of the salivary glands. Reality had to decide whether elaboration of the new phenomena was possible in that direction. I make bold to say that the following account will convince you, as I am convinced, that a boundless field of fruitful research opens before us in the given case; it is another and immense part of the physiology of the nervous system, a system which mainly establishes the correlation not between the separate parts of the organism, our main subject so far, but between the organism and the surroundings. Unfortunately, to date the influence of the surrounding world on the nervous system has been studied mainly in relation to subjective reactions—the content of the modern physiology of the sense organs.

In our psychical experiments we have before us definite external objects, exciting the animal and evoking in it a definite reaction, in the given case—secretion of the salivary glands. As has been said, the effect of these objects is substantially the same as in the physiological experiments, when they come into contact with the oral cavity. Consequently, we have before us simply further adaptation—the object acts on the salivary glands the moment it is being brought close to the mouth.

What are the specific features of these new phenomena compared with the physiological ones? Above all, the difference seems to be that in the physiological form of the experiment the substance come into direct contact with the organism, while in the psychical form it acts from a distance. But this circumstance in itself, if we reflect on it, does not, obviously, signify any essential difference between these, in a way specific, experiments, and the purely physiological ones. The point is that in these cases the substances act on other special receiving surfaces of the body—nose, eye, ear—through the medium in which both the organism and the stimulating substances exist (air, ether). How many simple physiological reflexes are transmitted by the nose, eye and ear, that is, originate at a distance! Hence, the essential difference between the new phenomena and the purely physiological does not lie here.

It lies much deeper, and should be sought, in my view, in a comparison of the following facts. In the physiological case the activity of the salivary glands is connected with the properties of the substance on which the effect of the saliva is directed. The saliva moistens dry substances and any ingested material; it neutralises the chemical effect of the substances. These properties constitute the special stimuli of the specific mouth surface. Consequently, in the physiological experiments the animal is stimulated by the essential, unconditioned properties of the object in relation to the physiological role of the saliva.

In the psychical experiments the animal is excited by the properties of the external object, which are unessential for the activity of the salivary glands, or even entirely accidental. The visual, acoustic and even purely olfactory properties of our objects, when they are present in other objects, do not of themselves exert any influence on the salivary glands which, in their turn, so to speak, have no business relations with these properties. In the psychical experiments the salivary glands are stimulated not only by the properties of the objects unessential for the work of the glands, but absolutely by all the conditions surrounding these objects, or with which they are connected one way or another—for example, the dish in which they are contained, the article on which they are placed, the room, the people who usually bring the objects, even the noises produced by these people, though the latter may not be seen at the given moment—their voices, even the sound of their steps. Thus, in psychical experiments, the connection of the objects acting as stimuli on the salivary glands becomes more and more distant and delicate. Here, undoubtedly, we have a phenomenon of further adaptation. We can admit in this case that such a distant and delicate connection as that between the step of the person who usually feeds the animal and the working of the salivary glands has no specific physiological significance other than its delicacy. But we need only recall those animals whose saliva contains protective poison, to appreciate the great vital significance of this timely provision of a protective means against an approaching enemy. The significance of the distant signs of objects producing a motor reaction in the organism, is, of course, easily recognised. By means of distant and even accidental characteristics of objects the animal seeks its food, evades enemies, etc.

If that is so, then the following questions are of decisive significance for our subject: can this seeming chaos of relations be included in a definite scheme? Is it possible to make the phenomena constant, to disclose the laws governing their development and their mechanism? It seems to me that the examples which I shall now present entitle me to give an emphatically positive answer to these questions, to find at the basis of all psychical experiments one and the same special reflex as the chief and most general mechanism. True, in its physiological form, our experiment, excluding, of course, all extraordinary conditions, always yields one and the same result; it is the unconditioned reflex. But the main feature of the psychical experiment is its impermanence, its obvious capriciousness. However, the results of a psychical experiment undoubtedly recur too, otherwise we would not speak of them at all. Consequently, the point is in the greater number of factors which influence the results of a psychical experiment compared with a physiological one. This, then, is a conditioned reflex. Here are facts which show that our psychical material may also be included in a definite scheme and that it is subject to certain laws. These facts were obtained in my laboratory by Dr. I. F. Tolochinov.[2]

It is not difficult to recognise during the first psychical experiments the chief conditions guaranteeing their success, i.e., their constancy. If an animal is stimulated (i.e., its salivary glands) by food placed at a distance, the result of the experiment depends solely on whether the animal has been prepared for it by a certain period of fasting. An animal experiencing keen hunger yields positive results; on the contrary, the most voracious and least fastidious animal, if it has just had a good meal, fails to respond to food placed at a distance. Thinking in terms of physiology we can say that we have here a different degree of excitability of the salivary centre—greatly increased in the first case, and greatly decreased in the second We may rightly assume that just as the carbonic acid contained in the blood determines the energy of the respiratory centre, so the different composition of the blood in a hungry animal and in one that is sated determines the above-mentioned fluctuations in the excitability and reactivity of the salivary centres. From the subjective point of view this could be designated as attention. When the stomach is empty, the sight of food easily causes the mouth to water; in sated animals the same reaction is either very weak or entirely lacking.

Let us proceed. If the animal is shown food or certain disagreeable substances, and if this is repeated several times, then with each repetition the experiment will produce a weaker result, and in the end there will be no reaction whatever. There is, however, a sure method of restoring the reaction; it can be achieved by giving the dog food or by introducing into its mouth substances which ceased to act as stimuli. This, of course, produces the usual strong reflex, and the object begins to act from a distance again. For the subsequent result it is immaterial whether food is placed in the mouth or any disagreeable substance. For example, if meat powder no longer stimulates the animal from a distance, its effect can be restored either by letting it eat the powder or by introducing into the mouth a disagreeable substance, e.g., acid. We can say that thanks to the direct reflex the excitability of the salivary centre has been heightened, and the weak stimulus—the object at a distance—has become sufficiently strong. Do we not experience the same thing ourselves when appetite comes with eating, or when, after unpleasant, powerful excitation, we begin to have the appetite that we previously lacked?

Here is a number of other facts of a constant character. The object placed at a distance stimulates the salivary glands not only by the entire complex of its properties, but also by its individual properties. If a hand smelling of meat or meat powder is brought into proximity with the dog, it often proves sufficient to induce a salivary reaction. Similarly the sight of food placed at a distance, and consequently the mere optical effect of the object, may also stimulate the activity of the salivary glands. But the combined, simultaneous action of all these properties of the object always produces a better and greater effect, i.e., the action of the sum of the stimuli is more powerful than each individual stimulus.

The object acts on the salivary glands from a distance not only by means of its inherent properties but also by means of incidental qualities deliberately imparted to it. If we colour the acid black, then even water to which the same colour is added will influence the salivary glands from a distance. However, all incidental qualities deliberately imparted to the distant object begin to act as stimuli of the salivary glands only when the object with its newly acquired properties is brought into contact with the oral cavity at least once. Black-coloured water began to stimulate the salivary glands from a distance only after preliminary introduction of black-coloured acid into the dog's mouth. The stimuli of the olfactory nerves belong to the same group of conditioned properties. The experiments carried out in our laboratory by Dr. A. T. Snarsky showed that simple physiological reflexes from the nasal cavity acting on the salivary glands are conducted only through the sensory nerves lying along the trigeminal nerve. Ammonia, mustard oil, etc., always produce an invariable effect even in a curarised animal. However, if the trigeminal nerves are severed, this action fails. Odours lacking a local stimulating effect have no influence on the salivary glands. If, for example, oil of anise is placed for the first time before a normal dog with constant salivary fistulae there will be no secretion of saliva. But if simultaneously with the odour the oil of anise (which produces a strong local irritation) is brought into contact with the dog's oral cavity, saliva secretion will be induced afterwards by the odour alone.

If food is combined with a disagreeable substance or with a certain property of the disagreeable substance, for example, if you show the dog meat moistened with acid, then, despite the fact that the dog reaches for the meat, a saliva secretion comes from the parotid gland (for meat alone there is no secretion from this gland), i.e., a reaction to the disagreeable substance. Moreover, if owing to repetition the action of the disagreeable substance placed at a distance becomes insignificant, then upon combining it with food which attracts the animal, the reaction always becomes intensified.

As mentioned above, dry food causes abundant saliva secretion, while moist food, on the contrary, produces either a weak flow of saliva or none at all. If one acts on a dog from a distance by showing it two extremes, for instance, dry bread and raw meat, the result will depend on the object which stimulates the dog more strongly, and this can be judged by its motor reaction. If, as usually happens, the dog is stimulated more strongly by the meat, then the only reaction will be the one peculiar to meat, i.e., there will be no saliva secretion. Thus, the bread, although it is before the dog's eyes, remains ineffective. It is possible to impart the smell of sausage or meat to dry bread so that the bread alone acts on the dog's eye, with the sausage or meat only leaving a smell, and yet the only reaction will be that induced by the sausage or meat.

The action of objects from a distance can be inhibited in other ways. If in the presence of a greedy, excitable dog we feed another dog, for example with dry bread, then the salivary glands, which previously evinced a most vivid reaction to the sight of bread, become inactive.

When the dog is placed on the stand for the first time, the sight of dry bread, which produced a very strong action on the salivary glands when the dog was on the floor, now has not even the slightest influence.

I have placed before you a number of easily and exactly recurring facts. It will be obvious that many striking instances of animal training belong to the same category as some of our facts. It follows, therefore, that they have long since testified to the strictly law-governed nature of certain psychical manifestations in animals. It is to be regretted that they have been left so long without science giving them the attention they merit.

So far in my exposition I have not mentioned any phenomenon corresponding to what in the subjective world we call desires. Actually we have not encountered such phenomena. On the contrary, the following fundamental fact constantly recurred before our eyes: the sight of dry bread, to which the dog hardly turned its head, produced an abundant secretion of saliva, whereas meat, to which the dog rushed with avidity, breaking from the stand and gnashing its teeth, failed to exert any influence on the salivary glands when placed at a distance. Thus, what in the subjective world we designate as desire, was expressed in our experiments only by the animal's motor reaction, but did not manifest any positive action on the salivary glands. Hence, the phrase that ardent desire stimulates the salivary or gastric glands in no way corresponds to reality. This sin of confusing what are obviously different things can be imputed also to me in my earlier articles. In our experiments we must, therefore, clearly distinguish between the secretory and the motor reactions of the organism; and in respect to the glands, if we compare our results with the phenomena of the subjective world, we must regard not the desire of the dog, but its attention, as the chief condition for the success of the experiments. The salivary reaction of the animal might be regarded in the subjective world as a substratum of elementary, pure notion, thought.

The above-mentioned facts, on the one hand, provide certain, and in my view, important conclusions about the processes taking place in the central nervous system; on the other hand, they make possible further successful analysis. Let us consider from the standpoint of physiology some of our facts, and first of all our fundamental fact. When a given object—a certain food or chemical irritant—is brought into contact with the special surface of the oral cavity and stimulates it by means of those of its properties on which the activity of the salivary glands is specially directed, then the other properties of the object that have nothing to do with the working of the salivary glands or even with the entire environment of the object, but simultaneously stimulating other sensory surfaces of the body, become connected, apparently, with the same nervous centre of the salivary glands to which the stimulation emanating from the essential properties of the object is conducted through a fixed centripetal path. It can be assumed in this case that the salivary centre acts in the central nervous system as a point of attraction for stimuli coming from other sensory surfaces. Thus, a certain path is opened from the other excited areas of the body to the salivary centre. But this connection of the centre with accidental points is very fragile and tends to disappear of itself. Constant repetition of simultaneous stimulation by means of the essential and unessential properties of the object is required to make this connection increasingly durable. In this way a temporary relation is established between the activity of a certain organ and the external objects. The temporary relation and its law—to become stronger as a result of repetition and to disappear when not repeated—play a big role in the well-being and integrity of the organism; by means of it the adaptability of the organism and the conformity of its activity to the surroundings become more perfect and delicate. The two parts of this law are equally important:

if the temporary relation to the object is of great significance for the organism, then the rupture of this relation is essential when it is no longer justified by reality. Otherwise the relations of the animal, instead of being delicate, would assume a chaotic character.

Let us turn to another point. From the standpoint of physiology how do we regard the fact that the sight of meat destroys in the parotid gland the reaction to the sight of bread, i.e., that the saliva earlier secreted at the sight of bread ceases to flow when there is a simultaneous meat stimulation? One could assume that strong excitation in a definite motor centre corresponds to the strong motor reaction provided by the meat, as a consequence of which, according to the above-mentioned law, the stimulation is diverted from other parts of the central nervous system and in particular from the salivary centres, i.e., their excitability is diminished. This interpretation is supported by another experiment in which the secretion of saliva at the sight of bread is inhibited by the sight of another dog. Here the motor reaction to bread is really greatly intensified. Even more convincing would be an experiment in which the dog would prefer dry food to moist and display a stronger motor reaction to it. We should be quite right in our interpretation of this experiment if in the dog in question the sight of dry food did not evoke secretion of saliva, or if the secretion should be much less than in usual dogs. It is a well-known fact that a very strong desire often inhibits certain special reflexes.

But among the above-mentioned facts there are some which, from the physiological point of view, can be explained only with great difficulty; for example, why does a conditioned reflex, when repeated, invariably become ineffective? The natural explanation of fatigue is hardly acceptable, since in this case we are dealing with a weak stimulus. Actually the repetition of a strong stimulus of an unconditioned reflex does not bring on early fatigue. Probably we have here altogether peculiar conditions for the excitation which is conducted along accidental centripetal paths.

From the above it is obvious that our new subject can be investigated quite objectively and that, in essence, it is a purely physiological subject. One can hardly doubt that analysis of this group of stimuli, coming into the nervous system from the external world will reveal to us laws of nervous activity and disclose its mechanism from aspects which so far have not been even touched upon by investigation of nervous phenomena in the organism, or have been touched upon only in rough outline.

Despite the complexity of the new phenomena, this investigation entails considerable advantages. In the present study of the mechanism of the nervous system, first, the experiments are conducted on animals that have just been injured by operations, and, secondly, and this is the chief thing, the nerve trunks of the animals are subjected to stimulation, i.e., the excitation extends simultaneously and in a uniform manner over a mass of highly diverse nervous fibres; such combinations, however, never occur in reality. Naturally, we experience great difficulty in discovering the laws of the normal activity of the nervous system, since we bring it to a state of chaos by our artificial stimulation. But in normal conditions, such as we maintained in our latest experiments, the stimulation is effected in an isolated manner, the correlations of the intensity being regulated.

Generally speaking, this applies to all psychical experiments, but in the case of our psychical phenomena, observed in the activity of the salivary glands, there is another special advantage. For successful investigation of a subject, complex by its very nature, it is important to simplify it in some way or other. In the given case we have this simplification. The role of the salivary glands is so clear that their relation to the external environment of the organism must be equally clear and accessible to investigation and interpretation. However, it must not be imagined that the physiological role of the salivary glands is confined to the above-mentioned functions. By no means. For example, saliva is used by the animals for licking and healing wounds, a thing that we constantly see. This is probably the reason why we can obtain saliva by stimulating various sensory nerves. And yet the complexity of the physiological relations of the salivary glands is much less than that of the skeletal muscles through which the organism is connected with the external world in an endless number of ways. At the same time a simultaneous comparison of the secretory, especially salivary, reaction with the motor reaction enables us, on the one hand, to distinguish between the particular and the general, and on the other hand, to get rid of our stock of routine anthropomorphic concepts and interpretations relating to the motor reaction of the animals.

Having established the possibility of analysis and systematisation of our phenomena we come to the next stage of our work—systematic division and derangement of the central nervous system in order to see how the previously established relations change. Thus, there will be an anatomical analysis of the mechanism of these relations. This will be the future and, I feel sure, the already approaching experimental psychopathology.

Here, too, the salivary glands as objects of investigation are of great value. The nervous system, which has a bearing on movement, is so highly intricate and predominates to such an extent in the brain that even the slightest damage to it often causes undesirable and very complicated results. The nervous system of the salivary glands, because of their inconsiderable physiological significance, comprises, it may be assumed, only a negligible portion of the brain substance, and is, consequently, so thinly distributed in the brain that its partial, isolated destruction does not bring about, even remotely, the difficulties which in this respect exist in the innervation motor apparatus. Of course, psychopathological experiments had their beginning at a time when the physiologists first removed these or other parts of the central nervous system and investigated the animals that survived these operations. In this respect the past twenty or thirty years have supplied us with a number of fundamental facts. We already know the drastic decline that takes place in the adaptive capacity of animals as a result of complete or partial extirpation of their cerebral hemispheres. But the investigation of this subject has not yet developed into a special branch, which could be studied without interruption and according to a definite plan. The reason for this, as I see it, is that the investigators still lack the more or less considerable and detailed knowledge of the animal's normal relations with the surrounding world that would enable them to make an objective and exact comparison of the state of the animal before and after the operation.

Objective investigation alone will gradually bring us to the complete analysis of that infinite adaptability in all its manifestations which constitutes life on earth. Are not the movements of plants towards light and the seeking of truth through mathematical analysis essentially phenomena of one and the same order? Are they not the last links of an almost endless chain of adaptation taking place throughout the living world?

We can analyse adaptation in its most elementary forms on the basis of objective facts. Is there any reason for changing this method in the study of adaptability in the higher orders?

Work in this direction has been started at different levels of life and has advanced effectively without encountering obstacles. The objective study of living matter, which begins with the theory of tropisms of elementary living things, can and must remain objective also when it reaches the highest manifestations of the animal organism, the so-called psychical phenomena in the higher animals.

Guided by the similarity or identity of external manifestations, science, sooner or later, will apply the objective facts also to our subjective world and thereby shed a bright light on our mysterious nature, elucidate the mechanism and the vital significance of that which occupies the human mind most—his consciousness and its torments. This explains why in my exposition I have some words which sounded as if they were contradictory. In the title of my paper and throughout my exposition I have used the term "psychical", at the same time bringing forward only objective investigation and leaving aside everything subjective. The vital phenomena that are termed psychical, despite the fact that they are objectively observed in animals, are only distinguished from purely physiological phenomena by degree of complexity. It makes no difference whether they are termed psychical or complex-nervous as distinct from the simple physiological, once it is realised and recognised that the naturalist should approach them only objectively, leaving aside the question of the essence of these phenomena.

Is it not clear that contemporary vitalism, that is, animism, confuses the different points of view of the naturalist and of the philosopher. The former always bases his grandiose success on the study of objective facts and their comparisons, disregarding on principle the question of the essence and final causes; the latter, personifying the highest aspiration of man for synthesis—although up to now it has been of a fantastic nature—and seeking to provide the answer to everything relating to the human being, must right now create an entity from the objective and the subjective. For the naturalist everything lies in the method, in the chance of obtaining an unshakable, lasting truth; and solely from this point of view, which for him is obligatory, the soul, as a naturalistic principle, is not only unnecessary but even harmful to his work, in vain limiting his courage and the depth of his analysis.

ON SLEEP[3]

Some of my young collaborators studying conditioned reflexes have now been complaining for a number of years of the drowsy state of their experimental animals, a state which hindered them from continuing their studies of the aforesaid phenomena for the simple reason that these phenomena disappeared. This difficulty made itself felt particularly when they chose as the conditioned agent for the thermal stimulation of the animal's skin either heat at about 45°C or cold of about 0° C.[4] The latter cases usually ended in the animal's deep sleep and cessation of all of its complex nervous activity. Even a prejudice against working with thermal agents has formed in the laboratory. However, we could only temporarily disregard the foregoing difficulty, but, essentially, it directly concerned our problem. Concentrated attention on this difficulty finally disclosed its mechanism. We had long and unwittingly been surprised at the contrasts between the great animation and mobility of the dog before the experiment and its drowsiness and sleep which developed soon after the beginning of the experiment. It occurred to us that something in our experiment was the cause of this drowsiness. And yet the experiment consisted only in the fact that the dog was either repeatedly given small portions of food or that several cubic centimetres of a weak solution of hydrochloric acid were poured into its mouth accompanied by thermal stimulation of the skin. Since neither the feeding hor the administration of the acid could have been the causes, the reasons for the drowsiness had to be sought only in the action of the thermal agent. In point of fact, as a result of various forms of the experiment, we found that the action of the same degree of heat or cold on the selfsame place of the skin, temporary but repeated, and the more so continuous for some time, infallibly led sooner or later to a drowsy state of a formerly lively and mobile animal and then to its deep sleep. It was becoming obvious that a definite agent of the external environment could condition in the same fatal and infallible manner the animal's peace, the depression of its higher nervous activity, as the other agents, on the contrary, evoked its particular complex-nervous functions. In other words, side by side with the various active reflexes there is also a passive sleep reflex. Once the external environment forces the animal to diverse activity infallibly connected with destruction of living substance, but at other times, when this activity is, according to the moment, superfluous, the same external environment with similar imperativeness dooms the animal to rest which ensures restoration of the living substance destroyed during the activity. And it is only thus that the physicochemical system of the animal's organism, which is always in motion, remains integral, remains itself. That sleep as a depression, inhibition of the higher nervous activity, besides the possible chemical reason in the form of accumulating products of activity, is also conditioned by a peculiar reflex stimulation, is confirmed by some of our other observations in which other types of obvious depression changed to drowsiness and sleep in a truly amazing manner. I am convinced that the solution of the still unclear phenomena of hypnosis and other related states lies along this path of research and that we do not face so many difficulties, at that. If ordinary sleep is a depression, inhibition of all of the activity of the higher division of the brain, hypnosis must be regarded as a partial depression of the different portions of this division. The episode with the sleep reflex is one of the numerous illustrations of how the study—by the objective method—of all the influences of the external environment on the animal organism, without exception and as fleeting and slight as they may be, gradually encompasses and will finally encompass the entire activity of the organism.

For us the sleep reflex is as yet but one of the inhibitors of our conditioned reflex. We call the inhibition conditioned by the sleep reflex a general inhibition because it depresses, in addition to ours, also the other complex-nervous phenomena.

ON INHIBITION AND SLEEP[5]

It has long been observed that under some conditions our dogs become sleepy and thus interfere with our work; under these conditions the conditioned reflexes weaken and disappear. We have particularly noticed that this onset of drowsiness occurred in dogs subjected to thermal stimulation when the thermal stimulation of the skin was connected with the stimulation of the salivary gland. It has developed that thermal stimulation calls forth sleep, that is, it conditions and evokes sleep, as other stimuli evoke other activities of the animals. It is interesting that to observe drowsiness requires stimulation with heat or cold at a certain spot and with the same degree of temperature. If you change the degree of heat or the place, the hypnotic influence is weak and does not attain the highest point of manifestation. On the basis of these experiments we had to speak of a sleep reflex and it became perfectly clear to us that this drowsy state was a form of depression of the activity of the cerebral hemispheres. Why depression? Because this drowsy state, the sleep reflex, acted on our other conditioned reflexes absolutely in the same manner as did the well-known inhibitors with all the details and peculiarities, as inhibitors act in general, i.e., there was a complete similarity of action. I shall give you facts where other forms of unquestionable depression gradually pass into sleep, apparently on the basis of their affinity.

I shall now consider other phenomena of depression. I obtain a trace reflex by mechanically stimulating the skin at a certain spot with a scratcher for a period of a minute; then I wait a minute and pour in the acid. It follows that my aim is to form a conditioned reflex from the trace of scratching, from what remains of this stimulation in the nervous system. After numerous repetitions I really get to the point where there is no effect while I scratch and, when the scratching is over and the minute between the scratching and the administration of the acid has ended, salivation appears; consequently, I have formed a trace reflex from the remainder of the mechanical stimulation of the skin in the nervous system. But if the experiment is continued, the following interesting phenomenon is observed: during the scratching the dog grows increasingly calmer and finally falls asleep, it even, so to speak, falls asleep demonstratively. Whereas the dog was wide awake before the scratching, as soon as you begin to scratch it, signs of sleepiness appear. Then the sleep grows increasingly deeper and lasts longer and longer.

Finally, the experiments have to be discontinued because the dog on the table has become a continuously sleeping animal. This seems to be an absolutely unsuitable, inappropriate process: you repeatedly administer to the dog acid which must greatly stimulate it and yet it all ends in sleep; the acid has become a hypnotic agent. The same dog with the same acid reflexes, only extant and not trace reflexes, manifests no drowsiness. How are we to understand it? During the scratching we never administer acid, consequently the process of depression must develop at this time. Thus, a paradoxical situation for the nervous system results. Depression must develop in response to the extant stimulus and a stimulus for acid must form from the trace of this stimulation. Since the depression is connected with intense stimulation, and excitation is connected with weak stimulation, the depression finally prevails, an exaggerated and very widespread effect of this depression results, this depression passing into a drowsy state and sleep, and these phenomena doing away with the conditioned reflex itself. If you observe these experiments many times and compare all the circumstances of the experiments, no other and more natural explanation of these curious relations can occur to you. At first these interpretations may appear somewhat far-fetched, but subsequently you will learn other facts which will incline you more towards our explanations.

I shall now consider another case in which the relation is simpler. You have before you some conditioned stimulus, say, a metronome which always evokes salivation. Now I add to the metronome an odour, say, that of camphor, and at this time I will not "reinforce" the metronome, i.e., I will not give the dog food when, in addition to the metronome, the dog is stimulated by the odour. At first, the metronome will evoke salivation despite the effect of the odour. But if this is repeated several times, this combination becomes ineffective: the metronome plus the odour of camphor does not evoke salivation. We call this fact a fact of conditioned inhibition and the added agent—a conditioned inhibitor.

The following are interesting details of conditioned inhibition. I start testing the stimulus—metronome in the morning; it produces at least ten drops. Then I try the metronome with camphor and the result is a zero effect. If I try the metronome alone one, two or three minutes after applying the conditioned inhibitor, it will yield very little: one or two drops. What does this mean? It means that the inhibition which has developed in the central nervous system when I used camphor together with the metronome has spread through the cerebral hemispheres and persists in them; it takes time for it to wear off. Therefore, if I try the metronome 10-30 minutes after the combination, the metronome acts well, as usual.

This fact of conditioned inhibition explained one thing to us which we could not fathom for a long time and which generally gave us great difficulties in our work. When our experimental animals included extremely mobile and lively dogs with which we expected to work rapidly and well, precisely these dogs, as soon as they were in the stand, drove us to desperation: in the stand they infallibly lapsed into sleep and no reflexes could be obtained from them. What was the matter? You have an animal which won't stay put, an animal that won't fail either to lick you, snap at you, spring on you, etc. You take this animal, place it in the stand and tie its legs; at first it behaves as it did on the floor; it tries to free itself, begins to reach for you, etc., you fight it, you tie the animal's paws, make fast its head, etc., and finally achieve what you wanted: the dog has grown calmer, but at the same time it has become sleepy, and the whole thing ends in deep sleep. What does this mean? You have inhibited the normal lively reaction of the animal to the surrounding world by various methods of violence. Depression has developed in the dog's nervous system and, continuously increasing, it has spread from the motor area to the entire hemisphere in the form of sleep. Thus the whole atmosphere was transformed into a conditioned inhibitor. This can be proved as follows: you may gradually reduce the elements of the situation and you will see that along with this the depression will also gradually diminish.

The following table (p. 38) demonstrates the results of one of the experiments conducted by Doctor N. Rozhansky.[6]

The first column shows the time of the experiment; the second column—the conditioned stimulus used; the third column—the number of drops received from the parotid gland, the measure of our salivary reflex; the fourth column—the time during which these drops were collected, and the last column—the position in which the dog was kept.

You let the dog down on the floor, applied a conditioned stimulus, and the dog gave you seven drops of saliva. You put the dog on the table, without the stand and straps

Experiment of February 22, 1911
(Kabill)

Time	Stimulus	No. of drops	Duration of its isolated action (in seconds)	Notes
3:50 P.M.	Metronome	1/2	30	In stand and straps
4:00 „	,,	2	30	In stand without straps
4:12 „	,,	4	30	On another table
4:25 „	,,	7	30	On floor
4:35 „	,,	3	30	On unusual table
4:47 „	,,	0	30	In stand without straps
4:56 „	,,	0	30	In stand and straps

and you got three drops. You placed the dog in the stand and the result is no salivation.

Thus we are faced with the following fact: by the situation you depress in the animal, as with a conditioned inhibitor, the muscular reaction to the usual external environment, but by doing it you also lose your conditioned salivary reflex. Consequently, you have a depression which is not confined to the limits you wanted, namely, the muscular division; the depression has progressed and has manifested itself in the form of general rest of the nervous system. These cases show us that the nervous depression produced in a certain spot has not remained at the one spot but has spread, has irradiated. Should this fail to be sufficiently convincing, we shall now consider, in conclusion, facts which will remove all doubts and which must be recognised as the best illustration of the law I have just discussed.

The experiment is demonstrated by Doctor N. Krasnogorsky,[7] who has made a study of this subject. In this case we have a dog with three stabbers: one stabber at the end of the left hind leg, another 3 cm upward from the end, and the third 22 cm away from the end. The lowest stabber is ineffective, because we did not accompany the stabbing of this spot with food and it ceased to act as a stimulus, whereas the stabbers three and twenty-two centimetres away from the end of the leg were continuously accompanied by food and are therefore effective. Earlier experiments convinced us that this differentiation of places is based on the development of depression at these places. If the stabber on the leg ceased to act, it did so because depression developed in this place and, consequently, does not permit the stimulation to spread. Now you see very clearly here that this process of depression irradiates over a certain distance and you watch the distance. We use the ineffective stabber and the result is zero. Then if you use the proximal stabber once and the distal stabber another time, you obtain an enormous difference. If, sometime after using the ineffective stabber you try the proximal stabber, you find that it is depressed. This means that the process of depression has spread to it, too. But if you try the distal stabber under absolutely identical conditions, you find that there is no depression. Thus, you follow with your eye the nervous process, the course of the wave of depression, and you see that it has stopped upon reaching a certain limit, has not gone any farther. Now it is possible to find out the speed with which this wave of depression spreads over the nervous system and how far it extends. If, after using the ineffective stabber, whose ineffectiveness is based on the development of depression at the given point, you try other stabbers within 1.5 minutes, you observe the aforesaid phenomenon, namely, that at a distance of three centimetres the depression is distinct, whereas at a greater distance (22 cm) it is imperceptible. Consequently, 1.5 minutes after the use of the ineffective stabber the process of depression does not spread over a long distance. But, if you try the stabbers not within 1.5 minutes, but within 15 seconds, the depression will also be on top so that you will quite clearly see how the wave of depression spreads over the nervous system and how it surges back. To me this fact appears as a most incontestable illustration of the law of irradiation of depression; this fact can be given no other interpretation.

Thus, after all the aforesaid experiments, we must say that depression also spreads over the cerebral hemispheres, like excitation.

But there are also many facts showing that depression likewise concentrates in the manner I have told you about excitation.

You have a conditioned reflex—metronome—and with it a conditioned inhibitor—camphor. If the latter is fresh and you try a short time (5-10 minutes) after it the stimulation alone, i.e., the metronome, there will be no reaction. But, if you continue the experiments, i.e., you reinforce the metronome alone with an unconditioned stimulus, and do not reinforce the metronome combined with camphor, you will see that the process of depression increasingly concentrates. Now, if you use, after the combination, the metronome alone, it will act exactly the same way 5-10 minutes later as it did before, i.e., in full measure. Apparently the same phenomenon is observed in the following facts. Say you have a tone of 1,000 vibrations and you differentiate from it, for instance 1/8 of a tone, that is, you accompany the tone of 1,000 vibrations by feeding and do not accompany the 1/8 of the tone by feeding. Finally, the stimulations will differ; one will act and the other will not. This differentiation is based on the process of inhibition. If you try the tone soon after the differentiated 1/8, it will prove depressed. But, if more time elapses after the elaboration of the differentiation, the depression will also concentrate, i.e., the trial of the differentiated tone after a short space of time will now no longer depress the active tone.

Entirely similar facts are also observed in the different dogs with which we work. So far, we do not control these facts, we are only observers of these facts, but the purport of these facts is apparently connected with the law of irradiation and concentration of depression.

Here is a number of dogs. You have one dog in which a drowsy state has developed under the conditions of our experiment, and this state has embraced the entire activity of the cerebral hemispheres. Then you have another type of dog which does not sleep in the stand. This means that depression has not reached the highest degree to be manifested in the general inactivity of the cerebral hemispheres. In this dog the depression is manifested in muscular rest, and the dog stands stock-still. But this depression has not confined itself to the muscular system; it has passed on to the salivary reflex. And now, the last dog. On the floor it is an extremely lively animal. It does not sleep in the stand but it is at muscular rest, it stands as though petrified, and yet this depression of the muscular system is limited and does not spread to the salivary reflexes which prove to be very intense. In different dogs we have different degrees of irradiation of the depression and a certain concentration of this depression from the very same depressing effect of our situation. The last dog has an ideally developed nervous system; in this dog the depression has remained at the spot where we wanted to retain it. It gave the dog muscular rest but did not go any farther; the salivary reflexes remained unaffected and intact.

What if this latter is only observational material, I repeat, the thing is perfectly clear: from the very same method you have a fact of conditioned inhibition and at the same time a fact of its definite limitation. I believe that all the foregoing facts give sufficient reasons to assume that depression is governed by the same basic laws as excitation. As excitation at first irradiates and then concentrates, so does also depression at first spread, and then concentrate.

These facts are at the same time an essential argument that excitation and depression are but different aspects, different manifestations of the selfsame process.

This is all we wanted to show you and tell you about today. In conclusion, I consider it rather interesting to let you in on some of the intimate facts which we observed in studying the phenomena we are now investigating by our method. These facts were finally elucidated not so long ago. When we decided about ten or eleven years ago to study the higher manifestations of the dog's nervous activity only objectively, ours was not an easy position. Like everyone else, we had the usual idea that the dog wanted something, thought something, etc. When we assumed the objective point of view, it seemed incredible that we could succeed. However, we had theoretical determination and started working by an objective method, while the field of phenomena we investigated was vast and, on the other hand, we were scarcely in possession of any of our simple facts. It stands to reason that we were in an awful position, because we had no actual proof that our decision was correct. We only had hopes that we would find something and, at the same time, doubts as to whether or not this would be recognised as scientifically adequate. This was followed by hours of success which encouraged us. In the course of time we accumulated many facts. Simultaneously we acquired greater conviction. We must confess, however, that our doubts also increased, and that these doubts persisted until very recently, although I did not disclose them to my associates. There were times when I asked myself the question: have we a correct attitude by viewing the facts only from the outside, or should we rather regard them from the old point of view? These cases recurred many times; naturally, they drew attention to themselves, and at last, this is what we found. Each time a new number of facts, especially a number of difficult facts, appeared, that is, facts hard to understand from our point of view, our doubts immediately increased. Why was it this way? What was the matter? It was quite simple, because in these new facts we did not as yet find causal relations, we could not explain the relations between the phenomena, and what was conditioned by what. Then, as we elucidated these relations, as we saw that a cause was followed by an effect, we immediately felt satisfied and reassured. Why had we before turned in a cowardly manner to the former subjective method? The answer is simple: because this is a method of causeless thinking, because psychological reasoning is a deterministic reasoning, i.e., I recognise a phenomenon as coming from neither here nor there. I say: the dog thought, the dog wants, and I am satisfied. And this is a fiction, and there is no cause for the phenomenon. It follows that the satisfaction of the psychological interpretation is also only fictitious, groundless. Our objective explanation is truly scientific, i.e., always turning to the cause, always seeking a cause.

CONDITIONS FOR ACTIVE AND RESTING STATES OF THE CEREBRAL HEMISPHERES[8]

I have entitled my report "Conditions for Active and Resting States of the Cerebral Hemispheres". By a resting state I imply a sleepy state to which I oppose the waking state. It stands to reason that this question is enormous and that I intend to formulate it only in its general outlines, to pose it before science. What I will say will be only small fragments relating to this immense subject which will sometime rise to its full stature for complete elaboration.

In his classical work *Reflexes of the Brain* 50 years ago Professor I. Sechenov envisaged with amazing intellectual power the main points of the question included in this subject and gave it the best formulation. He said that the active state of the higher division of the cerebral hemispheres required a certain minimal sum of stimulations coming to the brain through the usual receptive surfaces of the animal's body. This assumption made by I. Sechenov was subsequently brilliantly confirmed by a certain clinical case. Professor Strümpell[9] happened to have in his hospital a patient whose nervous system was impaired to such an extent that of all the receptive surfaces only the two eyes and one ear remained, and as soon as these last intact windows into the external world closed, the patient immediately fell asleep. This furnished complete confirmation of the fact that a certain minimal inflow of stimulation was necessary for the waking, active state of the cerebral hemispheres.

Quite recently I happened to see a similar case by courtesy of Dr. Shenger. It was a patient who had sustained a cranial and cerebral injury by falling off a tramcar. This person has become quite an invalid. He walks very slowly and carefully, speaks very slowly, and yet is quite a sane person who understands all questions and answers them sensibly. He has completely lost the vision of one eye and the hearing of one ear, but as for the sense of smell and the sense of touch he has not been examined. The following fact was reproduced on this patient. When his intact ear and eye are open, he understands everything and can read and write. But the moment you close either his ear or eye—these last windows into the external world—he infallibly lapses into oblivion and does not remember anything that happened to him during this interval.

I chanced to have suitable material in the laboratory when operating on dogs; I am referring to material on the same subject of the necessity of a certain minimum of stimulations for the active state of the cerebral hemispheres.[10] For example, the following is a very vivid case which recurred several times. You have a very lively dog, quickly reacting to everything, and you remove the greater posterior half of its cerebral hemispheres, i.e., the part where the centres for the eye and ear are located. I mean, of course, such cases when the operation is successful, without complications, without great injury and haemorrhages. When you remove this posterior part of the cerebral hemisphere on one side, and the operation is successful, the animal feels almost normal the very next day. As always, upon your appearance it wags its tail, becomes lively, lets you know it wants to eat, and this happens, I repeat, if not on the day after the operation, then by all means the day following. However, this occurs only if you have removed but half of the posterior divisions of the cerebral hemispheres. The situation changes entirely if you remove a similar half of the other hemisphere some time later. In this case, the animal lapses for several days, a week and even longer, into continuous sleep and it has to be awakened to be fed. This case is entirely similar to the two other cases I mentioned above. Since the bulk of the stimulations reaches the cerebral hemispheres through the eye and the ear, the elimination of these stimulations by some means or other leads to reduced activity of the cerebral hemispheres even to the point of their temporary complete rest.

And so, the first condition essential for the active state of the cerebral hemispheres, established by I. Sechenov, is a certain minimum of external stimulations; without this condition the animal sinks into sleep, because its brain passes into a state of rest. But the same stimulations which are necessary to maintain the brain in an active state under certain conditions evoke precisely the opposite state, they cause sleep. And this fact, an amazing fact, we, who are working with conditioned reflexes, have observed for many years.

As is well known to all who are present here, conditioned reflexes are formed as follows: you take some indifferent stimulus, for example, sound, light, etc., and repeat it with some constant reflex, say, the one the animal has to food, the food reflex. If you repeatedly combine this indifferent stimulus with an unconditioned, constant stimulus, this new agent itself becomes the cause of the same reaction which is produced by the unconditioned stimulus, i.e., in our case, the food reaction. When this formerly indifferent stimulus, for example, some sound, appears, the animal reacts to it as it would react to food. The animal turns to the side from which it is given food, licks its lips and salivates, although there is no food before it. It therefore follows that a new reflex, or as we call it, a conditioned reflex, has formed. It stands to reason that this conditioned reflex forms gradually and, in the course of time, the stimulus you have chosen becomes increasingly more effective.

And yet the following interesting fact subsequently comes to the fore. In all cases, despite the constant reinforcement of this reflex, i.e., its accompaniment by the unconditioned reflex, it sooner or later, within several weeks or months, disappears. And this is the amazing part of it. You constantly strengthen the connection and yet this connection seems to be destroyed. At first, it forms, then strengthens and, finally, disappears.

How is this connection destroyed then? You observe that the longer you repeat the experiments, the more the animal lapses into a sleepy state and finally falls asleep and sleeps under the most unsuitable circumstances. You take the animal which has not eaten for a day or two, and feed it according to signal, that is, after the beginning of the conditioned stimulus, for perhaps a whole year, and yet, as soon as you bring this signal into play, the animal falls asleep and the positive reaction to this signal is eliminated.

What is this state then into which the animal lapses? It would not be enough to call this state sleep. In many cases it is really distinct sleep with relaxed muscles, so that the dog passively hangs on the straps, falls, snores and does not react to external stimuli. But in many cases we have to extend this definition of the dog's state and say that this is not only sleep, but a state which resembles what we call hypnotic sleep. This will include such cases in which the animal does not exhibit the usual signs of sleep; it does not hang on its straps, does not snore and yet its reflexes disappear and the animal itself seems to be in a state of torpor. Then there is another fact. Hypnotism, as is well known, engenders dissociation in the functions of the brain. You have a hypnotised subject and you can ask him questions or order him to do something; the subject understands, but at the same time he has lost control over his skeletal muscles and cannot change the position of the parts of his body, much as he may want to do so. Something similar can also be observed in dogs. It happens that the dog retains its salivary reaction: as soon as the signal begins to act, saliva is secreted. When food is subsequently brought, the flow of saliva increases. And yet the dog will not take the food, it just can't take it. This fact is very similar to the one we encounter in man. There is yet another fact. There is something that resembles what we call suggestion; but if we speak about this, it will take us too far afield.

And so, our conditioned stimuli, despite the fact that they are confirmed every day, in the long run, as strange as it may appear, fatally lead to this sleepy, hypnotic state. It should be noted that the onset of this sleepy state makes no exception for any stimulus, however strong it may be. For example, you may use the strongest electric current as a conditioned stimulus. A conditioned food reflex forms to this current; it does so without any difficulty, but the thing still ends the same way. In the course of time, the food reaction will grow weaker and at last you will be altogether unable to obtain it.

Now some details. This state appears the sooner, the more often you repeat the feeding with your conditioned stimulus. In the beginning you always succeed in forming a conditioned reflex. But sometimes, as soon as you have formed the reflex, the sleepy state develops; at other times the disappearance of the reflex is delayed, as before stated, for a very long time. One thing is clear, however, the time at which the sleepy state appears depends on the number of repetitions of your conditioned reflex.

But this is not the only condition. This state sets in the sooner, the longer the interval between the beginning of the conditioned stimulation and the food, i.e., the longer the conditioned stimulus acts alone, without the unconditioned stimulus. For example, if I form a reflex to a sound and feed the dog fifteen seconds after turning on the sound, the sleepy state will develop relatively late. If I prolong this interval from fifteen seconds to two minutes in the same animal in which this arrangement of the experiment produces no signs of a sleepy state, the animal will very soon fall asleep.

The onset of this sleepy state also depends on other factors, namely, the quality of the conditioned stimulus and the individuality of the dog. The dependence on the quality of the stimulus is as follows. When this subject was only being outlined in the laboratory, those who were working with it were prejudiced against using thermal stimuli of the skin as conditioned stimuli, because the experiments with them for some reason or other were always extraordinarily difficult and unsuccessful. Later, when this question attracted attention to itself and was tackled seriously, it was found that of all stimuli thermal stimuli evoked this sleepy state the most readily. It is precisely thus with thermal stimulation, i.e., as soon as you have formed a reflex, the sleepy state begins to develop and you have to relinquish the experiments. Next in order after thermal stimuli are mechanical skin stimulations which also soon evoke a sleepy state. However, a very great difference is observed between the thermal and mechanical skin stimuli, and the more so between all the others. Thermal stimulations produce sleep within about ten days, whereas, for example, with an acoustic stimulus you will produce no sleep, much as you may try, even within a month. The mechanical skin stimuli will occupy an intermediate position. Thus, as optimum stimuli evoking a sleepy state, we must recognise the stimuli acting on the animal's skin, in the first place thermal and then mechanical.

The other condition on which the rapidity of the appearance of the sleepy state depends is the individuality of the dog. One animal lapses into sleep easily, another does so with greater difficulty. It should be noted that in this case we were somewhat mistaken. Formerly when this occurrence greatly hampered the experiments, we wanted to make sure and usually chose the liveliest dogs for our work. It turned out quite the contrary, these were precisely the dogs in whom the sleepy state developed with particular ease, whereas the calmer dogs with a more balanced nervous system did not succumb to sleep so easily.

Lastly, we feel that there is one more important factor. If you take our stimuli by themselves, without connecting them with an unconditioned stimulus, they do not prove under those conditions to be hypnotic. If you simply apply heat to the dog's skin for the same period of time, the sleepy state will not develop. It will develop only when you transform this stimulus into a conditioned stimulus, when you connect it with an unconditioned reflex.

How are we to understand this? It seems to me that the cell of the cerebral hemispheres, if the stimulation is concentrated in it and then frequently repeated, sooner or later gets into a state of special inhibition, unreceptiveness. As long as the external stimulus has not become conditioned, it is not concentrated and the stimulation spreads over the cerebral cortex. But as soon as it has become a conditioned, specific, concentrated stimulus, it attaches itself to one point and each time acts on the very same nerve cells. This concentration of stimulation at one spot, or, as we say in the laboratory, the hacking away at one cell, leads to the fact that this cell passes into a refractive state, a state of inhibition, unexcitability, and from here this state spreads over the entire cerebral hemispheres and becomes sleep, or, in cases of hypnosis, is somewhat delayed at the different stages of diffusion.

Thus we see, on the one hand, that the first condition for the active state of the cerebral hemispheres is a certain minimum of external stimulations, and on the other hand, we have found that prolonged accumulation of stimulation in one spot, the hacking away at one cell, in the long run, produces a resting state of the cerebral hemispheres, a state of sleep.

When we obtained this sleepy state, not counting the cases in which we especially worked with it, we asked ourselves how we could dispel it, how we could do away with it in order that it may not interfere with our work and how we could again produce an active state of the cerebral hemispheres. At first we tried to act so that instead of one reflex we produced several reflexes. In this case, we used reflexes to loud sounds, high tones and intense stimulation of the skin, for example, by electricity, thus hoping to do away with the sleepy state. However, we could not attain our aim and our efforts failed in every instance. As strong as the stimulus may have been, the thing always ended in sleep just the same. And yet, adhering to the point of view that there must be such a maximum of stimulation at which this sleepy state will be overcome, we continued our experiments. And only when we made the enormous world of sounds our conditioned stimulus (experiments of Dr. M. Petrova)[11] did we succeed in overcoming sleep. We had at our disposal about 40 phonograph records, which reproduced singing, music, and speech, and we used now one and now another record. Thus, if it is a question of overcoming sleep by a variety of stimuli, it requires an incredible number of stimuli, and if it is a question of sounds we must have at hand almost the whole world of acoustic phenomena. If boredom is regarded as something analogous, closely related to sleep, sleep with open eyes, it should be said, that he, who seeks to dispel it only by a variety of impressions, will attain very little.

We discovered one more condition which hinders the development of the sleepy state. As is often the case, the facts pointing in this direction were at first noticed accidentally and were systematised only later. A much more reliable way to eliminate the sleepy state is a variety of nervous processes either in the form of different unconditioned reflexes or in the form of different conditioned, now positive and now negative, i.e., inhibitory, reflexes. We have long since noted that during the experiments the dogs of some of our collaborators were asleep while those of the others remained awake. When we attended to this fact, we observed that this was conditioned by the nature of the experiments. For example, each time the experiments were conducted only with processes of excitation, repeating the positive conditioned stimulations, a sleepy or hypnotic state resulted. But if, in addition to stimulation, processes of inhibition were used, there was either no sleepy state at all or it was very easily overcome.

One of the dogs gave us particular trouble because of the ease with which it lapsed into sleep. This happened before our experiments with the phonograph records. We applied a host of various stimuli, but to no avail. However, this sleepy state disappeared when, in the course of the experiments, we decided to use the following combination: with the stimulation with cold we formed an acid reflex, and with the heat we connected the food reflex (experiments of Dr. P. Vasilyev[12]). The dog had a hard time of it; the reflexes formed very slowly. When we finally succeeded in forming these reflexes, the dog lost sleep despite the fact that precisely thermal stimulations most easily dispose to sleep. Following this Dr. Vasilyev worked with this dog for several months, applying these thermal stimuli with absolute impunity.

Thus we see that a variety of nervous processes is of much greater significance to the active condition of the cerebral hemispheres than is a variety of stimuli, however great it may be.

It must be assumed that the aforesaid conditions for the active and resting states of the cerebral hemispheres are the basic or, at any rate, some of the fundamental conditions. A complete analysis of these conditions will probably lead to enormous control over the activity of our cerebral hemispheres and to their extensive practical application. The mechanism of the work of the cerebral hemispheres is apparently opening up before us in its capital features.

SOME FACTS ABOUT THE PHYSIOLOGY OF SLEEP[13]

(Jointly with Dr. L. N. Voskresensky)

In our study of the so-called conditioned reflexes we often had to deal with the phenomena of sleep. Since these phenomena greatly complicated our experiments, disturbing them and deflecting them from their normal course, we were, naturally, compelled to devote special attention to them. In addition to accumulating isolated facts, two of our colleagues—N. A. Rozhansky and M. K. Petrova—elaborated this problem most systematically. N. A. Rozhansky investigated that form of sleep, or somnolent state, which apparently results from the influence of monotonous, indifferent stimuli, for example, the isolated environment in which the experimental animal is placed. When the animal is enclosed in an isolated chamber and placed in the stand, it gradually becomes drowsy, and then goes into deep sleep. Sleep also occurs under the influence of definite, active stimuli from which strong conditioned stimuli have been elaborated. Under the influence of these stimuli there arises a sleeping hypnotic state in all dogs, and in some of them with particular ease. Recently Dr. L. N. Voskresensky had a case of this somnolent state which for us was somewhat unexpected, since numerous experiments had already been performed on this dog by Dr. A. M. Pavlova and no marked signs of sleep had been observed during those experiments. But now in the course of our research, sleep unexpectedly intervened and constantly disturbed our experiments with conditioned reflexes; as a result, the usual phenomena were sometimes entirely absent and sometimes distorted. How did this come about? At first we were not quite sure whether this state was really sleep, and attributed the disturbances to other causes. But thorough observation and various tests excluded all other suppositions. All that remained was to admit the development of a state of sleep in the dog. But what caused it? When we closely considered all the details of the recent experiments performed on the dog, it appeared that the sleep was due to the following reasons. Prior to this peculiar period the experiment was usually begun the moment the dog was placed in the stand—it was subjected to the action of special conditioned stimuli and food was given as an unconditioned stimulus. These conditions did not produce a sleeping state. Now, however, due to certain circumstances, the dog was left in the stand for a relatively long time, waiting for the beginning of the experiment. And it was the continuously acting, monotonous surroundings which caused the gradual onset of a state of sleep. This interpretation proved to be perfectly reasonable. As the particulars relating to the development of a state of sleep were of great interest to us, we decided to investigate the question with the utmost thoroughness.

First of all it appeared that from the quantitative point of view the environment acts with surprising precision, i.e., if immediately after the necessary preparations (fixing the different funnels, fastening the apparatus, etc.) you begin the experiment, the usual stimulations of the animal, there are no signs of the phenomena of sleep at all. But should a minute pass between the completion of the preparations and the beginning of the stimulation the first phase of sleep becomes manifest. If ten minutes pass you observe the next stage of sleep and so forth. Thus the sleep-producing influence of the environment can be truly dosed. This made possible an easy study of the course of sleep, of the somnolent state which develops under these conditions. And here are the results of our observations. During the experiments we usually had before our eyes two reactions of the animal; on the one hand, there was a secretory reaction, a flow of saliva; on the other—a motor reaction—the dog seized the food offered to it. In other words, these were the motor and secretory reflexes. It turned out that the strictly law-governed development of the observed phenomena depends on the quantitative influence of the soporific environment; this is shown in the following table:

State of the dog	Phases of sleep	Reflexes*		Remarks
		Secretory	Motor	
Awake		+	+	
Asleep	I	—	+	
	II	+	—	
	III	—	—	Deep sleep
	II	+	—	
	I	—	+	
Awake		+	+	

* The sign + signifies the presence and the sign — the absence of a reflex.

In the wakeful state both the secretory and the motor reflexes are present. Immediately after the conditioned stimulus begins to act a secretion of saliva appears, and the dog takes the food as soon as it is offered. Thus both reflexes are effective. Now we keep the dog under the influence of the surroundings at least for two minutes, i.e., when the preparations for the experiment are finished, we let two minutes pass, and then apply the conditioned stimulus. The *first phase of the state of sleep* is then observed. It is manifested thus: the secretory reflex disappears; the conditioned stimulus no longer acts; but when the dog is offered food it immediately seizes it, which shows that

55

the motor reflex persists. Now you augment the influence of the surroundings, i.e., for example, you keep the dog waiting ten minutes before the experiment begins. Then its sleep deepens, and another kind of reaction is observed, which, strange as it may seem, is of a reverse nature and represents the *second phase of the state of sleep*; the dog exhibits a secretion of saliva, but does not take the food, and even turns away from it. Thus the salivary reaction which is absent during the first phase of sleep, reappears in the second, while the motor reaction disappears or even passes into a negative reaction; the dog not only refuses food but even turns away from it. If the dog is left in the soporific surroundings for a period lasting from half an hour to one hour before the beginning of the experiment, a *complete, deep sleep* sets in, and both reflexes vanish. Now let us wake the dog from its deep sleep. This can be done at once, and the simplest method is to apply a strong sound stimulus. In our laboratory we use a very loud rattle, which wakens the dog instantaneously. The animal immediately returns to a normal alert state. However, a more delicate stimulus may be used.

One of the customary methods of gradually dispelling sleep is to feed the dog at definite intervals; feeding may be even begun with the forcible introduction of food into the mouth. Then you can observe the phases described above but in reverse order. After the deep sleep the secretory reflex is present but the dog does not take the food. Later on, the secretory reflex fails to appear; however, the dog eats. And finally, after frequent repetitions of the feeding, both reflexes reappear. Now I shall call your attention to some authentic figures. Take, for example, a dog that has just been fastened in the stand; we begin at once to apply certain conditioned stimuli and a secretion of saliva appears. Our scale shows thirty-seven divisions, which indicates a normal salivary reaction. It should be added that the following precaution was observed by us in order to ensure strict precision in our investigation. The chamber itself had a hypnotising effect on the dog; the moment the lively, mobile and responsive animal was brought into the experimental room, it changed entirely. It goes without saying that the state of sleep deepened when the dog was placed in the stand and prepared for the experiment. In order to determine exactly the moment of the passage from the wakeful to the sleeping state, we did everything to prevent sleep while the dog was being fastened and the apparatus attached to it; we called it by name, stroked it and patted it. When everything was ready, we would quickly leave the chamber and begin the experiment immediately. In this way we obtained the above-mentioned normal secretory reaction, equalling thirty-seven divisions of our scale; the motor reflex was also present. In the next experiment we allowed the surroundings to act on the animal for a space of two minutes, and the following was observed: the secretory reflex failed to appear at all, not a drop of saliva was secreted in response to our conditioned stimulus, but the dog took the food at once. Next time we let the surroundings act for four minutes; we obtained twenty divisions of saliva but the dog took the food only in forty-five seconds, and even then only when the food was brought into contact with its mouth. Finally, when we allowed the surroundings to act for half an hour or an hour, all the reflexes disappeared.

The procedures were, of course, varied by us, so that we were able to obtain both phases of sleep in one and the same experiment. For example, the dog remained in the chamber for seventy-five seconds; as a result, the secretory reflex was zero, but the food was taken at once. Then we let an hour pass, leaving the dog alone. The excitation produced by a single meal neutralised to some extent the soporific influence of the surroundings, and only the second phase was observed: the secretion of saliva equalled twenty-two divisions, and the dog ate the food only for about half a minute after the food had been brought into contact with the mouth. Here is another concrete instance of how sleep is dispelled. The dog is in a deep sleep and in order to arouse it we apply, among others, a weak stimulus: someone enters the chamber where the dog is kept in the stand. The noise produced by the person entering the chamber, and perhaps his odour, slightly disturb the animal's sleeping state. If we now apply the conditioned stimulus we obtain twenty-four divisions of saliva, but the dog takes the food fifty seconds later, not of its own accord, however, but only when it is put into its mouth. We then feed the dog once or twice, thereby stimulating it; we dispel the state of sleep and observe a transition to the following phase: the secretory effect is diminished, there are only ten divisions of saliva and the food is taken by the dog after twenty seconds. Whereas in the preceding case the dog ate the food after fifty seconds and from the experimenter's hand, now it takes the food of its own accord and only after twenty seconds. With a fresh stimulus applied after twenty minutes, the secretory reflex is zero, and the dog eats the food almost immediately. Finally, when the next conditioned stimulus is applied, thirty-five divisions of saliva are secreted, and the dog takes the food right away. This signifies the presence of a perfectly alert state.

Hence, we must recognise as a thoroughly established fact that the processes of falling asleep and of awakening influence our two reflexes in a strictly definite way. We witnessed a very interesting fact which is, above all, of practical importance, since it enabled us to control the animal and to remove the influences which interfered with the experiment. It sufficed to feed the dog two or three times, or to prevent the surroundings from acting on it at the beginning, to make us masters of the situation; sleep did not disturb our experiments with the conditioned reflexes. Now the question arose: How to interpret this phenomenon? Certainly it is a complicated question and for the time being only an approximate answer can be given. Our colleagues N. A. Rozhansky and M. K. Petrova, on the basis of their experimental data, have come to the conclusion that both states of sleep observed by them represent an inhibitory process and that in one case it spread from several points of the cerebral hemispheres (case of Rozhansky), and in another case—from one definite point (Petrova). Our fact, it would seem, confirms this conclusion, since in our experiments there was actually in evidence a localisation and even a movement of the somnolent state in the cerebral hemispheres.

How can this movement of sleep inhibition be better traced in the cerebrum? A similar question arose and was successfully investigated in connection with another kind of inhibition, the so-called internal inhibition. A few months ago one of us addressed you here on this subject.[14] This investigation gives us reason to hope that we may achieve the same with regard to sleep inhibition. The simplest way would be to trace the movement of this sleep inhibition in a definite part of the cerebral hemispheres, since, as shown by our experiments concerning the irradiation of, say internal inhibition *over the entire hemisphere*, certain circumstances greatly complicating the picture are met with in this case (probably, the border-line layers between different parts of the hemispheres, various degrees of energy of stimulation, etc.). Experiments in this direction are now performed in our laboratory. It is more convenient to trace the movement of sleep inhibition in that part of the cerebral hemispheres which relates to the skin, being, as it were, its projection in the brain. Moreover, the conditioned stimulation of the skin provokes a sleeping state quite easily. If we assume that this sleeping state arises precisely at the point of stimulation, we see how this inhibitory movement spreads from this point over the entire cutaneous area of the brain; it will then be possible to determine how far and how quickly this process spreads. But, for the time being, this is only a hope.

PSYCHIATRY AS AN AUXILIARY TO THE PHYSIOLOGY OF THE CEREBRAL HEMISPHERES[15]

My earlier researches on the circulation of the blood and on digestion led me to the firm conviction that the physiological mode of thinking may derive great help from the study of clinical cases, i.e., from the countless number of diverse pathological variations and combinations of the functions of the human organism. For this reason, during many years of work on the physiology of the cerebral hemispheres I often thought of making use of the world of psychiatric phenomena as an analytical auxiliary to this physiological study. Indeed, instead of applying our usual method which, as a mode of analysis, consists in destroying certain parts of the brain, and is very crude compared with the complexity and delicacy of the mechanism under investigation, one might expect in some cases to achieve a more distinct, precise and detailed decomposition of the work of the brain as a whole into its separate elements, to obtain a delimitation of its functions resulting from pathological causes, which sometimes reach a very high degree of differentiation.

In the summer of 1918 I had at last the opportunity to study a number of cases of insanity. And as it seems to me my former hopes have not been in vain. In some instances, I saw excellent demonstrations of points more or less explained in physiology; in others, new aspects of the work of the brain were brought to light, new questions and unusual problems for laboratory investigation arose.

My attitude towards the psychiatric material, however, differed greatly from the usual attitude of specialists. Due to a definite inclination of thought developed during years of laboratory practice, I always reasoned on a purely physiological basis and constantly explained to myself the psychical activity of the patients in definite physiological concepts and terms. This did not present any great difficulty for me, since my attention was concentrated not on the details of the subjective state, but on the principal features and phenomena of one or another state of the patient. How this was achieved will be partly seen from the following account.

In this article I shall describe and analyse the symptoms observed in two patients. One was an educated, well-bred girl, twenty-two or twenty-three years old. We find her lying motionless in bed in the hospital garden, her eyes half closed. At our approach she does not speak of her own accord. The physician accompanying me tells me that this is now her usual state. She refuses to eat without assistance and is untidy. She appears to understand our questions about her family, and remembers everything perfectly; she answers correctly, but with great effort and after considerable delay. The patient exhibits a strongly pronounced cataleptic state. She has been ill for years, at times almost fully recovering, at others relapsing and manifesting a considerable variety of symptoms; her present state is one of these relapses.

The second patient is a man aged sixty. He spent twenty-two years of his life in hospital, lying like a living corpse, without the slightest voluntary movement and absolutely speechless; he was fed artificially and was untidy. During the past few years, as he was approaching sixty, he began more and more often to make voluntary movements. At present he is able to get up and go to the lavatory; he talks volubly and quite reasonably, and sometimes eats without assistance. Recalling his former state, he said that he had been conscious of his surroundings, but had experienced such extreme and insuperable heaviness in his muscles that he could hardly breathe. And this was the reason why he could neither move, eat, nor speak. The disorder began to develop when he was thirty-five. Tonic reflexes were recorded in the history of the case.

How should one assess the physiological state of the two patients?

In order to answer this question let us consider the strongly pronounced motor symptoms which are observed in both cases: the catalepsy of the first patient and the tonic reflexes of the second. When do these symptoms manifest themselves in animals? A long time ago Schiff[16] observed cataleptic phenomena in a rabbit deprived of the cerebral hemispheres. Decerebration introduced by Sherrington[17] is a simple method of obtaining distinct tonic reflexes in cats. Intoxication by certain narcotics, for example, urethan, also produces cataleptic phenomena. In all these cases there occurs an elimination of the activity of the cerebral hemispheres *without the suppression of the lower parts of the brain*; in the first two cases this is due to a specific property of the brain tissue of the given animals, as well as to the freshness of the operation, i.e., to the absence of subsequent reactive phenomena; in the case of intoxication by urethan it is due to the presence in the latter of an ammoniac grouping which produces a stimulating action on the lower motor centres. Such an isolated exclusion of the cerebral hemispheres, the nervous organ of the so-called voluntary movements, reveals the normal activity of the lower parts of the nervous motor apparatus. This activity is designed first of all for equilibrating the organism and its parts in space, which represents the equilibration reflexes, always functioning under normal conditions and at the same time constantly disguised by voluntary movements. Thus, catalepsy is a normal and permanent reflex which manifests itself in a distinct and patent way only when the action of the cerebral hemispheres is excluded as in the above-mentioned case. As for the tonic reflexes, they are the elements of this complex reflex.

Consequently, the existence of the same mechanism must be assumed in our patients, i.e., exclusion of the activity of the cerebral hemispheres. It is clear, however, that here only the activity of the motor region of the cerebral hemispheres is excluded, since our patients, unable to make any voluntary movements or suffering extreme impairment of this function, are able, at the same time, as can be seen or as they themselves acknowledge, to understand perfectly well what they are told; they also remember everything and are conscious of their state, i.e., the work of all the other parts of their cerebral hemispheres is quite satisfactory.

The strictly isolated inhibition of the motor region of the cerebral cortex is observed also in other cases, in other definite states inherent in man and animals. A subject in a certain degree of hypnosis understands your words quite well, remembers them and is willing to do something in connection with the conversation, but he has no power over his skeletal muscles and remains in the posture imparted to him, even though it is uncomfortable and he does not like it. Apparently, this phenomenon is essentially accounted for by a fully isolated inhibition of the motor region of the cerebral cortex, an inhibition which does not spread either over other parts of the hemispheres or to the lower levels of the brain mass. I have often observed a similar state in dogs when I worked in the laboratory with the so-called conditioned reflexes. Jointly with Dr. Voskresensky I studied these relations with particular precision and in a most systematic way on one of our dogs.[18] For weeks and months this dog was often left alone in the room for a long time, strapped in the stand without being subjected to any experimental influence. As a result, the entire environment of the room became for the dog a soporific agent, to the degree that the moment it entered the room, its behaviour immediately changed. Strictly measuring the influence of this agent by varying the duration of its action we could clearly see the separate phases in the development of the sleeping state. The following phenomena were observed. The so-called conditioned food reflex for sound (association) was elaborated in the dog, i.e., at a definite sound the dog exhibited an alimentary reaction: it secreted saliva and made appropriate movements, licking its lips, turning in the direction from where the food was usually offered, and eating the food the moment it was offered. With the first signs of the sleeping state the conditioned salivary reflex to the sound disappeared, but the motor reflex to the sight of food remained quite normal, i.e., the dog began to eat without any delay. This first phase was followed by another one, which was quite unexpected and of considerable interest. Now the conditioned salivary reflex to the sound reappeared and became intensified with the addition of the natural conditioned stimuli proceeding from the food itself. But the motor reflex was absent—the dog did not take the food, even turned away from it and resisted its forcible introduction. In the following phase—the phase of profound sleep—all reactions to food, naturally, vanished. When the animal was deliberately awakened (by means of strong stimuli) the phases indicated above manifested themselves in reverse order as the sleeping state gave way. The second phase, naturally, could be interpreted as follows: the motor region of the cortex was already embraced by sleep inhibition while all other parts of the cerebral hemispheres still functioned quite satisfactorily and manifested their activity on an organ fully independent of the motor region—on the salivary gland. It is impossible not to see here a complete analogy with a person who is being awakened by you; he understands and even admits that you are rousing him at his own insistent request, but he cannot overcome the influence of sleep, begs you to leave him alone or he becomes angry and even aggressive when you persist in fulfilling his request and continue to disturb his sleep.

The first phase and its replacement by the second when the sleep becomes more profound, can be explained thus: since in our case the entire environment of the room, i.e., all the stimuli affecting the eyes, ears and nose, acts as a soporific agent, the parts of the cerebral hemispheres corresponding to these stimuli were the first to be subjected to sleep inhibition, the latter, though still superficial, was strong enough to suppress the conditioned action of the stimuli. At the same time the soporific influence was not yet sufficient to inhibit the more powerful part of the cortex—the motor region. But when monotonous cutaneous and motor stimuli (due to the limited movement in the stand) were added to the sleep-producing action of the room, sleep inhibition extended also to the motor region. And now this part of the cortex, being the strongest, attracted sleep inhibition from all other parts in accordance with the law of concentration of the nervous process; it thereby once more liberated them temporarily from this inhibition, until with the ever-increasing action of all soporific agents the sleep inhibition embraced all parts of the cerebral hemispheres with an equal and sufficient intensity.

And so we have sufficient grounds for granting the existence in the above-described patients of a concentrated and isolated inhibition of the motor region of the cerebral cortex as a result of the pathogenic cause.

What objections, from the clinical point of view, can be raised against our interpretation of the symptoms in our above-mentioned patients? I shall cite the arguments or the seeming inconsistencies with clinical cases which were pointed out by the psychiatrists when we informed them of the results of our analysis. Some of them were inclined to see in the cases cited by us a state of stupor evoked by strong emotions. But in the first place, this concerns the cause of the symptoms and not their mechanism. Evidently cases of stupor, i.e., of similar cataleptic states, may occur under the influence of strong, unusual stimulations caused by sounds of extraordinary intensity, by uncommon pictures, etc.; a very strong stimulation of certain parts of the hemispheres may lead to the inhibition of their motor region and thus create favourable conditions for the manifestation of the equilibrating reflex. In the second place, in the above-mentioned patients there are no indications of the existence of such a mechanism, and nothing reveals the presence of any extraordinary stimuli; one of the patients plainly points out the extreme difficulty, the impossibility of voluntary movements.

Further, it was stated that in progressive paralysis a destruction of the cerebral hemispheres is proved even on a pathological anatomical basis, although catalepsy is absent. However, in this case there is no complete elimination of the motor activity of the cerebral hemispheres either. The patients are able to make many voluntary movements though they are badly co-ordinated; besides, they often exhibit phenomena of extreme motor excitability of the cortex in the form of convulsions. Consequently, here the main condition for the manifestation of a pure equilibrating reflex is absent.

Reference was made to cases of thrombosis and haemorrhage in the cerebral hemispheres, which are accompanied by paralysis and not by catalepsy. But again this is not a condition which provokes catalepsy. In these cases one observes the absence of even spinal reflexes. It is clear that the inhibitory action of the destruction extends even to the spinal cord. And this inhibition must manifest itself all the more in the parts of the brain adjacent to the cerebral hemispheres.

Thus, the clinical cases of cerebral diseases do not reveal any actual inconsistencies with our analysis of the pathological state of the patients; therefore, in definite cases the mechanism of the pathological activity of the cerebral hemispheres suggested by us must be acknowledged as quite real. The fact that after more than twenty years of illness the patient described in our second case shows signs of returning to normal state, also leads us to interpret the general symptoms as an inhibition of the motor region of the cortex. This means that all the time his state was of a functional rather than of an organic, pathologico-anatomic nature.

Analysing further the state of our patients we must point to another essential circumstance. Although, according to present-day physiology, the cortical motor elements controlling different movements (skeletal, verbal, ocular, etc.), are localised in different parts of the cerebral hemispheres or, so to speak, scattered over them, nevertheless, in our patients they are all united by a common inhibition contrary to all other elements of the hemispheres which remain at the same time more or less free. This leads us to the important conclusion that all the motor elements possess common features in respect of their structure or chemical constitution, or, most probably, of both. Therefore, their relation to the cause originating the pathological symptoms is the same, and in this respect they differ from other cortical elements—visual, auditory, etc. This difference between certain elements of the cortex naturally manifests itself also in the above-mentioned phases of hypnosis and sleep when, influenced by one and the same cause, some elements are in one state and others in a different state.*

---

* This difference between the cellular elements of the cerebral cortex must be regarded as being incontestable, especially since in the physiology of the peripheral nerves we constantly meet with a strongly pronounced individuality (excitability, relative strength, etc.) of the nerve fibres (and of their peripheral endings) of different functions. This individuality underlies the methods by means of which the differentiation of these different fibres of one and the same anatomic trunk can be effected. Let us recall, for example, the methods used in separating vasoconstrictor from vasodilator fibres.

Let us now answer the following question: What cause actually determines the given symptoms? Different assumptions are, of course, possible. There may be a definite toxic action, the sphere of influence of which is naturally limited by the individual peculiarities of the separate cortical elements that have just been mentioned. One can also assume exhaustion of the elements of the cortex resulting either from the general exhaustion of the organism, or only from overfatigue of the brain, from exhaustion concentrated in definite elements of the brain either because of the predominant part of these elements in the work producing the exhaustion, or again as a result of their specific nature. Finally, there is the possibility of direct or indirect (the last resulting from local changes in blood circulation or in general nutrition) reflex influences which may effect injuriously and also in an elective manner different elements of the cortex. Hence, in different cases, in spite of the similarity or even identity of the mechanism of the given complex of symptoms, the causes producing them may not be the same.

Finally, the following question is also of definite interest to us: what is the explanation for the case of our second patient, in whom the inhibition of the motor region of the cerebral cortex, having remained for twenty years almost at the same level of intensity, at last began drastically to diminish? This can be accounted for only by the patient's age. Approaching the age of sixty, when a sharp decline in the strength of the organism and the process of its aging usually becomes pronounced, he began to return to his normal state. How is this connection to be interpreted? If a certain toxic agent acted in this case then, with the senile transformation of the body's chemism, there could take place a weakening, diminution of the agent producing this action. If the principal cause of the disease was chronic exhaustion of the nervous substance, then, with the senile transformation of the brain (lesser reactivity and lesser functional destructibility of the brain which is manifested in a sharp weakening of the memory for current events), this cause could now be less pronounced. Since sleep and hypnosis should be regarded as a kind of special inhibition, it may be admitted that our second patient presented an example of chronic partial sleep or hypnosis. With the advent of old age there is in evidence a relatively greater decline of the inhibitory processes, expressed in senile talkativeness, fantasticality, and in extreme cases, in dotage. In view of this, the recovery of the patient may be attributed to the senile decline of the inhibitory process.

It can hardly be disputed, I think, that the physiological analysis of the above cases raises before the physiology of the brain many new problems which can be investigated in the laboratory.

CONCERNING THE SO-CALLED HYPNOTISM IN ANIMALS[19]

The so-called hypnotism of animals (the experimentum mirabile of Kircher) consists in the fact that by means of energetic action, overcoming all resistance, the animal is brought to an unnatural posture (laid on its back) and kept thus for a brief space of time. Afterwards, when the hands are removed from the animal, the latter remains motionless for many minutes and even hours. Different authors, noting one or other detail of this phenomenon, have explained it in various ways. At present, thanks to the systematic study of the normal activity of the brain, I am in a position to indicate the biological significance of this phenomenon and to give an exact and full explanation of its physiological mechanism; thus I am able to combine all the separate facts of the different authors. The phenomenon represents a self-protecting reflex of an inhibitory character. Faced with an overwhelming power, from which there is no escape in struggle or in flight, the animal's only chance of salvation is to remain immobile in order not to be noticed, since moving objects attract particular attention, or not to provoke by fussy, restless movements an aggressive reaction on the part of this overwhelming force. Immobility is brought about in the following manner. Extraordinary external stimuli highly intense or very unusual in form, first of all cause a rapid reflex inhibition of the motor region of the cerebral cortex which controls the so-called voluntary movements. Depending on the intensity and duration of the stimulus, this inhibition is either confined to the motor region and does not pass to other regions of the cerebral hemispheres and to the mid-brain, or it irradiates over all these parts. In the first case there are present reflexes of the eyes muscles (the animal follows the experimenter with its eyes), of the glands (when food is offered, there begins a secretion of saliva, although no skeletal movements in the direction of food are observed), and finally tonic reflexes from the mid-brain to the skeletal muscles in order to retain the position into which the animal has been brought (catalepsy). In the second case all the above-mentioned reflexes gradually disappear, and the animal passes into an absolutely passive, sleeping state accompanied by a general relaxation of the musculature. This course of the phenomena is further confirmation of the conclusion which I reached at a previous meeting of our section, namely, that the so-called inhibition is nothing more than sleep, but partial and localised. It it clear that the rigidity and stupor which seize us in cases of great fear is nothing else but the above-described reflex.

P.S. It should be added that during the period when I did not have physiological literature at hand, which I managed to get only in the spring of 1922 in Helsingfors, a number of other authors came to this same conclusion concerning hypnosis in animals.

RELATIONS BETWEEN EXCITATION AND INHIBITION, DELIMITATION BETWEEN EXCITATION AND INHIBITION, EXPERIMENTAL NEUROSES IN DOGS[20]

Dedicated to the memory of my best friend, Professor Robert Tigerstedt, to whom physiology owes so much for his investigations and for his work in promoting physiological knowledge and physiological research.

All the factual material which follows relates to the work of the cerebral hemispheres and has been obtained by the method of conditioned reflexes, i.e., reflexes formed in the course of the animal's individual life. Since the concept of conditioned reflexes is not yet generally known and recognised among physiologists I shall, for the purpose of avoiding repetition, refer the reader to my articles recently published in these archives (1923).

Proceeding from the big difference between the phenomena, we had to distinguish two kinds of inhibition in the work of the cerebral hemispheres—external and internal—according to our terminology. The former appears in our conditioned reflexes at once; the latter develops with the passage of time and is elaborated gradually. The first is an exact repetition of the well-known inhibition in the physiology of the lower part of the central nervous system, which appears when stimuli acting on the various centres and evoking different nervous activities, meet; the second can be inherent only in the cerebral hemispheres. It may be, however, that the difference between these kinds of inhibition is connected only with the conditions of their emergence and not with the essence of the process itself. This question is still being investigated by us. The present article deals only with internal inhibition; further, I shall call it simply inhibition, without the adjective, although each time implying internal inhibition.

There are two conditions, or to be more precise, one condition, the presence or absence of which determines whether the impulse brought into the cells of the cerebral hemispheres from the outside chronically provokes a process of excitation or a process of inhibition. In other words, the impulse will in one case become positive and in the other negative. This fundamental condition consists in the following: if the stimulation coming to a cerebral cell coincides with another extensive stimulation of the cerebral hemispheres, or of a definite lower part of the brain, then it will always remain positive; given the reverse condition it will, sooner or later, become a negative, inhibitory stimulus. Of course this indubitable fact gives rise to the question: Why is this so? But so far there has been no answer to this question. Thus, we must proceed from this fact without having analysed it. Such is the first basic relation between excitation and inhibition.

Physiologists have long been aware of the irradiation of the excitatory process. The study of the higher nervous activity led us to the conclusion that the inhibitory process, too, spreads, under certain conditions, from the point where it originated. The facts underlying this conclusion are perfectly plain and obvious. Now, if the excitatory process spreads from one point, and the inhibitory process from another, they limit each other and confine each other to a definite area and within definite bounds. In this way a very delicate functional delimitation of separate points of the cerebral hemispheres can be obtained. When these separate points are subjected to excitation under corresponding conditions, it can be easily explained by the scheme of the cellular construction. But this interpretation meets with certain difficulties when there is an excitatory or inhibitory process related to various intensities or other similar variations (for example, to different frequencies of the metronome beats) of one and the same elementary external stimulating agent. In order to explain this on the basis of the same simple cellular scheme, it would be necessary to assume as a point of application of this agent not a single cell but a group of cells. In any case, it is actually possible to associate the excitatory process with one intensity of a certain elementary agent and the inhibitory process with another. Thus, the second general relation between excitation and inhibition consists in their mutual spatial limitation, in their delimitation. A clear demonstration of this is obtained by the experiments with mechanical stimulation of various points of the surface of the skin.

Thus, we have to assume that a certain conflict takes place between two opposing processes which normally ends in the establishment of a definite equilibrium between them, in a definite balance. This struggle and this equilibrium confront the nervous system with a difficult task. We have seen this from the very outset of our research, and we are seeing it now. This difficulty is often manifested in the animal in the form of motor excitation, whining and dyspnoea. But in most cases equilibrium finally sets in; each process is allotted its place and time, and the animal becomes perfectly quiet, reacting to respective stimuli now by the excitatory, now by the inhibitory process.

Only under certain conditions does this conflict end in disturbance of the normal nervous activity; then a pathological state sets in which lasts for days, weeks, months and perhaps even years, and either gradually returns to the normal of itself after the experiments have been discontinued for a time and the animal has been allowed rest, or it must be eliminated by definite treatment.

These special cases at first emerged spontaneously, unexpectedly, but later they were deliberately produced by us for research purposes. We describe them here in chronological order.

The first of these cases was obtained by us a long time ago (experiments of Dr. Yerofeyeva[21]). It consisted in the following. The conditioned food reflex was elaborated in the dog not from an indifferent agent, but from a destructive one, provoking an inborn defensive reflex. The animal's skin was irritated by an electric current, and at the same time the animal was fed, at first even forcibly. In the initial phase a weak current was applied, but later it was increased to the maximum. The experiment ended thus: the strongest current, as well as the severe burning and mechanical destruction of the skin, provoked only a food reaction (a corresponding motor reaction and a secretion of saliva) without any sign of a defensive reaction, or even of any change in respiration and heartbeat—the usual accompaniments of this reaction. Evidently this result was obtained by transferring the external excitation to the food centre and simultaneous inhibition of the centre of the defensive reaction. This specific conditioned reflex persisted for months, and probably would have remained unchanged under the given conditions had we not begun to modify it, systematically transferring the electric irritation to new points of the skin. When the number of these points became considerable, the picture suddenly and abruptly changed in one of our dogs. Now only a very strong defensive reaction manifested itself everywhere, even in the first location of the skin stimulus and under the action of the weakest current; there was no trace of the food reaction.

The old result could not be reproduced. The dog which had previously been quiet became greatly excited. In another dog a similar result was obtained only when—notwithstanding the large number of points on the skin from which we could produce only an alimentary reaction under the application of a strong current—we frequently and quickly, in the course of one and the same experiment, transferred the irritation from one place to another. We had to allow rest to the dogs for several months, and only in one of them were we able, acting slowly and cautiously, to restore the conditioned food reflex to the destructive agent.

The second case of a similar character was observed somewhat later (experiment of Dr. N. R. Shenger-Krestovnikova[22]). A conditioned food reflex was brought about in a dog by a circle of light projected on a screen placed in front of the animal. We then began to elaborate a differentiation of the circle from an ellipse of the same size and intensity of light, i.e., the appearance of the circle was accompanied each time by feeding, whereas that of the ellipse was not. In this way the differentiation was obtained. The circle evoked a food reaction, but the ellipse remained ineffective, which, as we know, is a result of development of inhibition. The ellipse which was applied first greatly differed in form from the circle (the proportion of its axes was 2:1). Then the form of the ellipse was brought closer and closer to that of the circle, i.e., the axes of the ellipse were gradually equalised, and thus sooner or later we were able to obtain an increasingly delicate differentiation. But when we applied an ellipse whose axes were as 9:8, the picture abruptly changed. The new delicate differentiation, which always remained incomplete, persisted for two or three weeks, after which it not only disappeared itself, but caused the loss of all earlier, even the least delicate, differentiations. The dog, which previously behaved quietly in the stand, was now constantly moving about and whining. All differentiations had to be elaborated anew, and the crudest one now demanded much more time than at first. When the final differentiation was reached, the same story was repeated —all the differentiations vanished, and the dog again became excited.

Some time after these observations and experiments we set ourselves the task of investigating this phenomenon more systematically and in more detail (experiments of Dr. M. K. Petrova[23]). Since it was possible to conclude from the above-mentioned facts that the derangement of normal relations was caused by a difficult collision between the excitatory and inhibitory processes, we carried out on two dogs of different types—one very lively and the other inactive and quiet—experiments first of all with various inhibitors and their combinations. Together with the conditioned reflexes, delayed for three minutes, i.e., when the unconditioned stimulus was added to the conditioned only three minutes after the beginning of the latter, owing to which the positive effect of the conditioned reflex appeared only after a preliminary inhibitory period of one or two minutes, other kinds of inhibition were applied (differentiation, etc.). But this task was accomplished by the different nervous systems without any derangement of the normal relations, although with a different degree of difficulty. Then we added the food reflex formed by means of a destructive agent. Now it was sufficient, having evoked this reflex, to repeat it for a certain period of time even on one and the same part of the skin, in order to obtain an acute pathological state. This deviation from the normal occurred in the two dogs in opposite directions. In the lively dog the elaborated inhibitions either suffered to a considerable degree or wholly disappeared and turned into positive agents; in the quiet dog it was the positive salivary conditioned reflexes that either weakened or completely vanished. And these states persisted for months without any spontaneous change. In the lively dog with the weakened inhibitory process a quick and lasting return to the normal was obtained in a few days by means of rectal injections of potassium bromide. It was worth noting that with the appearance of normal inhibition the strength of the positive conditioned action, far from decreasing, was even somewhat increased; consequently, on the basis of this experiment we can assume that the action of bromide does not consist in diminution of nervous excitability, but in regulating nervous activity. In another dog permanent and more or less considerable salivary reflexes could not be restored despite the different means applied for this purpose.

Shortly after these experiments similar results, and even with more instructive details, were obtained with a dog subjected to experimental investigation for quite a different purpose (experiments of Dr. I. P. Razenkov[24]). Many positive conditioned reflexes were elaborated on the animal from various receptors, or several reflexes from one and the same receptor by a certain stimulating agent of varying intensity. Among others there was obtained a reflex to a definite frequency of mechanical stimulation of a certain point on the skin. We then began to elaborate a differentiation from the same place on the skin by means of a mechanical stimulation of another frequency. This differentiation was also obtained without difficulty, and no change in nervous activity was observed. But when, after application of a completely inhibited rhythm of mechanical skin stimulation, we tried without any interval to effect stimulation by a positively-acting rhythm, a peculiar disturbance was manifested in the dog, lasting for five weeks and only gradually ending in a return to the normal, perhaps somewhat accelerated by our special measures. A few days after the collision of the nervous processes occurred, all the positive conditioned reflexes disappeared. This lasted for ten days, after which the reflexes began to reappear, but in a peculiar way: contrary to normal, the strong stimuli remained ineffective or produced the minimum effect; considerable effect was shown only by the weak stimuli. This state persisted for fourteen days and was again superseded by a peculiar phase.

Now all the stimuli acted equally, approximately, with the same force as strong stimuli under normal conditions. This lasted seven days, and then came the last period before the return to the normal; this phase was characterised by the fact that the stimuli of average strength greatly exceeded those in the normal state, the strong stimuli became somewhat weaker than in the normal and the weak stimuli lost their action altogether. This, too, lasted for seven days, and then, finally, came the return to the normal. Repetition of the same procedure which was responsible for the disturbance described above, i.e., repetition of direct, without any interval, transition from the inhibitory mechanical stimulation of the skin to the positively-acting stimulation, resulted in the same disturbance with the same variation in phases, but of considerably shorter duration. With further repetition the disturbance became more and more fleeting, until the same procedure no longer evoked any derangement. The decline of the pathological disturbance was manifested not only in the shortened duration of the abnormal state, but also in a reduction in the number of phases, and in the disappearance of the more abnormal phases.

Thus, the difficult collision between the excitatory and inhibitory processes leads now to a predominance of the excitatory process disturbing the inhibition, or, one may say, to a prolonged increase of the tonus of the excitation, and now to a predominance of the inhibitory process, with its preliminary phases, disturbing the excitation, and increasing the tonus of the inhibition.

But then we witnessed the same phenomena also under other conditions, besides those mentioned above.

Under the action of extraordinary, directly inhibiting stimuli on the animal a chronic predominance of inhibition takes place. This manifested itself with particular force in a number of dogs after the unusual flood that occurred in Leningrad on September 23, 1924, when our experimental animals were rescued with great difficulty and under exceptional conditions. The conditioned reflexes disappeared for some time and only slowly reappeared. For a considerable period after rehabilitation any more or less strong stimulus, which earlier would have been regarded as a very strong conditioned stimulus, as well as the application of a previously elaborated and thoroughly concentrated inhibition, again provoked this chronic state of inhibition either in the form of complete inhibition or of its above-mentioned preliminary phases (experiment of Dr. A. D. Speransky[25] and Dr. V. V. Rikman). To a lesser degree and for a shorter time the same thing is often observed in more normal conditions, such as transferring the animals to a new environment, to a new experimenter, etc.

On the other hand, a slight change in the application of a well-elaborated positive conditioned reflex, namely, an unconditioned stimulus administered directly, without any interval, after the conditioned stimulus, increases the tonus of the excitation to such a degree that elaborated inhibitions, now under investigation, either fully disappear or greatly lose in constancy and regularity. And often a frequent interchange of positive and inhibitory reflexes brings the dogs, especially the lively ones, to the highest pitch of general excitation (experiments of Dr. M. K. Petrova and Dr. Y. M. Kreps).

However, what has been said above does not exhaust all our facts concerning the relation between excitation and inhibition. In the course of our work we encountered other peculiar cases of the same kind.

We frequently noticed that a distortion of the action of conditioned stimuli took place in certain phases of drowsiness in normal animals.

The positive stimuli lost their effect, while the negative inhibitory ones assumed a positive character (for example, in the experiments carried out by Dr. A. A. Shishlo). In the light of this relation we can explain the frequently recurring fact that in the drowsy state of the animals there begins as it were a voluntary secretion of saliva not observed in the waking state. The explanation is that at the beginning of the elaboration of the conditioned reflexes in a given animal the entire mass of accessory stimuli, one can say, the entire laboratory surroundings, enter into conditioned connection with the food centre, but later all these stimuli become inhibited owing to the specialisation of the conditioned stimulus applied by us. It can be assumed that in a state of drowsiness these inhibited agents temporarily recover their original effect.

The temporary transformation of the elaborated inhibitory stimulus into a positive one is also observed in pathological states of the cerebral cortex in intervals between the convulsive fits caused by post-operative cicatrisation in the cortex. It is interesting to note that along with this elaborated inhibitory stimulus, only the weakest of all the positive conditioned stimuli, viz., light, acts, also positively, during this time, whereas all other moderate and strong positive conditioned stimuli remain ineffective (experiments of Dr. I. P. Razenkov).

Related to this is the fact, frequently reproduced by us, that accessory stimuli evoking certain reflexes of moderate strength transform in the course of their action the inhibitory reflexes into positive ones (we call it disinhibition).

On the contrary, during disturbance of the cortex, caused by extirpation, the positive conditioned stimuli belonging to the disturbed part of the cortex become inhibitory, a point mentioned in my last article on sleep. This phenomenon is particularly manifest and has been best studied in the cutaneous region of the cerebral hemispheres. (Earlier experiments of Dr. N. I. Krasnogorsky and recent experiments of Dr. I. P. Razenkov.) If the lesion is insignificant the effect produced by the previous positive conditioned mechanical stimulation of the skin is less than normal, and if repeated during one and the same experiment soon becomes inhibitory; being added to other effective stimuli it weakens their effect and when applied alone induces a state of sleepiness in the animal. If the lesion is more severe, it does not, in normal conditions, produce any positive effect, being of a purely inhibitory nature; its application leads to the disappearance of all positive conditioned reflexes in the other parts of the cerebral hemispheres.

But this agent, now inhibitory, may, in certain circumstances, manifest a positive effect. If the animal becomes sleepy of itself, this stimulus, as well as the elaborated inhibitory agent, as mentioned above, produces a slight positive effect. But afterwards this effect can be obtained by other methods. If we repeatedly apply this stimulus several times with a brief intermission, for example, of five seconds instead of the usual thirty (i.e., if the unconditioned stimulus is added five seconds instead of thirty seconds after the beginning of the conditioned stimulus), then, upon delaying it again for thirty seconds, we may obtain a positive effect, although a fleeting one. Setting in very soon after the beginning of the stimulation, it quickly diminishes in the course of stimulation and finally disappears altogether (pure excitatory weakness). A similar transitory effect can be obtained by means of a preliminary injection of caffeine and by other measures (experiments of Dr. I. P. Razenkov).

Of a somewhat different character, but still related to our subject, are the following facts. Given a very weak general excitability of the cortex, as observed in aged animals (Dr. L. A. Andreyev's experiments) or in animals with removed thyroid glands (experiments of Dr. A. V. Valkov), as well as in certain states brought on in the animals by convulsions during post-operative scarring in the cortex (experiments of Dr. I. P. Razenkov), the inhibitory process either becomes impossible or is greatly weakened.

In such cases only an increase of the tonus of cortical excitability, achieved by application of stronger unconditioned stimuli, can sometimes provoke an inhibitory process.

The phenomenon of reciprocal induction, mentioned by me in the previous, above-mentioned articles (experiments of D. S. Fursikov, V. V. Stroganov, Y. M. Kreps, M. P. Kalmykov, I. R. Prorokov and others), is also related to our subject. Finally, the last fact: if separate points of the cortex are reinforced for a prolonged period by a corresponding procedure, some of them as points of excitation and others as points of inhibition, they become highly resistant to attacks, to the influence exerted by opposite processes, and at times call for exceptional measures in order to change their functions (experiments of Dr. B. N. Bierman and Dr. Y. P. Frolov).

All the foregoing facts allow us, it seems to me, to systematise the states to which the cortex is subjected under different influences in a definite consecutive order. At one pole there is the state of excitation, an exceptional increase of the tonus of excitation, when an inhibitory process becomes impossible or is greatly impeded. Next comes the normal, wakeful state, the state of equilibrium between the excitatory and inhibitory processes. This is followed by a long, but also consecutive, series of states transitory to inhibition; the most typical of these are: the equalisation state when in contrast to the wakeful state all stimuli, irrespective of their intensity, act with an absolutely equal force; the paradoxical state, when only the weak stimuli act, or when the strong stimuli act, too, but produce a barely noticeable effect; and finally, the ultra-paradoxical state when only the previously elaborated inhibitory agents produce a positive effect— a state followed by complete inhibition. There is yet no clear explanation of the state when excitability is so low that inhibition is utterly impossible or greatly impeded, just as in the case of the state of excitation.

At present, among other things, we are engaged in the experimental solution of the following question (for which we now have some clues): are there not in evidence the transitory states so sharply expressed in pathological cases also in all cases of normal transition from an active state to a state of inhibition, such as the process of falling asleep, the process of elaborating inhibitory reflexes, etc.?

Should this be so, then only the retardation, certain isolation and fixation of the states which normally develop and change quickly, or almost imperceptibly, bear a pathological character.

The above facts open the way to an understanding of numerous phenomena relating both to the normal and pathological higher nervous activity. I shall give some examples.

I have already shown in previous articles how normal behaviour is based on the elaborated delimitation of the points of excitation and inhibition, on their grandiose mosaic in the cortex, and how sleep represents irradiated inhibition. We are now in a position to give some details showing how certain variations of normal sleep, as well as separate symptoms of the hypnotic state, can be easily understood when regarded as different degrees of extensiveness and intensiveness of the inhibitory process.

Cases of sleep setting in while walking or riding horseback are not unknown. This means that the inhibition is confined only to the cerebral hemispheres and does not spread to the lower centres established by Magnus. We know also of sleep accompanied by partial wakefulness in relation to definite stimuli, for instance, the sleep of the miller who wakes when the noise of the mill stops, the sleep of the mother awakening at the faintest sound coming from her sick child, but who is not disturbed by other and much stronger stimuli, i.e., in general a sleep with easily excitable points on guard. Catalepsy in hypnosis is, apparently, an isolated inhibition only of the motor region of the cortex, not affecting all the other parts of the cortex and not spreading to the centres of equilibrium of the body. Suggestion in hypnosis can be rightly interpreted as such a phase of inhibition when weak conditioned stimuli (words) produce a greater effect than the evidently stronger direct and real external stimuli. The symptom established by Pierre Janet—loss of the sense of reality during sleep lasting for many years, can be explained as chronic inhibition of the cortex which is interrupted only for a short time and only under weak stimuli (usually at night); this inhibition particularly concerns the cutaneous and motor regions which are most important for the influence of the external world on the organism, on the one hand, and for the real action of the organism on the external world, on the other. Senile talkativeness and dementia are easily explained by the extreme weakening of inhibition in cases of very low excitability of the cortex. Finally, our experiments on dogs entitle us to regard chronic deviations of the higher nervous activity from the normal, produced in the animals by us, as pure neurosis; to a degree they also explain the mechanism of the origin of these deviations. Similarly the action of exceedingly strong, extraordinary stimuli (for example, unusual flood) on dogs with a weak nervous system and a predominance of the inhibitory process under normal conditions, in other words, with a constantly increased tonus of inhibition, reproduces the aetiology of a special traumatic neurosis.

As for a theory that would cover and generally substantiate all these phenomena, it is obvious that the time has not yet come for it, although many hypotheses have been advanced, each one of them justified to a degree. It seems to me that as things are at present it is possible to make use of the different concepts which actually systematise the factual material and advance new and detailed problems. In our experiments so far we think of different phases, from extreme excitation to deep inhibition, which develop in the nervous cells of the cortex under the influence of effective stimuli, and which depend on the intensity and duration of these stimuli and on the conditions under which the latter are formed. We incline to this view because of the obvious analogy between the changes observed in the activity of the cerebral cortex and the changes taking place in the nerve fibre under various strong influences, which have been described in the well-known work of N. E. Vvedensky—*Excitation, Inhibition and Narcosis*. We do not share his theory,[26] but we have grounds for relating all the observed transitions from excitation to inhibition to one and the same elements—to the nerve cells—just as Vvedensky rightly did in the case of the nerve fibre.

One can hardly doubt that only the study of the physicochemical process taking place in the nerve fibre will provide us with a real theory of all nervous phenomena, and that the phases of this process will give us an exhaustive explanation of all external manifestations of the nervous activity, of their sequence and interconnections.

NORMAL AND PATHOLOGICAL STATES OF THE CEREBRAL HEMISPHERES[27]

I have the great honour of claiming your kind attention to the report on the results of my recent investigations conducted jointly with my collaborators. I hope the subject of the investigations is capable of arousing considerable interest. These investigations were carried out on animals, namely, on the dog, this friend of man since pre-historic times. For the last 25 years we have endeavoured to understand the animal's entire higher nervous activity purely physiologically without using any psychological ideas or terms.

Of course, the cerebral hemispheres are the chief organ of higher nervous activity.

The central phenomenon in the activity of the cerebral hemispheres around which all our experimental material is concentrated is, what I call, the conditioned reflex. The idea of reflex in physiology, the gift of Descartes' genius, is, of course, a purely natural-science idea. Today we can regard it as adequately established that the so-called instincts are the same reflexes only often of a somewhat more complex composition. It is therefore preferable to leave the one term "reflex" for all of these regular reactions of the organism, while we add to it the adjective "unconditioned".

Let us take one of these unconditioned reflexes, the most usual, daily reflex—the food reflex. To the food as a stimulus, when it is before the dog and later in its mouth, the dog responds with a certain motor and secretory reaction. If several seconds before the food gets into the dog's mouth, the dog's ear begins to be stimulated, for example, by metronome beats and this coincidence is repeated once or several times, the metronome beats will evoke the same reaction as does the food, i.e., the dog will perform the same movements and will similarly secrete saliva and other digestive juices. This food reaction may become just as precise as it is to food and may exist for an indefinitely long time. This is just what I call a conditioned reflex. Why should not this be a reflex? The mechanism is apparently the same: a certain external agent, motion of the stimulation along a certain afferent nerve, and a central connection with certain efferent nerves of the muscles and glands. The difference is not in the mechanism, but in its consummation. The mechanism of the unconditioned reflex is completely ready since the day of birth. The conditioned reflex is completed in the course of individual existence at one of its points—the central nervous system, namely, the cerebral hemispheres, since with the removal of the hemispheres the conditioned reflexes disappear from the activity of the nervous system. Since this completion of the reflex mechanism in the normal animal necessarily takes place under certain physiological conditions, there is absolutely no reason to regard it as anything but physiological. The consummation of the mechanism in the conditioned reflex clearly consists in a coupling, formation of a connection on the way of the motion of stimulation. At the present time we have facts which warrant the assumption that the act of coupling is even an elementary physiological process.

Conditioned reflexes are formed to all manner of agents in nature, for which the given animal has receptor apparatus, and with all unconditioned reflexes. Their biological significance is enormous, since only because of them can the most precise and finest equilibrium be established between the complex organism and its environment, in vast regions of the latter. Innumerable conditionally acting agents signal, as it were, the relatively few and close agents directly favourable or harmful to the organism. Minutest and most remote conditioned stimuli, acting on the eye, ear and other receptors, cause the animal to move towards food, the opposite sex, etc., on the one hand, and away from all harmful and destructive agents, on the other hand.

From the aforesaid points of view the physiological role of the cerebral cortex is, on the one hand, coupling (according to its mechanism) and, on the other hand, signalling (according to its significance), at the same time with variable signalling in precise conformity with the external conditions.

Before I proceed, I should like to say a few words about our method. For the formation of conditioned reflexes we used almost exclusively two unconditioned reflexes—food and defensive—to nonalimentary, disagreeable substances introduced into the animal's mouth; we poured a weak acid solution into the dog's mouth. In this case we recorded not the motor component of conditioned reflexes, but the secretory component, namely, salivation, since this offers greater convenience for measuring the reaction.

Above we have cited a positive conditioned reflex in which the conditioned stimulus evokes a process of excitation in the cerebral cortex. But side by side with the positive reflex there are always also conditioned negative, inhibitory reflexes, in which the conditionally acting agent evokes not the process of stimulation, but the process of inhibition. For example, we formed a positive conditioned reflex to a tone of 100 vibrations per second. When we afterwards tried for the first time other tones, these, too, began to exert the same positive conditioned action. But, if we repeat them without accompanying them by the unconditioned stimulus, they will gradually not only lose their positive effect, but will be transformed into inhibitory agents. Their inhibitory effect is apparently revealed in the fact that after their application for some immediate period of time (minutes and even many minutes) the positively acting tone also becomes entirely ineffective or weakened.

Our studies of the conditioned reflexes have now greatly expanded and I am unable to set them forth in any detailed manner. After this necessary introduction I must briefly dwell on two or three more details in order that I may only then deal with the special subject of my present report.

Both, the process of excitation and the process of inhibition move through the cerebral cortex, at first irradiating rather far from the initial point and then concentrating in it. During concentration these processes are very subtly localised, owing to which the entire cortex is transformed into a vast mosaic of closely following each other stimulated and inhibited points.

This mosaic is formed and strengthened partly by the mutual impact of the antagonistic processes of excitation and inhibition evoked directly by appropriate external stimuli, and partly because of the internal relations, i.e., mutual induction, in which one process leads to the strengthening of the other.

My recent article printed in the *Skandinavisches Archiv für Physiologie (Scandinavian Archive of Physiology)* cites a long series of our experiments which, I am convinced, prove beyond any doubt that sleep is the same inhibition which alway coexists with excitation in the waking state of the cerebral hemispheres, but only that it is not scattered as it is there, but is continuous, and irradiates not only to both hemispheres, but also to the underlying parts of the brain.

Of late we have been studying the transitional phases between the animal's waking state and sleep. Under our experimental conditions, when the dogs are in the stand, restrained and alone in the experimental room, i.e., even isolated from the experimenter and exposed to our specific stimuli, they easily lapse into a special state in the direction, so to speak, of sleep. Partly because of the individual properties of the nervous systems of the different dogs and partly because of the measures we adopt we can observe and study, as it were, fixed definite phases in the transition from the waking state to complete sleep. Several such phases can be clearly distinguished. I shall dwell on two of them.

When conditioned reflexes are formed from different external agents by means of the same unconditioned stimulus, the effects produced prove to differ very greatly quantitatively despite the final elaboration of all the reflexes. To our usual thermal and mechanical stimuli of the skin, as well as optic stimuli, the conditioned reactions are less intense than they are to acoustic stimuli. As our recent special experiments have shown, this is conditioned by the absolute energy of each stimulus, i.e., the greater the energy of the stimulus, the greater its effect. During a certain phase in the transition from the waking state to sleep this normal relationship between the effects disappears and is replaced either by an equalisation of the effects (equalisation phase), or by their perverted relationship, i.e., the effects of weak stimuli become greater than those of the strong stimuli, or even only weak stimuli remain effective (paradoxical phase). Here are examples. A dog formerly responding by conditioned reflexes of different intensity, in accordance with different stimuli, began to lapse into a barely visible drowsy state, as the experiments with this dog continued, and all its conditioned reflexes were equalised as regards the intensity of the effect. As soon as this dog was administered a small amount of caffeine subcutaneously it became quite alert and all its reflexes arranged themselves in the proper sequence with respect to the intensity of the effect.

In another dog which always remained quite awake during the experiment we ourselves induced a sleepy state by repeated and prolonged application of inhibitory stimuli in the course of the given experiment. On testing a weak positive conditioned stimulus we now found it ineffective, although we gave the dog a little food. This, of course, made the dog somewhat less sleepy. By repeating the conditioned stimulus once more we began to obtain some effect from it. We fed the dog again. The third time the conditioned reflex to the same stimulus attained its usual intensity and even exceeded it. This time the conditioned stimulation was also accompanied by food. Then we applied one of the strongest conditioned stimuli and its effect turned out to be less intense than that of the weak stimulus applied prior to this. As our experiment was continued in the same manner, the normal relationship between the stimuli was finally quite restored in accordance with their strength. Apparently, the stimulation with repeated acts of eating gradually overcame the sleepy, inhibitory state of the hemispheres produced by us in the beginning of the experiment and this state passed again into a completely waking state only by successive phases.

Another example. To a dog in which many reflexes to agents of different strength had been rapidly elaborated, one more weak stimulus was applied several times running in each experiment and for several days at that. This decisively changed the animal's general condition. The animal became less lively in the stand; at times it stood stock-still; at the same time, of the old elaborated stimuli, only the weak ones retained their effect. Weak stimuli produced the complete secretory effect as long as they were applied and the dog began to eat the moment it was given food. The strong stimuli elicited little salivation only in the beginning of their action; then salivation ceased and the dog did not touch the food it was offered. If, on entering the room, we stimulated the dog in every possible manner, stroking it, calling it by name, etc., all the conditioned reflexes were immediately restored and the stimuli ranged in the normal sequence as regards the effect. But, if the dog was left in the stand for several days without special stimulation, all its conditioned reflexes finally disappeared and, while in the stand, the dog did not take the food it was offered. However, the moment the dog was released from the stand it very greedily devoured the food.

It can hardly be disputed that in the foregoing experiments we have a definite hypnotic phase. I think that our paradoxical phase is a real analogue of the particularly interesting phase of human hypnosis, the suggestion phase, when the strong stimuli of the real world yield to the weak stimuli furnished by the words of the hypnotiser. The paradoxical phase also renders intelligible many cases of short and protracted, often of many years standing, abnormal sleep, when man sometimes, and only for a short time, returns to the waking state, precisely when the strong (daytime) stimuli are eliminated, mainly at night. (The case of sleep lasting five years, observed by Professor Pierre Janet and the Petersburg case of such sleep which lasted 20 years.)

Thus the transitional phases between the waking state and sleep are different degrees of the extent and intensity of the inhibitory process in the cerebral hemispheres. The long-known so-called animal hypnosis is real hypnosis, one of the transitional phases between waking and sleep, inhibition concentrating mainly on the motor area of the cortex in virtue of a certain peculiarity of the procedure by which it is obtained. The cataleptic state taking place at this time apparently occurs because of the activity of the balancing centres of the brain, discovered by Magnus and de Kleijn, which now free themselves from the camouflaging influence of the motor area of the cortex. Our experiments have shown that different transitional phases and sleep may be obtained from weak as well as strong and unusual stimuli so that the waking state is, so to speak, generally established in response to usual stimuli of medium strength, particularly, of course, for certain nervous systems.

Of particular interest is also the fact that we observed the paradoxical phase apart from the states in which the aforesaid dogs were. After each single application of the conditioned inhibitory reflex, especially, soon after its elaboration, a long subsequent period of inhibition is observed all through the hemisphere. During this period it is also possible clearly to observe the paradoxical phase. This once more confirms our former conclusion that sleep and inhibition are the selfsame process.

Now another series of our experiments. At first we accidentally encountered, and then purposely produced in our dogs, pathological functional changes in the nervous system similar to human neuroses.

In two dogs the conditioned reflex was gradually elaborated not to an indifferent stimulus, but to very strong electric current applied to their skin. During application of the current the dog did not howl or defend itself but turned to the place whence it was usually given food, licked its lips, etc.; in a word, it exhibited a vigorous food reaction with abundant salivation. The electric current was sometimes replaced with cauterisation and injury to the skin, but the effect remained the same. This conditioned reflex persisted unchanged for a long time. We began to apply the electric current to ever new points. The state of affairs long remained the same. Then, when the current was applied to a certain new point (I do not remember its ordinal number), everything at once radically changed in one of the dogs. The conditioned food reflex to electric current disappeared without leaving a trace, and now the weakest current evoked only the strongest defensive reaction even at the initial point. In the other dog with the same reflex the transition to new points alone did not produce the same effect. But, when we stimulated these different points one after another in the selfsame experiment, exactly the same thing happened as did in the former dog. Both dogs generally became very excitable, restless. We had to suspend all experiments with them for three months and then it was possible, after that long rest, very slowly, beginning with very weak current, to form the same reflex again only in one of them. In the other dog it failed.

A conditioned reflex to a lighted circle projected on a screen was elaborated in another dog. Then we differentiated from this circle an ellipse which at first also acquired a positive conditioned effect, but repeated unaccompanied by an unconditioned stimulus also became a conditioned inhibitory agent. This first differentiated ellipse, having the same area and the same lighting as the circle, differed very much from the circle in shape. Then ellipses with a continuously decreasing ratio of semi-axes were successively differentiated. The new differentiations also formed and persisted. But when one of the ellipses, closest to the circle in shape, was introduced into the experiment, the differentiation formed at the outset was not strengthened by its repetition, but was weakened, i.e., this ellipse began to act positively and, with the passage of time, increasingly so. Together with this all the formerly firmly elaborated, coarser differentiations also disappeared. We had to resume the whole thing from the ellipse which was the remotest from the circle in shape, and act more cautiously and slowly than we had the first time. When the ellipse which proved to be marginal on first application was applied, the old story repeated itself. The general behaviour of this dog also sharply changed after many experiments: from a quiet animal it was transformed into a very excitable one.

In both cases—the experiments with the conditioned food reflex to the electric current and in the experiment of differentiating the ellipses from a circle—it was the inhibitory process that clearly suffered chronically. In the first case, for the food reaction to the current to exist, the defensive reaction to the current had to be inhibited. In the second case, as was shown above, the differentiation was based on inhibition.

The foregoing observations were made at an earlier stage of our work and long remained unutilised. Only of late have we made them a special subject and have expanded this subject in many respects.

In some dogs we obtained the same results. Under the effect of such methods their nervous system lost very much of its inhibitory function. Of the many different cases of inhibition only a few of the simplest ones remained intact, but even they were defective. This pathological state sometimes lasted for months, often remaining quite stationary. It is interesting that in some of these cases administration of bromides for several days very quickly and radically cured the animal. But on other dogs, apparently of a different nervous type (I shall have a pleasant occasion to speak of the different types of nervous system in the dog at your Psychological Society) we obtained entirely different results. In these cases, despite the fact that we used the same methods, the inhibitory process prevailed. The positive conditioned reflexes either disappeared altogether or presented peculiarities characteristic of the afore-described transitional phases from waking to sleep. Here is a relevant experiment.

A conditioned reflex was formed in a dog to a rhythmic mechanical stimulus applied to the skin with a certain frequency. From this conditioned stimulus we differentiated a stimulus almost identical with the former one and differing from it only in the frequency of the rhythm, i.e., one frequency of the rhythmic mechanical stimulation of the skin was made a conditioned positive stimulus and the other—a conditioned inhibitory stimulus. When these two reflexes became quite stable, we applied a positive stimulus directly, i.e., without any pause, after the action of the inhibitory stimulus; in other words, one frequency of mechanical stimulation of the skin was substituted for another. This led to an acute pathological state of the nervous system which became normal only after many weeks and, perhaps, partly under the effect of some of our measures. We observed the animal continuously, day in and day out. It all began with a complete disappearance of all the conditioned reflexes. Then they were gradually restored, going through the phases we are already familiar with, each characteristic phase persisting for several, even up to ten days. Between these phases the paradoxical and equalisation phases again clearly came to the fore.

Thus, in our pathological cases we had the same nervous phenomena as in the normal cases. But normally they quickly alternate, whereas here they become chronic. This is true of the prevalence of the excitatory, as well as the inhibitory process.

What common factor underlies all our pathological cases? In a word, what conditions protracted deviation from normal during the application of our methods? We think we are justified in saying that a difficult encounter, an unusual collision, whether as regards time or intensity, or both, of the two antagonistic processes, excitation and inhibition, leads to a protracted disturbance of the normal balance between them.

We must add, however, that some of the methods by which we produced a pathological state are not effective for all dogs. There are some which endure them without any harm. We cannot say the same for the electric current as a conditioned stimulus because we have had but few experiments with it.

We now encompass the entire foregoing factual characteristics of the physiological work of the cerebral hemispheres in the following preliminary conception by which we are guided in the performance of our subsequent experiments. We ascribe coupling, formation of new connections, to the functions of a dividing membrane, if it exists, or merely ever finer ramifications between neurons, between individual nerve cells. We ascribe the variations in excitation and the transition to an inhibitory state to the cells themselves. This distribution of functions seems probable to us in virtue of the fact that, while new connections, well elaborated, persist for a very long time, the changes in excitability, transition to an inhibitory state, are very mobile phenomena. We regard the phenomena of excitation and inhibition as different phases in the activity of the cells of the cerebral cortex. These cells must be recognised as possessing the highest degree of reactivity and, consequently, destructibility.

This precipitate functional destructibility serves as the main impulse for the appearance in the cell of the special process of inhibition, an economical process which not only limits further functional destruction, but also fosters restoration of the expended excitable substance. This is the most natural way of conceiving the most constant and most vivid fact with which we have to do during our work with conditioned reflexes. This fact consists in the following. A conditioned stimulus, if it is applied alone even for a couple of dozen seconds, will sooner or later in all cases, and in some dogs amazingly soon, reduce the cell to an inhibited state and, after the cell, the entire cortex and some underlying parts of the brain to a state of complete sleep. The fact that this does not occur, if an unconditioned stimulus is soon added in the beginning of the action of the conditioned stimulus, does not contradict our conception of these facts. Our latest experiments show that during the action of the unconditioned stimulus the positive conditioned stimulus loses its effect, becomes inhibited. The most vigilant signaller has played its important role and, for a time, while it is not needed, its rest is carefully guarded.

The value of the excitable substance of the cells of the cerebral cortex and its limited reserve are attested by the following experiments. Several years ago, when we were very short of foodstuffs, our experimental animals, of course, also very greatly suffered from hunger. With such animals it was almost impossible to work on conditioned reflexes. A positive conditioned stimulus rapidly became inhibitory despite all our efforts. All our work was confined to the single subject of the effect of hunger on conditioned reflexes. It should be noted, that the extraordinary tendency to transition to the inhibitory state made itself equally felt in both the food and acid conditioned reflexes. This fact once more denotes greater sensitivity of the conditioned reflex method in the physiological studies of the cerebral hemispheres.

From the point of view I have set forth we can easily understand the existence of the different types of nervous systems in the dogs with which we had to deal in our work. Of course, we must entertain similar ideas of our own nervous systems. We can easily conceive of nervous systems which, either from the very day of birth or under the effect of life's difficulties, possess a small reserve of excitable substance in the cortical cells and which therefore easily lapse into the inhibitory state, its different phases, or are even always in one of these phases.

I have finished and I should be very happy to have any of my highly esteemed listeners to come to me either for explanations or with objections, since I hardly could have discussed satisfactorily so vast and complex a subject of our work reported so briefly.

INHIBITORY TYPE OF NERVOUS SYSTEM IN DOGS[28]

I wish to express my sincere gratitude for the high honour you have shown me (by electing me a member of your Society) and for your readiness to hear my report, which also gives me great pleasure. I am convinced that sooner or later the physiologists who are studying the nervous system and the psychologists will have to unite in friendly work. Now let each of us try in his own way to marshal his special resources. The more approaches, the greater are the chances that we will finally come together, useful and necessary to each other.

As you know, in studying the activity of the brain of higher animals (the dog in particular) my collaborators and I have adopted a purely physiological point of view and operate with exclusively physiological conceptions and terms.

The more we have studied the higher nervous activity of dogs by our method, the more frequently we have come upon distinct and considerable differences in the nervous systems of different dogs. On the one hand, these differences rendered our investigations difficult and often hindered us from completely reproducing our facts on different animals and, on the other hand, gave us a great advantage in that they brought forward, emphasised, so to speak, certain aspects of nervous activity. At last we are in a position to distinguish several definite types of nervous systems. To one of these types I shall take the liberty of calling your attention. These are dogs which everybody, by observing their behaviour, especially in new surroundings, would call timid and cowardly animals. They walk cautiously, tail tucked in and legs half-bent. Should we make a sudden movement or slightly raise our voice, they draw back and crouch on the floor. We now have in our laboratory an extreme representative of this type. The dog—a female, was born in the laboratory and has lived there for five or six years. We have never given this dog any trouble. The only thing we have required of her was to eat periodically in the stand the food we offered her in the presence of certain signals, our conditioned stimuli. And yet, at the sight of any of us, permanent members of the laboratory staff, she starts and slinks away as if we were her most dangerous enemies. An animal of this type is very useful for work on conditioned reflexes, but not right away. It is exceedingly difficult to form conditioned reflexes in such dogs from the very outset: an animal of this type resents being placed in the stand, the attaching of various pieces of apparatus, the special form of feeding, etc. But when all the difficulties have at last been overcome, the dog becomes a model experimental object, a good machine. Particularly notable in the case of such dogs is the stability of the conditioned inhibitory reflexes, i.e., when conditioned agents evoke not the process of excitation but the process of inhibition. In the dogs of all other types it is, on the contrary, precisely the process of inhibition that proves more labile and especially easily disturbed. When the dog of this type is exposed, under the usual experimental conditions, to some new inconsiderable stimulation, for example the cautious presence of new persons behind the door of the experimental room, only the positive conditioned reflexes are immediately affected; they disappear or weaken, while the inhibitory reflexes are fully retained.

I shall now tell you about a dog of this type on which

Dr. Speransky, my collaborator, experimented. Six positive reflexes were elaborated in this dog: to a bell, metronome beats, a certain tone, increased general lighting of the room, the appearance of a circle of white paper and a toy rabbit. Differentiations from these stimuli were formed, i.e., metronome beats of another frequency, reduced general lighting, the form of a square and a toy horse were made inhibitory stimuli. The intensity of the positive reflexes varied as follows. All the auditory reflexes were 50-100 per cent more intense than the visual. Of the sounds, the bell occupied first place and was followed by the metronome beats, the tone being the weakest. The visual reflexes were all of about the same intensity. As has already been stated in general, and this dog also worked perfectly, all the afore-mentioned relations were always reproduced uniformly.

In September of last year (1924) Leningrad suffered a great flood. The dogs were saved only with considerable difficulties, and under extraordinary circumstances. Within five or ten days, when everything was put in order again, our dog, to all appearances perfectly healthy, greatly perplexed us in the experimental room. All the positive conditioned reflexes had completely disappeared: the dog did not salivate at all and did not take the food offered to it in the usual manner. For a long time we could not guess what was wrong. None of our initial suppositions about the reason for this phenomenon could be substantiated. Finally it dawned on us that the strong effect produced on the dog by the flood persisted. Then we did the following. We now usually conduct our experiments with conditioned reflexes so that the dog is alone in the experimental room, while the experimenter is in another room from where he acts on the dog, gives it food and records the results of the experiments. For our dog we now made certain changes. Dr. Speransky sat quietly in the room together with the dog and did nothing, while I performed the experiment for him from the other room. To our great satisfaction the conditioned reflexes reappeared and the dog began to take the food. By repeating this method for a considerable period of time, at first infrequently and then more often, gradually weakening it, i.e., sometimes leaving the dog alone in the room, we finally restored the dog in a certain measure to its normal condition. Then we tried the effect of various, so to speak, components of the flood in the following miniature form.

We let a stream of water trickle into the dog's room from under the door. Perhaps the soft sound of the flowing water or the watered surface of the floor returned the dog to its former pathological state. The conditioned reflexes disappeared again and they had to be restored by the former method. Moreover, when the dog recovered, we could not use the bell, formerly the strongest conditioned stimulus. The bell itself acted as an inhibitor and afterwards all the other reflexes were also inhibited. A year had passed since the flood and during that time we did everything to protect the dog from any extraordinary stimulation. Finally, last autumn (1925), we were able to obtain the old conditioned reflex also to the bell. But after its very first application this reflex gradually began to diminish, although it was used only once a day; at last it disappeared altogether and along with it all the other reflexes were also affected, now disappearing and now presenting various hypnotic phases ranging between waking and sleep, although this dog had never been sleepy before. While the animal was in this condition, we tried two more methods to restore the normal reflexes. In this dog, as was already mentioned above, the inhibitory reflexes were unusually stable. We knew that good inhibitory stimuli could induce and strengthen the process of excitation. We therefore applied to the dog the inhibitory stimuli, i.e., the differentiated agents, which I enumerated above. And, as a matter of fact, we saw many times that after that the reflexes appeared and the dog took the food, whereas formerly the reflexes had been absent and the food had been refused, or the phases were transposed toward the normal state during transitional hypnotic phases, under the influence of induction. The other method was only a variation of the one just described. We placed in the dog's room only part of the experimenter's clothing, rather than the experimenter himself, and this was enough markedly to increase the reflexes. The dog did not see the clothing and, consequently, it was the odour that acted.

To the experimental part which I have purposely kept clear of all suppositions I must add the following. If we observe the movements of the dog when the conditioned reflexes disappear and the dog refuses food, we see in this case not the motor food reaction but a passive-defensive, as we call it, reaction which would ordinarily be called the reaction of fear. It produces a particularly strong impression on the observer, when the dog is in one of the hypnotic phases, the phase we call paradoxical, i.e., when only the weak conditioned stimuli are effective and the strong ones are not. To weak visual stimuli the dog responds with a distinct motor food reaction, while to auditory stimuli it responds with a markedly passive-defensive reaction. The animal moves its head from side to side, crouches on the floor with head hanging low and does not make the slightest movement in the direction of the apparatus with food.

To all this I must add that our animal is very well nourished, very lively and has an excellent appetite when out of the experimental room or the stand.

However, the afore-described animal was in no way exceptional. As I have already mentioned, we had several dogs of this type which had similarly, although with some variations, been affected by the flood. Now I can pass to our interpretation of all the foregoing facts. To us it is perfectly clear that our type must be the opposite of all the other types in which it is often absolutely impossible to elaborate full inhibitory reflexes or in which, even if they may be well elaborated, they are very unstable and are easily impaired. This means that in the afore-described type the inhibitory process predominates, whereas in all the other types the process of excitation either prevails or is more or less balanced by the process of inhibition.

How can we approach an understanding of our type and of its, so to speak, deeper mechanism?

We know, as the most constant and general fact concerning the physiology of conditioned reflexes, that an isolated conditioned stimulus obviously addressed to the cortical cells will sooner or later, and often strikingly rapidly, lead to an inhibited state of the cells and to its extreme limit, i.e., to the animal's sleep. This fact can best be understood thus: these cells, as extremely reactive structures, extraordinarily rapidly expend their excitable substance during stimulation, and another process, to a certain extent protective and economical—the process of inhibition, sets in. This process stops the further functional destruction of the cell and thus aids in the restoration of the expended substance. Our fatigue after the day's work speaks in favour of this, the fatigue being eliminated by sleep, which, as I have already demonstrated earlier, is diffuse inhibition. The same thing is apparently proved by our precise fact that after injury to certain parts of the cerebral cortex it is for a long time impossible to obtain any positive conditioned reflexes from the receptors connected with them, the stimulation of these receptors producing only an inhibitory effect. But, if later stimulation produces a positive effect, this effect is only temporary and is quickly replaced by an inhibitory effect, which is a typical phenomenon of so-called stimulatory weakness. Here we must also mention the observations of our dogs made during the recent difficult years of my country when the state of exhaustion which the animals shared together with us caused them uncommonly quickly to lapse into different stages of inhibition and, finally, into sleep, in response to our conditioned stimulation in the stand, so that it was impossible to carry on any research in positive conditioned reflexes.

We may therefore conclude that the cortical cells of the type of dog being described have a very small reserve of excitable substance, or especially easily destructible substance.

An inhibitory state in the cells may be evoked either by very weak or very strong stimuli. With stimuli of medium strength the cells may remain for the longest time in a state of excitation without passing into various degrees of inhibition. During weak stimulation inhibition replaces the process of excitation slowly, during strong stimulation—rapidly. Of course, these degrees of the strength of stimuli are entirely relative, i.e., what is a strong stimulation for one nervous system is only of medium strength for another nervous system. The extraordinary flood made itself felt by inhibition only in the type we have so far discussed, producing no perceptible effect on the others. A bell did not act as an uncommonly strong stimulus, i.e., inhibitory, on our dog until the appearance of its neurosis after the flood (we may justly compare this neurosis with the so-called human traumatic neurosis), but after the dog had developed the neurosis the bell clearly became a strong inhibitory stimulus. The same can apparently be said of one of the normal hypnotic phases—the paradoxical, when only weak stimuli act positively and the strong ones lead to inhibition.

Then we cannot but note the clear resemblance of the passive-defensive reflex in dogs to the inhibitory process. Our dog, as we observed, had a nervous system in which the inhibitory process predominated. Its general behaviour was characterised by the constant presence of the passive-defensive reflex. At the height of the development of its neurosis with all conditioned stimuli, during the paradoxical phase, when only the strong stimuli, i.e., inhibitory stimuli, act, the passive-defensive reaction always comes to the fore. A surprising thing! Even in dogs, of which the passive-defensive reaction is usually not characteristic, this reaction clearly occurs during their paradoxical phase in response to strong conditioned stimuli.

I think that on these grounds we may assume that normal timidity, cowardice, and especially pathological phobias, are based on a mere predominance of the physiological process of inhibition, as an expression of weakness of the cortical cells. Please, recall the afore-cited case of induction in which a purely physiological method temporarily eliminated the inhibition and with it the passive-defensive reflex.

As I gradually analysed the types of nervous system of different dogs it seemed to me that they all fitted in well with the classical description of temperaments, especially their extreme groups—the sanguine and the melancholic. The first of these is the type which constantly requires varying stimuli; this type untiringly seeks such stimuli and is in this case capable of manifesting extraordinary energy. Contrariwise, with monotonous stimuli it very easily sinks into a state of drowsiness and sleep. The melancholic type is the type with which we experimented. Let us recall the extreme representative of this type which I mentioned in the beginning of my lecture. Is it not natural to consider and call this type melancholic, if at every step, at every moment, the environment evokes in the animal the same persistent passive-defensive reflex?

Between these extremes are variations of the balanced type in which the process of excitation and process of inhibition are both of equal strength and interchange promptly and exactly.

Lastly, we have encountered in our dog a definite social reflex, the effect of an agent of the social environment. The dog, like its wild ancestor—the wolf, is a herd animal, and man, owing to old historical association, represents a "Socius" for it. Dr. Speransky,[29] who always brought this dog to the experimental room, treated it kindly and fed it, became a conditioned positive stimulus for the dog, which enhanced the excitatory tone of the cortex that eliminated, overcame the inhibitory tone. That Dr. Speransky was for the dog only a synthetic external stimulus consisting mainly of visual, auditory and olfactory components was demonstrated by our last experiment when even the scent of Dr. Speransky alone produced the same effect on the dog's nervous system as he did himself only, of course, much weaker.

This experiment together with one of our earlier experiments at last brings us into the field of social reflexes which we now include in the programme of our future experiments.

Now it can hardly be doubted that vast prospects present themselves for purely physiological investigations of the activity of the cerebral hemispheres with the aid of conditioned reflexes.

INTERNAL INHIBITION AND SLEEP ARE ESSENTIALLY THE SAME PHYSICOCHEMICAL PROCESS[30]

In the last lecture we arrived at the very important proposition that the cortical cell under the influence of conditioned stimulations inevitably, sooner or later, and with frequent repetitions very rapidly, passes into an inhibited state. And this had to be most legitimately understood thus: this cell as, so to speak, the sentry post of the organism possesses the highest reactivity and, consequently, is subject to precipitate functional destruction, rapid fatigue. The inhibition which then develops, while itself not being fatigue, plays the role of a safeguard of the cell, preventing further excessive, dangerous destruction of this exceptional cell. During the inhibitory period, remaining free from work, the cell restores its normal composition. This applies to all the cells of the cortex and, consequently, with numerous working cells of the cortex the entire cortex must develop the same inhibited state which we saw in individual cortical cells when they were acted upon by our conditioned stimuli. And this is a daily occurrence. It is our sleep and the sleep of all animals. All of our twenty-five years of work with the cerebral hemispheres have been a continuous and constant proof of this conclusion. Today this is one of the firmest propositions in the physiology of the cerebral hemispheres as we study it by our method. Sleepiness and sleep of our experimental animals have accompanied our work from its very beginning and we still always have to do with them. Thus, we have accumulated vast factual material which during the different stages of our research naturally gave grounds for many assumptions which somewhat differ from each other. But several years ago all these assumptions merged into a final proposition, which harmonises with absolutely all of our facts, that sleep and what we call internal inhibition are the selfsame process.

The basic condition for the onset and development of this inhibition and sleep is absolutely the same. It is a more or less continuous or many times repeated, isolated conditioned stimulation, that is, stimulation of the cortical cell. In all the cases of internal inhibition, which we considered in the fourth, fifth, sixth and seventh lectures, we always encountered the sleepiness and sleep of our animals. If we effect extinction, we observe in some animals even for the first time, in addition to cessation of the conditioned salivation and the corresponding motor reaction, extreme sluggishness compared with their state prior to the extinction. With the extinction repeated for a number of days, even if alternated with application of reinforced conditioned stimuli, the thing almost always ends in distinct sleepiness and sleep in the stand, although this had not happened to the animal until then. The same thing is still more clearly observed during elaboration of differentiations. For example, we have for the animal a number of conditioned stimuli, including a definite tone. The animal is always wide awake in the stand. Then we start differentiating one of the marginal tones. Together with the differentiating inhibition which begins to develop, there appears a sleepiness which keeps increasing and which ends in deep sleep with complete relaxation of the skeletal muscles and snoring of the animal so that during the following positive conditioned stimulation and feeding we have to shake the animal out of sleep or even put the food into its mouth in order that it may begin to eat. We find the same thing during the formation of a long delayed reflex (three minutes) so that formerly, when we still had very little knowledge of the thing, we were unable to elaborate the reflex we needed because of the sleep developing in some of the animals at that time. Lastly, the same thing takes place during elaboration of conditioned inhibition. It should be noted that the degree of interference of sleep somewhat differs in the different cases of internal inhibition. It makes itself felt the least, precisely in conditioned inhibition.

This happens in all cases in which internal inhibition develops rapidly, owing to the fact that the conditioned stimulus is not accompanied by an unconditioned stimulus; but the same thing also occurs during slowly increasing inhibition of the reinforced but many times repeated conditioned reflexes, inhibition which was given special consideration in the last lecture. Here, too, months or years later, the thing ends in various transitional stages between waking and sleep (which will constitute the content of the next lecture) and complete sleep, depending on the animal. The animals differ from each other as much in this respect as they do with regard to the rapidity of the onset of inhibition.

Our work with conditioned reflexes is so replete with cases of inhibition passing into sleep that there is no need citing separate examples. Thus, inhibition is really closely connected with sleep and directly passes into sleep, if no suitable measures are taken.

It is interesting that there is hardly a stimulus for either internal inhibition or sleep which does not produce them under certain conditions. The strongest electric current applied to the skin as a conditioned food stimulus revealed in Yerofeyeva's experiments after many months increasing inhibition during reinforced reflexes and in Petrova's experiments demonstratively evoked sleep. On the other hand, various external agents playing the role of conditioned stimuli are arranged entirely alike as regards the rapidity with which they develop both internal inhibition and sleep. In the last lecture it was observed that inhibition developed the most readily in response to thermal stimuli and with greatest difficulty in response to acoustic stimuli. Strictly parallel with this, sleep develops rapidly in thermal conditioned reflexes, and more slowly and more rarely in acoustic reflexes. With thermal conditioned stimuli the interference of sleep is so insistent and deranges the work to such an extent that in the beginning of our research it was difficult to find people willing to work with these stimuli.

Lastly, as has already been mentioned, the duration of the conditioned stimulation is of decisive significance to inhibition and the onset of sleep. Some dogs, if the conditioned stimulus is delayed 10-15 seconds, retain a perfectly alert state during a long period of work. But as soon as the reflex is delayed 30 seconds and longer, the dog immediately develops sleepiness and sleep. This form of experiment is often truly amazing. The rapid transition from complete waking to actual sleep with such apparently insignificant changes in the experimental conditions appears entirely unexpected. Our work contains numerous such examples with different periods of delay and different degrees of distinctness.

All the methods without exception, cited in the last lecture as retarding the onset of increasing inhibition of the long repeated, although constantly reinforced conditioned reflexes, as well as those eliminating inhibition, are equally suitable for the struggle against sleep.

After all we have just said, the following most natural question arises: if sleep coincides to such an extent, in its appearance and disappearance, with internal inhibition, how can the latter be the most important factor of the waking state, the basis for the finest balancing of the organism with the environment? The facts reported in the earlier lectures must, in my opinion, entirely eliminate the seeming, at first sight, difficulty of the answer. Internal inhibition in the waking state is partial sleep, sleep of separate groups of cells, like sleep is internal inhibition, irradiated, spread over the entire mass of the hemispheres and the underlying divisions of the brain. It is, consequently, a matter of spatial limitation of inhibition, its enclosure within a definite framework. And this is, of course, done by the antagonistic nervous process, as we saw it in the lectures on the mosaic nature of the cortex and on its analysing activity.

During extinction sleep does not appear, is precluded only when, after the already achieved extinction, we systematically apply reinforced conditioned stimuli and do not repeat the extinction too often. During differentiations the developing inhibition, at first accompanied by sleep, remains, so to speak, a business-like inhibition without being complicated by untimely sleep only when, intermittently with the non-reinforced agent, we use, and usually more often, our conditioned stimulus, the positively acting agent, i.e., the process of stimulation continuously counteracts the spread of the process of inhibition. The same thing occurs during conditioned inhibition and during depression. In all these cases, if the experiment is conducted expediently, sleepiness and sleep appear only as a phasic phenomenon, when an exact delimitation between the regions of the excitatory and inhibitory processes has not yet been established. As soon as the conditions of the experiment favour prevalence of inhibition, sleep sets in. Here is a vivid example. In the lecture on mosaic I mentioned a dog in which a positive conditioned reflex was elaborated to a definite tone, and the twenty neighbouring tones, upward and downward, were differentiated, i.e., were negative conditioned stimuli. The dog was generally very much disinclined to sleep when a certain ratio in applying the positive and negative stimuli was observed, and always fully reacted to all the positive stimuli. But as soon as the differentiated tones were brought into play several times in succession, the dog lapsed into such deep sleep that even very strong outside stimuli were unable to awaken it. Contrariwise, sleep does not develop despite frequent application of negative conditioned stimuli, if they alternate with positive stimuli. Very instructive in this respect are the already mentioned experiments with mosaic and, especially, the experiments with the mechanical skin mosaic. Despite the fact that conditioned mechanical stimulation of the skin greatly disposes to sleepiness and sleep, Kupalov's dog, on which only the mechanical skin mosaic has been practised for more than two years, displays no inclination towards sleep, apparently because the inhibitory process is constantly isolated, enclosed in a narrow framework by the stimulatory process. We also counteract the widely irradiating inhibition by increasing the number of positive conditioned stimuli which limit the spread of inhibition from its starting-points. I shall cite a more complex example from the work of Petrova, an example which is partly related to this case. Elaboration of a greatly delayed (three minutes) food reflex to metronome beats was at once started in a dog. The dog soon began to lapse into a sleepy state and ended in complete sleep. Inhibition, which had to develop during the first period of the action of the metronome, as very remote from the time the unconditioned stimulus was added, apparently prevailed, meeting with no due counteraction on the part of the process of stimulation, which had not yet manifested itself, during the second period of the metronome action as directly preceding the action of the unconditioned stimulus. Five new agents to be elaborated as conditioned stimuli were then introduced, the food being added to them only five seconds later. The sleepy state quickly disappeared and all the reflexes were easily formed; then the act of eating was gradually delayed, five seconds every day from the beginning of application of the conditioned stimuli. The latent period of the reflexes was also correspondingly prolonged, and, finally, without the least interference of sleep, six reflexes were obtained with a latent period of 60-90 seconds, i.e., with a preliminary inhibitory process. Thus, the process of stimulation, which initially arose at six points of the cortex and only gradually gave place to the process of inhibition, limited it in time and space and precluded sleep.

Here we must also include the influence of the limitation of movement in our stand on some, though not many, dogs, especially inclined to inhibition and sleepiness. In these cases it is sometimes expedient to conduct the experiments, at least temporarily, on the floor, with the dogs unrestrained. It is to be assumed that the stimuli coming during movement from the motor apparatus and from the skin form alternately appearing foci of excitation in the cerebral cortex which also to a certain extent counteract the spread of inhibition, although here there is probably also another factor of greater importance, which will be discussed below.

What we saw in the cortical cell as regards the appearance of inhibition in it in cases of conditioned stimulation, recurs in it during stimulation with any agent which is of no special conditioned physiological significance. As has already been mentioned, among the reflexes there is an investigating reflex. This reflex has as its points of application the cells of the cerebral hemispheres, as well as the underlying parts of the brain. In the presence of the hemispheres it apparently takes place with the participation of the cells of the cerebral hemispheres. This is clearly demonstrated by its greatest finesse, when it appears during the slightest variation in the environment, which is possible only with the higher analysing function of the cerebral hemispheres and is absolutely inaccessible to the underlying parts of the brain. The investigating reflex, as we all know, infallibly weakens by repetition and, finally, completely disappears despite the continued existence of the agent which has evoked it. Special experiments conducted in our laboratory by N. Popov have shown that the disappearance of the investigating reflex is based on the development of inhibition and is quite analogous, as regards details, to the extinction of conditioned reflexes.

Whereas the given agent of the investigating reflex applied repeatedly at short intervals ceases in the course of the experiment to evoke the corresponding motor reaction, at longer intervals in the same experiment this reaction is restored, as is the case with the extinguished conditioned reflex. The investigating reflex which has disappeared in the experiment because of repetition appears for some time, if immediately after its disappearance a new outside stimulus is used, i.e., another investigating reflex is produced. Consequently, it becomes disinhibited like the depressed conditioned reflex. If the investigating reflex to a certain agent is repeated for a number of days, it disappears chronically as a systematically non-reinforced conditioned reflex. Lastly, the extinguished investigating reflex is temporarily restored under the influence of stimulants (caffeine), as is the case, for example, with conditioned differentiated agents. This inhibition of the investigating reflex infallibly, and even more readily than the inhibition of the conditioned reflex, leads to sleepiness and sleep. I shall now cite experiments from S. Chechulin's work in which inhibition and sleep during the investigating reflex were combined with application of conditioned stimuli.

A conditioned food reflex to a whistle was elaborated in a dog. Agents used for the first time—hissing, gurgling, mechanical stimulation of the skin, etc.—are employed as stimulators of the investigating reflex.

Time	Conditioned stimulus applied for 30 seconds	Salivation (in drops) in 30 seconds	Latent period (in seconds)	Notes
4:07 P. M.	Whistle	3	3 }	reinforced
4:15 „	„	4	3 }	

Then, beginning on the twenty-first minute, the sound of gurgling is used for thirty seconds and repeated every two minutes. During the first three repetitions movements in the direction of the sound occur and gradually weaken. The fourth repetition reveals sleepiness. The sleep is interrupted by different factors of the stimulation until the eighth repetition. During the eighth and ninth repetitions there are no more movements in response to the stimulus; the sleep is uninterrupted. At 4:43 P.M. gurgling alone is at first used for ten seconds and then a whistle is added to it for thirty seconds. There are no reactions, either motor or secretory; the sleep continues. Food awakens the dog, the dog begins to eat but remains sleepy also after eating. The experiment with the conditioned stimulus continues as follows.

Time	Conditioned stimulus applied for 30 seconds	Salivation (in drops) in 30 seconds	Latent period (in seconds)	Notes
4:53 P.M.	Whistle	2.5	8	reinforced
5:02 "	"	3	7	

Prior to this experiment the dog never slept in the stand. During the subsequent experiments, new agents evoking the investigating reflex were either repeated until the onset of sleep or only until the movements in response to them disappeared, but before the appearance of sleepiness. Twenty-one days after the foregoing experiment, an experiment with mechanical stimulation of the skin was performed. The experiment was conducted as follows:

Time	Conditioned stimulus of different duration	Salivation (in drops) in 30 seconds	Latent period (in seconds)	Notes
2:05 P.M.	Whistle 5 seconds	—	—	
2:12 "	Whistle 30 seconds	6	5	reinforced
2:21 "	Whistle 5 seconds	—	—	

117

Mechanical stimulation of the skin starts at 2:25 P.M., continues for thirty seconds each time and is repeated every minute. During the first three repetitions, the head moves in the direction of the stimulated spot. During the fourth and fifth repetitions there are no more movements. At 2:32.5 P.M. the mechanical stimulation of the skin alone is used for 10 seconds and then a whistle is added to it for thirty seconds. Salivation begins in the fifteenth second after the addition of the whistle and during the thirty seconds of its action two drops of saliva are secreted. The experiment is continued as follows.

Time	Conditioned stimulus applied for 30 seconds	Salivation (in drops) in 30 seconds	Latent period (in seconds)	Notes
2:45 P.M.	Whistle	5	7	reinforced

In the beginning of the experiment the conditioned stimulus was reinforced now five and now thirty seconds later in order to preserve the normal value of its effect to the end of the experiment.

We see that with repetitions of the agent which evokes the investigating reflex its motor effect keeps gradually diminishing and then with continued repetitions now sleepiness and sleep directly occur and grow deeper and now the agent remains for some time as though without any effect. However, the conditioned stimulus added to it (in the second of the just described experiments) attests that during this period it produces an inhibitory effect. That the inhibitory effect on the conditioned stimulus is now not based on the mechanism of what we call external inhibition is proved by the fact that (as we saw it in the sixth lecture studying the effect of the investigating reflex on the delayed conditioned reflex) the investigating reflex, when it happens to be very small, disinhibits rather than inhibits the conditioned reflex. It follows that here we have the effect of inhibition developing during the repetition of the investigating reflex and later passing into sleep during which the conditioned reflex disappears altogether (in the first of the just described experiments).

We see the same thing particularly clearly marked in pups (I. Rozental's experiment). During monotonous repetition of some stimulus and generally invariable environment pups often lapse into sleep with amazing precision and rapidity. On the other hand, isn't it a commonly known truth, although heretofore unelucidated scientifically, that all people, especially those who have no strong inner life, irresistibly lapse into sleepiness and sleep in response to monotonous stimulations, however untimely and out of place this may be? It means that certain cortical cells which react to the given long-continued external agent spend themselves, pass into an inhibited state and in the absence of counteraction on the part of the other active points of the cortex the inhibitory process spreads and conditions sleep. The extraordinarily rapid exhaustion of the cortical cell with passage of the cell into an inhibited state sharply contrasts with the endurance of the cells of the lower parts of the brain under the same conditions. The experiments conducted by Zelyony in our laboratory have shown that, whereas in the normal dog the investigating reflex quickly disappears in response to a certain sound, the same sound in the same situation stereotypically evokes this reflex a great number of times in the dog deprived of the cerebral hemispheres.

Now back to the conditioned reflexes.

The following facts which we have repeatedly encountered also prove that exhaustion of the cortical cell and its weakening in general serve as the basis for the development of inhibition and the following onset of sleep. When we impaired some analyser surgically, by an operation on a hemisphere, the positive conditioned stimuli pertaining to it either could hardly be applied isolated for even a very short time (they were quickly transformed into inhibitory stimuli) or even altogether lost their positive effect, becoming only negative, inhibitory. This is particularly easily and constantly observed during impairment of the cutaneous analyser.

When the *gyri coronarius* and *ectosylvius* are extirpated in the dog, its positive conditioned cutaneous mechanical reflexes from the extremities and the shoulder and pelvic girdles disappear for a considerable period of time (often for many weeks) and are replaced with negative inhibitory reflexes. The latter is proved by the fact that the positive conditioned stimuli from the other analysers act well prior to the application of the cutaneous mechanical stimuli and lose their effect after their application. At the same time these mechanical stimuli applied to the skin extraordinarily easily and rapidly evoke sleep in such dogs which never before slept, when thus stimulated during our work with them. This fact often assumes the following pronounced form. A conditioned cutaneous mechanical stimulus applied to the part of the skin surface impaired by an operation on the brain leads to inhibition and sleepiness, while the same stimulus applied to unimpaired places produces a positive effect and leaves the animal perfectly awake (experiments of N. Krasnogorsky, I. Razenkov and V. Arkhangelsky).

Here, too, we can justly mention the fact observed in the laboratory during the period of famine several years ago. Conditioned reflexes could not be studied on the emaciated animals because all the positive conditioned stimuli extraordinarily rapidly changed to negative stimuli and at the same time the dogs fell asleep precisely in connection with the application of conditioned stimuli. The general emaciation of the animals made itself felt particularly in the cortical cells (experiment of Frolov, Rozental, et al.).

In the very many cases heretofore enumerated we always saw that inhibition passed into sleep, but we could also observe the reverse—sleep passing into inhibition. We elaborated a conditioned reflex delayed for three minutes. The separate experiment sometimes proceeds as follows. We place the animal in the stand. The animal is awake. But as soon as a conditioned stimulus is applied, the animal immediately becomes sleepy, the salivary effect is absent during all the three minutes and, when food is given, the animal does not at once eat the food and then eats it sluggishly. We repeat the conditioned stimulus in the experiment several times at usual intervals. Each time, our dog becomes more awake during stimulation and at the end of the three minutes of stimulation salivation appears. Salivation increases with repetition. At last the three-minute period of stimulation is divided approximately into two halves: during the first half there is no salivation, although the animal remains entirely awake; during the second half there is abundant salivation and the dog very rapidly and greedily eats the food given to it. Here the irradiated inhibition—sleep—which emerged in virtue of predominance at first of the inhibitory process during the first half of the action of the conditioned stimulus gradually passes into limited, concentrated inhibition under the pressure of the continuously increasing process of stimulation connected with the second half of the action of the same conditioned stimulus. In similar cases we sometimes also see outright replacement of inhibition with sleep. The following relationship is sometimes observed during a prolonged (three minutes) and a shorter delay (thirty seconds). The animal usually remaining awake in the stand falls asleep during the experiment each time precisely in the beginning of the action of the recurring conditioned stimulus: the eyes close, the head drops, the whole body relaxes and hangs in the straps, and even snoring is sometimes heard. But a certain period passes (1.5-2 minutes during a prolonged and twenty-five seconds during a shorter delay), the animal awakens by itself, salivation appears and a sharp food motor reaction is observed. It is clear that in this case concentrated inhibition is chronically replaced with diffuse sleep. Lastly, we can sometimes observe how summation of two inhibitions produces sleepiness.

One of the dogs (Fursikov's experiment) had a well-elaborated conditioned reflex, delayed for three minutes. During the first two minutes the dog did not salivate, then salivation began and reached its maximum towards the end of the third minute. In the given experiment an outside agent—soft hissing—was used together with the conditioned stimulus. It disinhibited the first half of the reflex, a slight motor reaction, investigating reflex, being observed in response to the hissing. The conditioned reflex was reinforced. When the same combination was repeated, there was no more orienting reaction to the hissing, the conditioned reflex disappeared altogether and the animal was very sleepy. The reflex was reinforced again. The result must, apparently, be understood as follows. The investigating reflex to hissing is extinguished during the second time, i.e., now it is inhibition that develops in response to hissing, as already mentioned in this lecture. This inhibition added to the inhibition of the first phase of the delayed reflex intensifies inhibition so much that the active phase of the reflex is discontinued and gives way to the animal's sleepiness. Continuation of the experiment attests that this interpretation of the experiment is correct. During the next repetition of the conditioned stimulation without the addition of hissing we obtain the proper delayed reflex with two phases. The combination of the metronome and hissing repeated once more again reproduces the sleepiness and the conditioned reflex disappears.

The following are the figures of this experiment.

Time	Stimuli applied for 3 minutes	Salivation (in drops) every 30 seconds	Notes
4:52 P.M.	Metronome beats + hissing	033.5 103.5	Slight movement in response to hissing
5:03 "	Same	000 000	No movement, sleepiness
5:15 "	Metronome beats	000 0.19	
5:28 "	Metronome beats + hissing	000 000	Sleepiness

In this case I deem it useful, for the sake of clarity, purposely to call your attention to the following. This experiment together with the afore-mentioned Chechulin's experiments apparently adds an extra new phase to the action of outside agents on a conditioned reflex. If we take a strong external agent, this agent, as you remember from the sixth lecture on the delayed reflex, first inhibits the entire delayed reflex by the investigating reflex it evokes, then, when the investigating reflex considerably weakens during repetition, it only disinhibits the first phase of the delayed reflex and, lastly, as you are learning now, it inhibits this reflex once more, but now on another basis, itself becoming the primary stimulator of the inhibitory process in the cerebral cortex. On the other hand, the weak external agent, as was the case in Fursikov's experiment, conditioning from the very beginning a weak and transitory investigating reflex, begins, during its first application, directly with disinhibiting action on the delayed reflex and ends with the same second inhibition.

The identity of the processes of inhibition and sleep is also attested by their common properties. In the preceding lectures we observed even too many facts incontestably demonstrating the motion of the inhibitory process through the mass of the cerebral hemispheres; moreover, this motion proved very slow, was measured in minutes, and even many minutes, and, besides, greatly varied as regards its speed in different animals and under different conditions. Sleep is obviously also a moving process. We all know how sleepiness and sleep gradually take possession of us and how often they retreat, are dispelled with difficulty and slowly. There is scientific information on the gradual cessation of the function of different sense organs and other more complex mental activities during the onset of sleep. On the other hand, we all know that people differ very greatly as regards the rapidity with which they fall asleep and awaken, and this rapidity differs under different conditions. The same thing was observed by us in the dogs.

Furthermore, we always saw in our work how inhibition, if it develops at first with difficulty, becomes an increasingly more easily reproduced process with practice, in connection with repetition and application of various cases of inhibition. Similarly conditioned stimuli, when they condition sleep under suitable conditions, as well as indifferent stimuli, evoke sleep more and more rapidly, the more often they are repeated.

The following is particularly interesting. As was shown before, inhibition induces excitation. In some dogs in which, as was reported somewhat earlier, during the delayed reflex the conditioned stimulus is replaced with sleep, instead of inhibition, in the initial phase of stimulation, the onset of sleep is sometimes preceded for a very short period by slight general excitement of the animal. This phenomenon comes to the fore still more clearly and constantly when the animal falls asleep under the influence of continued or repeated indifferent stimulation. This was often observed in Rozental's afore-mentioned experiments. When the indifferent stimulus clearly begins to make the pup sleepy, the latter, before finally falling asleep, for some time becomes excited: it begins to move uneasily, scratch and bark without any reason into the air. I happened to observe the same thing in children falling asleep.

A perfectly strange and unexpected picture. We can justly see the phenomenon of induction in it. The well-known excitation in the beginning of narcotisation could be interpreted the same way.

I think that the aggregate of the afore-mentioned facts must be considered sufficient to prove conclusively the truth of our proposition that sleep and internal inhibition are the selfsame process. Personally I do not now know, do not see a single fact in our work that seriously contradicts our conclusion. It is a matter of regret that we have not as yet a good graphic method for picturing sleep. Only rarely have we used for this purpose descriptions of the position of the animal's head. Of course, the reports of our experiments concerning sleep accompanied by some picture of sleep would greatly add in your eyes to the cogency of our arguments.

All the details of our normal, usual sleep apparently quite harmonise with our conclusion. Our daily work, very monotonous for some and, on the contrary, greatly varied for other people, must in the end equally condition the onset of sleep. Prolonged stimulation of the same points of the cortex leads to their very deep inhibition which, naturally, extensively irradiating, embraces the hemispheres and descends to the underlying parts of the brain. On the other hand, in varied activity, although individual points of the cortex do not reach a considerable state of inhibition, their greater number creates, even without wide irradiation, a diffuse inhibited state which also descends. Of course, a very large number of rapidly changing stimuli may often long resist the general involvement of the hemispheres by the inhibitory process and delay the onset of sleep. And vice versa, a strictly established order of alternation between waking and sleep, a fixed rhythm may enhance the insistence of sleep without sufficient fatigue of the cortical cells. In our experiments we had enough examples of analogous relations between the excitatory and inhibitory processes for both cases.

TRANSITIONAL PHASES BETWEEN THE ANIMAL'S WAKING AND COMPLETE SLEEP (HYPNOTIC PHASES)[31]

Last year I cited an imposing number of facts proving that sleep is internal inhibition, continuous (and not partial, constantly alternating with the process of excitation), spread over the entire mass of the hemispheres and descended also to some underlying parts of the brain. It was to be expected that, since inhibition spreads gradually, there would be a different extensiveness of sleep, a gradual involvement by it now of larger and now of smaller regions. Consequently, there must be different transitional forms to complete sleep. This is actually what takes place, and we observed and produced them. In our experiments we had to do not only with the usual form of sleep characterised in the absence of normal activity of the hemispheres by relaxation of the skeletal muscles (closed eyes, head dropped low, half-bent limbs and body passively hanging in the straps and loops for the legs), but also with an entirely different form as regards the state of the skeletal muscles. In this form the hemispheres are also inactive, all the conditioned stimuli fail to act and there is no reaction to any outside stimuli if the latter are not strong enough, but the animal retains quite an active pose. It stands with open fixed eyes, raised head, on taut limbs without resting on the loops for the legs, and stands motionlessly for minutes and hours. If the position of its limbs is changed, the animal retains the position imparted to them. The jerking-away of the paw on contact with its sole assumes the character of a contracture. When given food the animal does not react, remains motionless and does not take the food. This form of inhibition is encountered quite infrequently and we do not as yet know with what special conditions in the situation of our experiment or with what peculiarity of the nervous system it is connected. Our collaborator N. Rozhansky who carefully observed the transition from waking to sleep in dogs has arrived at the conclusion that the aforesaid state always exists under these conditions, but is usually a very fleeting and transient phenomenon. It is not particularly difficult, as it seems to me, to understand this state physiologically. Here we have the inhibited activity only of the cerebral hemispheres, but the inhibition has not descended to the centres which regulate the balancing, the fixing of the body in space (the Magnus-de Kleijn centres), i.e., we have a *cataleptic* state. It follows that in this form the line of demarcation between the inhibited part of the brain and the part free from inhibition lies directly under the cerebral hemispheres. But it may also divide large regions of the hemispheres. We encounter this form more frequently and can even purposely reproduce it. We observed it for the first time under the following conditions (L. Voskresensky's[32] experiments). One of the dogs which had never before fallen asleep during work with it was frequently left alone in the stand and the experimental room for hours without any influences exerted on it and therefore began to lapse into a sleepy state. Evidently, the monotonous stimulation produced by the environment, as was shown in the preceding lecture, finally conditioned a strong continuous inhibition of the brain. The inhibitory effect of the environment became so strong that bringing the dog into the experimental room alone apparently immediately transformed it, especially when it was placed in the stand. The animal had to be purposely stimulated in every possible manner to prevent it from falling asleep towards the end of the preparations for the experiment.

When the experimenter later left the room to conduct the experiment from the next room and immediately, without losing a moment, began to act with conditioned food stimuli, the normal conditioned reflex was always present: the dog salivated and immediately began to eat the food it was given. But if four or five minutes elapsed after the experimenter had left the room, the result was entirely different; the dog salivated in response to the conditioned stimulus, the salivary reaction increased when the dog was given food, but the animal did not take the food and had to be fed by force. At that time the skeletal muscles were not yet relaxed. If the experimenter waited with the application of the conditioned stimulus for ten minutes after leaving the room, it now produced no effect at all and the animal turned out to be completely asleep, muscles relaxed and snoring. What other explanation of this fact can there be except that during the initial spread of inhibition the latter involved for some time only the motor region of the cortex, as yet leaving unaffected all the other regions of the cortex whence the conditioned stimuli spread to the organ (gland) unconnected with the motor region. And only somewhat later did continuous inhibition involve the entire mass of the hemispheres and descend to the underlying parts of the brain resulting in complete sleep. In the given case this stage of the developing sleepy state took place under the influence of indifferent stimuli acting for a long time on the cerebral hemispheres. Usually we have it during the action of negative conditioned stimuli repeated many times in the same experiment, as well as positive conditioned stimuli, especially weak, also during their frequent and continuous application. I shall cite two examples.

The first example refers to a dog already mentioned in the earlier lectures; for this dog a tone of 256 vibrations per second was a conditioned food stimulus, while ten tones upward and downward from it were differentiated (Bierman's experiments[33]).

Time	Conditioned stimulus applied for 30 seconds	Salivation (in drops) in 30 seconds	Notes
3:50 P.M.	Tone of 256 vibrations	13	Eats the food given to it
4:00 "	Tone of 426 vibrations	0	Gradually becomes sleepy
4:05 "	Tone of 160 vibrations	0	
4:10 "	Tone of 640 vibrations	0	
4:13 "	Tone of 256 vibrations	9	Does not eat the food given to it

I am taking the second example from the work (Rozental's) with a dog which at first had many and constant conditioned food reflexes. But, when one more reflex was elaborated in the dog in response to the appearance of a gray paper screen before its eyes and it was repeated many times and often continuously, one after another, in the same experiment, the following state of the dog developed: the dog frequently secreted a considerable amount of saliva in response to the conditioned stimuli, but did not touch the food.

Here is such an example.

Time	Conditioned stimulus applied for 30 seconds	Salivation (in drops) in 30 seconds	Notes
3:15 P.M.	Metronome beats	5	Does not eat the food given to it
3:18 "	Flash of a bulb	7	
3:21 "	Gurgling sound	7	
3:24 "	Bell	7	

In this case the dog only scarcely moves, but there is no visible sleep as yet. Without application of the conditioned stimuli and in the same stand the dog greedily eats the same food.

The following casual observation also belongs here. One of the dogs, which had long served for experiments with conditioned reflexes, had never exhibited dissociated secretory and motor reactions in a conditioned food reflex and had never slept in the stand, was for the first time brought before a large audience to demonstrate certain experiments with these reflexes. The unusual and very complex situation apparently greatly affected the animal: it grew torpid and slightly trembled. When the conditioned stimulus was tested, it evoked the secretory effect, as usual, but the dog did not take the food given to it and within a rather short time fell asleep in the stand, its skeletal muscles completely relaxed, right there in the room. This time the strong, unusual stimulus apparently directly inhibited the cerebral hemispheres, at first partly, only in the motor region, and then completely with transition to the underlying part of the brain. This case should be considered perfectly identical with the usual form of experiment with the so-called hypnosis of animals when abrupt immobilisation of the animal and turning it over on its back also leads to inhibition in different degrees of its diffusion, now only to catalepsy and even partial (body motionless but eyes and head moving), and now to complete sleep. In our laboratory we also had a case in which a very disobedient animal greatly resisted being equipped for the experiment and immediately lapsed into complete sleep in the stand when its movements were suddenly limited by strong hands which applied a considerable mechanical stimulus to it.

Thus both partial and complete sleep are produced by weak, long-continued general stimulation, as well as short but strong conditioned inhibitory and positive stimuli. I shall come back to some of the details concerning this case in my next lectures.

But, in addition to the different extensiveness of diffuse inhibition, our factual material has acquainted us with different variations, different stages of the very process of inhibition, with a different, if I may say so, intensity of diffuse inhibition, sleep.

Before treating this subject I must touch upon a point which is of paramount importance to many of our experiments concerning variations of the diffuse inhibitory process. In one of the lectures I raised the question of what underlies, in the simultaneous complex stimulation, the disguise of the stimulus from one analyser by a stimulus from another analyser, and voiced the assumption that it may be connected with the different strength of the agents used by us and belonging to different analysers. The intended experiments were performed during these lectures of ours and quite confirmed my assumption. When we purposely very greatly changed the relative intensity of our usual stimuli: considerably weakened the acoustic stimuli and either left the others as they were usually employed or intensified them, the acoustic agents now, on the contrary, participated less than the others in the effect of the complex stimuli, i.e., in individual tests the conditioned action belonged much more to the latter than to the former.

Here are our experiments. The simultaneous complex stimulation of one dog consisted of our usual mechanical stimulus of the skin and an acoustic, extraordinarily weakened stimulus (V. Rikman's experiments). The firmly elaborated stimulus produced 4-4.5 drops of saliva in 30 seconds of isolated action. A separately tested acoustic component produced 0.5-1.5 drops and mechanical skin stimulus 2.5-5 drops. The complex, also simultaneous, stimulation of another dog consisted in a rhythmic flashing of a 400-watt bulb and the sounding of a greatly dampened tone. The elaborated complex stimulus produced 7-8 drops of saliva in 30 seconds. A separately applied optic stimulus produced 5 drops and an acoustic stimulus 2.5 drops. Similarly combined stimulation with cold at $0°$ C applied to the skin and a very weak sound, when broken up into components, showed that the cold produced a much greater effect than did the sound (W. Horsley Gantt's and Kupalov's experiments).

Thus, the difference in the effect of our usual conditioned stimuli belonging to different analysers is conditioned by the different strength of the stimuli and is not connected with the quality of the cells of the different analysers.

With this proposition we can attack our next theme of the stages of the diffuse inhibitory process. This investigation was occasioned by the pathological state of a dog's nervous system under the influence of one of our methods of a functional rather than surgical character. The pathological changes experimentally produced by us in the nervous system will occupy our attention in the next lecture. Here I shall only describe the initial pathological experiment which gave rise to our further studies of healthy animals.

Positive conditioned food reflexes to a whistle, metronome beats, rhythmic mechanical stimulation of the skin (24 contacts per minute), flashing of an electric bulb, as well as several differentiations, including a differentiation for another frequency of contacts (12 per minute) during mechanical stimulation of the skin at the same site were elaborated in a dog (Razenkov's experiments[34]).

The following is the normal effect of the positive conditioned stimuli.

Time	Conditioned stimulus applied for 30 seconds	Salivation (in drops) in 30 seconds
2:03 P.M.	Mechanical stimulation of the skin (24 contacts)	3
2:10 "	Whistle	5
2:21 "	Flashing of bulb	2
2:32 "	Metronome beats	3.5

From the foregoing it follows that the stimuli ranged in strength, from the strong to the weak, thus: whistle, metronome beats, mechanical stimulation of the skin and flashing of the bulb.

This was followed by an experiment in which among the other stimuli a differentiated mechanical stimulus (12 contacts per minute) was used for 30 seconds and was directly replaced by a positive mechanical stimulus (24 contacts per minute) also for 30 seconds.

The day after this experiment and during the subsequent nine days all the conditioned reflexes disappeared and were manifested only very rarely and to a minimal extent. This period was followed by a very special period. Here it is.

Time	Conditioned stimulus applied for 30 seconds	Salivation (in drops) in seconds
11:10 A.M.	Whistle	0
11:19 „	„	0.3
11:32 „	Flashing of bulb	3
11:48 „	Metronome beats	1
0:06 P.M.	Mechanical stimulation of the skin (24 contacts)	5.5

The result, as you see, is quite the reverse of what formerly occurred normally: strong stimuli either failed to act or barely acted, while the weak stimuli produced an effect even greater than normal. Following the example of N. Vvedensky[35] we named this state of the hemispheres the paradoxical phase. The paradoxical phase lasted 14 days and passed into the following phase of this form:

Time	Conditioned stimulus applied for 30 seconds	Salivation (in drops) in 30 seconds
10:40 A.M.	Mechanical stimulation of the skin (24 contacts)	4
10:48 „	Metronome beats	4.5
10:58 „	Whistle	4
11:10 „	Flashing of bulb	4

We named this phase the equalisation phase, because during this phase all the stimuli proved equal in effect. The equalisation phase lasted seven days and was replaced by another new phase in which the intermediate stimuli became greatly strengthened, the strong stimulus slightly weakened and the weak stimulus produced no effect at all. The normal state was restored seven days later. In this work, as also in our subsequent experiments concerning this subject, we used, for the sake of greater incontestability, the same stimuli but of different intensity, so that it was obvious that it was all a matter of the reaction of the cells precisely to the different strength of stimulation.

Thus, we found for the first time in our experiments that the cells of the hemispheres pass through a number of special transitional states, from the normal state of excitation to that of complete inhibition, revealed in the unusual reactions of these cells to the different strength of stimulation.

After acquainting ourselves with these transitional states in a clearly pathological case we asked ourselves the next question: Do not these states perhaps also exist normally during transition from waking to sleep and vice versa? It appeared probable that in the afore-described case the pathological state consisted only in the fixation of these states for a long time, whereas normally they could be very transient, without striking the eye, as was the case with catalepsy. Our investigations were directed along this line and led to an affirmative answer. The following are some of our experiments.

Here is a dog already mentioned in this lecture before: in addition to one positively acting tone, this dog had 20 differentiated neighbouring tones. Among many other positive conditioned reflexes this dog had additionally elaborated reflexes to soft and loud crackling sharply differing as to the intensity of the effect.

The following are their normal ratios.

Time	Conditioned stimulus applied for 30 seconds	Salivation (in drops) in 30 seconds
2:10 P.M.	Loud crackling	12.5
2:20 "	Soft crackling	4.5
2:30 "	Loud crackling	11

The experiment was continued as follows. By repeated application of the differentiated tones we brought the dog to a state of apparent sleep and applied the soft crackling. There was no secretory effect. By offering the dog food we awakened it and the dog began to eat. Somewhat later the soft crackling was repeated. Now it produced an effect, although a small effect as yet. The dog was fed again. The third time the crackling produced a normal and sometimes even a greater effect. Reinforcement was employed again. The next time a loud crackling was used. Its effect was somewhat inferior to that of the preceding soft crackling. And only somewhat later, when the waking state was completely restored, did loud crackling produce its normal effect and with this the usual quantitative relations between these two stimuli generally appeared.

Here are the figures of one of these experiments.

Time	Conditioned stimulus applied for 30 seconds	Salivation (in drops) in 30 seconds
2:48 P.M.	Loud crackling	13

Then the dog was put to sleep by application of the differentiated tones.

3:17 P.M.	Soft crackling	8
3:22 "	" "	3.5
3:26 "	" "	7
3:32 "	Loud "	6
3:40 "	Soft "	5.5
3:50 "	Loud "	10

Sometimes, when these stimuli are repeated in such experiments, their equality, rather than the initial predominance of the soft crackling over the strong, is observed. As the sleepy state is gradually dispelled under the influence of the recurring short act of eating, the cortical cell, returning to the waking state, apparently, now passes through the paradoxical and equalisation phases.

Consequently, we have the same thing as in the pathological case with the only difference that what then lasted for days now lasts for minutes (Bierman's experiment).

In one of our other dogs, owing to protracted work with it, a light drowsy state developed in the stand and affected the conditioned reflexes in that the formerly distinctly different stimuli, as regards the extent of their conditioned effect, were now all equalised. Injection of a suitable dose of caffeine put the dog into the initial waking state and with it restored the normal relations between the conditioned stimuli (N. Zimkin's experiments).

Time	Conditioned stimulus applied for 30 seconds	Salivation (in drops) in 30 seconds
0:50 P.M.	Loud metronome beats	8
0:57 „	Flashing of bulb	7 5
1:04 „	Loud bell	8
1:11 „	Choked metronome beats	8

The next day, 18 minutes before the experiment, 8 cm^3 of a two per cent solution of *Coffeini puri* was administered to the dog subcutaneously; the dog was perfectly awake.

Time	Conditioned stimulus applied for 30 seconds	Salivation (in drops) in 30 seconds
0:18 P.M.	Flashing of bulb	7
0:25 „	Loud metronome beats	10
0:32 „	Soft bell	6
0:39 „	Choked metronome beats	7.5
0:46 „	Loud bell	8 5

In the dog already mentioned in this lecture as exhibiting the stage of dissociation of the secretory reaction from the motor reaction, we frequently observed that, in this stage, of all the stimuli only the weakest (flashing of a bulb) sometimes produced the most positive effect by evoking the complete normal reflex: the dog salivated and ate the food it was offered. Thus, such cases with a certain degree of extensively diffused inhibition also included the paradoxical phase (Rozental's experiments).

The following, also perfectly strange, phenomenon was observed during a clearly drowsy state, but as yet before the onset of complete sleep. When the conditioned positive stimulus either completely or almost completely lost its effect, the well-elaborated negative stimulus, on the contrary, produced a distinct positive effect. Here is an example (Shishlo's experiments).

Positive conditioned food reflexes to mechanical stimulation of the skin of the shoulder and thigh and to application of heat (45° C) to the skin, as well as a constant negative conditioned reflex to mechanical stimulation of the skin on the back were elaborated in the dog. The effect of the positive mechanical stimulation of the skin normally gave 15-18 drops per minute. The thermal conditioned stimulus quite soon began to evoke sleepiness and sleep. The thermal stimulus was the first to be used in the given experiment. Sleepiness developed. Then the experiment proceeded as follows.

Time	Conditioned stimulus applied for 1 minute	Salivation (in drops) in 1 minute	Notes
0:29 P.M.	Mechanical stimulation of the shoulder	2	The dog is constantly sleepy despite reinforcement
0:39 „	Mechanical stimulation of the thigh	1.5	
0:50 „	Mechanical stimulation of the back	12	

We repeatedly observed the same thing during some pathological states of the hemispheres. We named these states the ultra-paradoxical phase.

While observing so many different states of the cerebral cells during the animal's transition from waking to complete sleep and being cognisant of the fact that sleep is continuous and diffuse internal inhibition, we should have expected to encounter some of these states also in what we call consecutive inhibition with which we thoroughly acquainted ourselves in the early lectures on internal inhibition. It seems to me that this had occurred in a single case as yet, which we were able to investigate precisely in conditioned inhibition (Bykov's experiments).

The dog had five positive conditioned stimuli: metronome beats, loud tone, the same tone greatly dampened, appearance of a cardboard circle before its eyes and mechanical stimulation of the skin. Conditioned inhibition was elaborated to a combination of mechanical stimulation of the skin and a gurgling sound. The conditioned stimuli, as regards the salivary effect (average of many experiments), ranged in the following order: 22 drops, 18.5, 16.5, 13.5 and 10 drops in 30 seconds. As soon as the conditioned inhibition was finally elaborated, all the conditioned stimuli were tested. Ten minutes after application of the conditioned inhibition, metronome beats produced 16.5 drops, the loud tone—16, the dampened tone—20 and the circle—18 drops. Considering the possible participation of the motion of inhibition, as well as induction in this fact, the only thing that could be ascribed to the point of interest to us is that the dampened tone produced a more than normal effect when the effect of the loud tone was below normal. Since this occurred at the same point of the cortex we could interpret this as a manifestation of the paradoxical phase. We are now continuing this investigation on other types of internal inhibition.

Then we dwelled on the following point. In the lecture on mutual induction we made the following assumption: Is not what we call external inhibition a phenomenon of negative induction, i.e., inhibition induced on the periphery of the region which is in a state of excitation? In other words, is not external and internal inhibition basically the same physicochemical process? We planned to obtain perhaps some confirmation of this assumption by investigating the following question: Does not external inhibition condition the same states of the cortical cell with which we have just acquainted ourselves in the cases of internal inhibition? Since this investigation required a rather long period of external inhibition, we conducted it by introducing into the animal's mouth various disagreeable substances which produce protracted external inhibition.

The experiments were conducted on two dogs with food reflexes.

In one dog (Prorokov's experiments), after a soda solution was poured into its mouth, when the salivation caused by it ceased, the strong as well as weak conditioned stimuli immediately tested were equally greatly inhibited, but later, during the nearest 15-20 minutes, the weak stimuli already acted normally and even more than normally and were equal in their effect to the strong stimuli or even considerably exceeded them if they were still greatly weakened. Here is an example.

A soda solution was poured into the dog's mouth at 9:41 A.M.

Time	Conditioned stimulus applied for 30 seconds	Salivation (in drops) in 30 seconds
9:46 A.M.	Flashing of bulb	0.4
9:51 „	Mechanical stimulation of the skin	6.2
9:56 „	Loud bell	3.0

The usual effect of the electric bell—about eight drops in thirty seconds; the effect of mechanical stimulation of the skin—about four drops.

In another dog (P. Anokhin's experiments) the results of the experiments partly coincided with the result obtained on the first dog and partly differed from them. Ofter administration of disagreeable substances into the dog's mouth and cessation of the salivation caused by it, immediately and up to the end of the experiment all the stimuli which formerly always differed as to the effect they produced (the loud bell produced the greatest effect and the light of the bulb—the weakest) became equalised in this respect. But side by side with this the reflexes declined step by step during the experiment. The experiment proceeded as follows.

A soda solution was poured into the dog's mouth. Salivation continued for 10 minutes.

Time	Conditioned stimulus applied for 30 seconds	Salivation (in drops) in 30 seconds
11:10 A.M.	Flashing of bulb	12.5
11:15 "	" "	10.5
11:20 "	Loud bell	10.5
11:25 "	Metronome beats	6.3
11:30 "	Soft bell	6.8

Although the result obtained on both dogs generally favours the assumption that internal and external inhibition are basically the same process, the complexity of the phenomena requires repetition and variation of these experiments with stricter attention to other possible interpretations of the facts.

Lastly, we thought it interesting to investigate the relation of our conditioned reflexes under the effect of hypnotics from the beginning of this effect to the complete lapse of the animal into sleep and the reverse, to the animal's return to the waking state. For this purpose we used urethane and chloral hydrate. Here another course of phenomena prevailed almost exclusively, namely, a gradual diminution of all reflexes so that the weak stimuli naturally became ineffective sooner than the strong stimuli. We named this state of the cells the narcotic phase. The following is one of these experiments (S. Lebedinskaya).

The dog reacted to the following positive conditioned stimuli: loud bell, metronome beats, soft bell, mechanical stimulation of the skin and intermittent flashing of an electric bulb before the dog's eyes. According to the effect, the stimuli ranged as they are listed. At 10:09 A.M. 2 g of chloral hydrate in 150 cm^3 of water was administered per rectum. The dog was in the stand. The experiment continued as follows.

Time	Conditioned stimulus applied for 30 seconds	Salivation (in drops) in 30 seconds	Notes
10:14 A. M.	Metronome beats	11	Eats
10:21 "	Flashing of bulb	3.5	Yawns and reels, eats
10:29 "	Loud bell	7	Hangs on straps, eats
10:38 "	Mechanical stimulation of the skin	0	" "
10:45 "	Soft bell	2	Slowly rises and eats
10:53 "	Loud bell	0	Sleeps, does not eat
11:06 "	Metronome beats	0	" "
11:13 "	Soft bell	0	" "
11:19 "	Loud "	5.5	Awakens, eats
11:26 "	Mechanical stimulation of the skin	0	
11:35 "	Flashing of bulb	0	
11:45 "	Metronome beats	5	
11:53 "	Soft bell	9.5	
12:00 Noon	Mechanical stimulation of the skin	4	
0:07 P.M.	Loud bell	8.5	Eats
0:15 "	Flashing of bulb	6	
0:24 "	Metronome beats	9.5	
0:34 "	Loud bell	13	
0:42 "	Soft "	10	
1:03 "	Mechanical stimulation of the skin	5.5)	

We see that during the development of the hypnotic effect all the stimuli gradually lost their effect, whereas during the return to the waking state all of them also gradually regained their normal effect. The only marked exception to the twenty stimuli was the soft bell which was sounded at 11:53 A.M. and produced a disproportionately great effect.

Thus, on different healthy animals and under different conditions we obtained many different states of the hemispheres as regards their reactions to conditioned stimuli. The following question arose: To what extent are all these states, including the narcotic phase, peculiar to each animal under the usual conditions of existence? While working on this question we found ourselves in a fortunate position. Among our dogs there was one (the experiments cited at the end of Lecture Fourteen were conducted on this dog) belonging to the extreme nervous type of which I shall speak in the next lecture. Under certain conditions this dog was often noted for the amazing conditioned reflex patterns of its higher nervous activity. It was repeatedly and deservedly called a "living tool" by us. This dog, as has already been reported, had ten conditioned reflexes: six positive—to a bell, metronome beats, whistle, increased general lighting of the room, appearance of a circle and a toy horse before its eyes, and four negative reflexes—to another frequency of metronome beats, decreased general lighting of the room, a square and a toy rabbit of about the same size and colour as the horse. Of late we have not, for some reasons, used the bell, and of the negative stimuli we used only differentiated metronome beats. Acoustic stimuli usually, and in the early experiments constantly, produced a much greater (30-50 per cent) salivary effect than did optic stimuli. After the dog's long laboratory service (more than two years) the positive conditioned stimuli began to display a tendency to a decreased effect and a change in the quantitative relations between them, as it often occurs with our dogs when the same conditioned stimuli are used for a long time. And now we could distinctly see in our dog all the states of the hemispheres described earlier in this lecture as variations of the oncoming diffuse inhibitory process. Each of these states of the hemispheres was either clearly marked throughout the entire experiment or, now by itself and now under the influence of our measures, passed into other states (Speransky's experiments). The only thing we did not observe in this dog was the ultraparadoxical phase. Nor was there any occasion for it, since the dog never became clearly sleepy.

The following are experiments performed on different days and during different periods.

Time	Conditioned stimulus applied for 15 seconds	Salivation (in drops) in 30 seconds
	Normal experiment	
10:30 A.M.	Metronome beats	8
10:40 "	Increased lighting of the room	5
10:50 "	Whistle	8
11:00 "	Circle	5
11:10 "	Metronome beats	9
11:20 "	Increased lighting of the room	5
11:30 "	Whistle	8
11:40 "	Circle	6
	Experiment with Equalisation Phase	
9:00 "	Metronome beats	7
9:10 "	Increased lighting of the room	5
9:20 "	Whistle	5
9:30 "	Circle	4.5
9:40 "	Metronome beats	5
9:50 "	Increased lighting of the room	5
10:00 "	Whistle	5
10:10 "	Circle	4

Time	Conditioned stimulus applied for 30 seconds	Salivation (in drops) in 30 seconds

Experiment with Paradoxical Phase Passing into Normal Phase

10:00	A.M.	Metronome beats	4
10:11	"	Increased lighting of the room	6
10:22	"	Whistle	4
10:33	"	Circle	7
10:43	"	Metronome beats	4
10:54	"	Increased lighting of the room	2.5
11:03	"	Whistle	9
11:12	"	Circle	4.5
11:22	"	Metronome beats	9.5
11:33	"	Increased lighting of the room	5

Experiment with Complete Inhibition Passing into Narcotic Phase

10:00	"	Metronome beats	0
10:09	"	Increased lighting of the room	0
10:19	"	Whistle	3
10:31	"	Circle	0
10:42	"	Metronome beats	3
10:52	"	Increased lighting of the room	0
11:03	"	Whistle	3.5
11:12	"	Circle	0

When the reflexes greatly diminished and were perverted we intensified and corrected them, as was indicated in Lecture Fourteen, by acting with conditioned stimuli to the point of addition of an unconditioned stimulus for a shorter time. Hence, the different duration of the isolated conditioned stimulation in the experiments cited there. Transition from one phase to another in the two last experiments occurred, it must be assumed, under the influence of the repeated act of eating. But we ourselves possessed two special methods by which we could immediately change the phases. These were—application of always complete differentiation (to another rate of metronome beats) as an agent concentrating inhibition or inducing the process of excita-

tion, as well as application of a social stimulus which was the presence of the experimenter, the dog's master, in the experimental room.
Here are examples.

Time	Conditioned stimulus applied for 30 seconds	Salivation (in drops) in 30 seconds	Notes
9:30 A.M.	Metronome beats	0	Does not eat
9:37 "	Toy horse	0	" " "
9:45 "	Differentiation	0	
9:52 "	Metronome beats	4	
9:59 "	Increased lighting of the room	9	
10:10 "	Whistle	6.5	Eats
10:18 "	Toy horse	11	
10:30 "	Metronome beats	12.5	
10:38 "	Circle	8.5	

The complete inhibitory phase (there is neither secretory nor motor reaction) after application of differentiation passes first into the paradoxical and then into the normal phase.

Time	Conditioned stimulus applied for 30 seconds	Salivation (in drops) in 30 seconds	Notes
10:00 A. M.	Metronome beats	0	Does not eat

Experimenter enters and stays in the room with the dog.

| 10:09 " | Metronome beats | 9 | Eats |
| 10:18 " | Increased lighting of the room | 3.5 | " |

The presence of the experimenter in the room with the dog immediately transforms the complete inhibitory phase into the normal phase.

The question whether it is possible to arrange the aforesaid transitional phases in the states of the hemispheres in a single series and, if it is possible, in what series is as yet completely unsettled for us. If we take all our cases, the succession of the phases proves to be quite diverse. Thus it is still unclear whether these states are strictly successive or parallel. Nor can we point out exactly why a given phase directly passes now into one and now into another phase. Consequently, further research is required.

It can hardly be doubted that the states of the hemispheres described in this lecture are what is known as hypnosis in its different stages and features. We shall deal in detail with the phenomena of human hypnosis in connection with the facts, obtained by us, in the next lecture.

DIFFERENT TYPES OF NERVOUS SYSTEM. PATHOLOGICAL STATES OF THE CEREBRAL HEMISPHERES AS A RESULT OF FUNCTIONAL INFLUENCES EXERTED ON THEM[36]

Until now we have studied the normal activity of the cerebral hemispheres. But the experiments to which we subjected our animals, in other words, the neural tasks which we gave them, without, of course, at first having any idea of the possible limits, so to speak, of the endurance of their brain, in our experiments sometimes produced chronic disorders of the normal activity of the cerebral hemispheres. Here I mean only the functional disorders and produced also functionally and not surgically. In some cases these disorders gradually passed by themselves under the influence of rest alone, owing to cessation of the experiments, and in other cases proved so stubborn that they required special therapeutic measures on our part. Thus the physiology of the cerebral hemispheres changed before our eyes into their pathology and therapy. The pathological states of the hemispheres were manifested very differently in our different animals under the influence of the same harmful conditions. Some animals fell ill seriously and for a long time, others lightly and for a short time, and still others endured the same influences almost without any effect.

In some dogs the deviations from normal proceeded in one direction, in others—in another direction. Since this diversity was apparently connected with the difference in characters, types of nervous system of the different animals, it is necessary to dwell on the types of nervous system of our dogs before dealing with the pathological states of the hemispheres. At the present time rather exact criteria are already beginning to show in our studies of the cerebral hemispheres and with these criteria we shall be able to produce strictly scientific characteristics of the nervous system of our different animals. Among other things we shall then be able to conduct on our animals a strictly scientific experimental study of the hereditary transmission of the various aspects of nervous activity. Now I shall describe these types as they appear to ordinary observation. Two types, and extreme types, it must be assumed, have come particularly definitely and distinctly to the fore.

One type has long since made itself known to us. I repeatedly mentioned this type in my early articles and reports as a type which we at first failed to understand when we used it for our experiments. When, because of our inexperience in our early work, we encountered considerable difficulties with the sleepiness of the animals while using some conditioned stimuli and some of our methods, we wanted to do away with this evil by choosing for our experiments particularly lively dogs. These were extremely fussy animals, which sniffed at everything, examined everything, quickly reacted to the slightest sounds, and were very impertinent when making the acquaintance of people (and they made this acquaintance very readily); they were animals which could not be easily pacified with either shouting or light whipping. And it is precisely these animals which, when placed in the stand, limited in their movements and, especially, left alone in the experimental room, despite the use of conditioned stimuli with feeding or pouring acid into the mouth, very quickly became sleepy and their conditioned reflexes either greatly diminished or completely disappeared. Our recurring agents, when no strong conditioned stimuli had as yet been elaborated from them, demonstratively at once caused sleepiness although the dog was still awake since the beginning of the experiment. Some of these dogs, even in experiments not in the stand but outside of it, if the experimenter remained impartial to them and did not, so to speak, amuse them, also soon began to close their eyes, reel and finally lay down on the floor. This often happened immediately after the dog was fed following the conditioned stimulus. At first we had to give up our work with such animals. But then we gradually found a way of handling them. If conditioned reflexes to many different agents were simultaneously elaborated in these dogs, if the same stimuli were not repeated in the course of the experiment, if no long intervals between the individual stimuli were made, if not only positive but also inhibitory reflexes were developed in the dogs, in other words, if the experiment was greatly varied in a, so to speak, business-like manner, they became quite satisfactory experimental objects. The question that still remains and that we are now trying to settle is whether this type has a strong or weak nervous system.

Offhand, before establishing a more scientifically substantiated system, I thought that the types of dogs, as I chanced to acquaint myself with them during experiments in the laboratory, in some measure corresponded to the ancient classification of the so-called temperaments. The dogs I have just described must then be recognised as true sanguine types. If the stimuli are rapidly changed, they are energetic and business-like, but, if the surroundings become in the least monotonous, they are sluggish, sleepy and, consequently, inactive.

The other type of dogs, also very clearly defined, must be placed at the opposite end of the classical series of temperaments. In any new, especially somewhat unusual circumstances they are greatly restrained in their movements and continuously inhibit them; they walk slowly along walls on rather stiff legs and frequently, with the least outside movement or sound, completely crouch on the floor. A shout or threatening movement of a human being immediately immobilises them in a passively sprawled pose. Whoever sees them immediately takes them to be very cowardly animals. It is but natural that they very slowly adapt themselves to our experimental situation with the different manipulations performed on them. But when all this finally gets to be the usual thing for them, they become model objects for our investigations. The animal praised at the end of the last lecture belongs to this type. Usually dogs of this type do not sleep in the stand. If the experimental situation remains more or less monotonous, all their conditioned reflexes, especially the inhibitory reflexes, prove highly stable and regular. We now have in our laboratory an extreme representative of this type which we are studying. This female dog was born in our laboratory and had never had any trouble with anybody. When she was about one year old she began to be brought to the experimental room where she was fed only a few times in the stand during the formation of conditioned reflexes in the course of the experiment. She is still the same she was five years ago when she first appeared in the experimental room. She has not yet become accustomed to the laboratory. On her way with her master (experimenter) to the experimental room, always with her tail between her bent legs, she invariably either precipitately leaps to a side or backs up and crouches on the floor when meeting the permanent members of the laboratory (some of them always pet her). She similarly reacts to the least unintentional livelier movement or louder word of her master. With respect to us she behaves as if we were her most dangerous enemies from whom she constantly and cruelly suffers. Despite all this, however, when she finally adapted herself to the situation in the experimental room, she formed many precise positive, as well as negative, reflexes. This was so unexpected that we gave her the flattering name of "Smarty". I shall come back to this animal later.

It would be no exaggeration to regard such animals as the melancholic type. We cannot help considering their life unhappy if they inhibit constantly and without any need the main manifestation of life—motion.

Both described types are apparently extreme types: the process of excitation excessively prevails in one and the process of inhibition in the other. They are therefore limited types with, so to speak, restricted boundaries of life. One of them requires constant change of stimulations, their novelty, which the surroundings may often lack. The other one, on the contrary, needs a very monotonous life's situation which, however, may be replete with variations and changes.

In relation to the afore-described types I deem it necessary briefly to dwell on the following. Some of you may, in view of what I have reported on these types, have some objection to the proposition of the identity of sleep and internal inhibition in that the type with the excitatory process prevailing is greatly inclined to sleep under the conditions of our experiments, while the type which is so easily inhibited, on the contrary, remains awake under the same conditions. But these, as has already been pointed out, are extreme types with special qualities of the nervous system and, hence, with special conditions of their existence. If we assume—and justly so—that functional exhaustion of the cells provides an impetus for the emergence of the inhibitory process in them, it will become clear that the extraordinarily irritable cortical cells, i.e., the cells with precipitate functional destruction, will particularly tend to develop the inhibitory process which will spread extensively as long as they are subjected to protracted monotonous stimulation. Only a quick change to the new stimulations addressed to other cells may neutralise the natural but, perhaps, biologically unprofitable result of the given property of the nerve cells. Similarly, if the so easily emerging inhibition of the motor area of the cortex (this passive-defensive reflex) were accompanied by a spread of inhibition over the entire mass of the hemispheres and further down the brain, this second type would be biologically impossible and would have no chances for a stable existence. There had to be a chance for restoring the vigorous activity of the organism, as soon as the cause evoking the initial inhibition had passed, and this is precisely what the cells of the hemispheres, remaining uninhibited, do. Consequently, the limited spread of inhibition is in this case a special, biologically elaborated property of a generally defective nervous system, a special adaptation, just as man can learn to sleep even on the move, i.e., to limit the inhibition only to the hemispheres without letting it go down lower.

Now about the other variations of the nervous system. Between the afore-mentioned extreme types there are numerous intermediate types in which the processes of excitation and inhibition are more or less balanced. However, some of them somewhat approximate to one extreme type and others to the other, while, on the whole, they are better adapted to life and, consequently, are viable. Some of these animals are lively, active and, for the most part, aggressive. Others are quiet, sedate and restrained. I remember one dog of the latter group with truly amazing behaviour. I never saw this dog, when brought to the laboratory from the kennel, to lie down on the floor in expectation of the experiment, but at the same time it seemed to take no interest in what was happening in its surroundings and did not establish either friendly or hostile relations with any of us, including even its experimenter. The dog was never sleepy in the stand and always manifested precise positive as well as negative conditioned reflexes, especially, the latter. In any event, a strong inhibitory process had to be ascribed to this dog. However, it was also capable of great excitement. Once I managed to disturb its usual tranquillity by making extraordinary sounds before it with the aid of a toy trumpet, while wearing an animal's mask. Only in this case did it lose its invariable composure; it began to bark loudly and rushed at me. A truly phlegmatic but strong nature.

Another group apparently belongs more to the excitable type, perhaps corresponding to the choleric temperament in ancient classification. In these animals the negative conditioned reflexes are not infrequently disturbed.

Of course, there are many animals of a less definite type. But, as a whole, the entire mass of our animals before our eyes is divided into two categories: with extraordinary or moderate predominance of the excitatory process and extraordinary or moderate prevalence of the inhibitory process.

Now I can deal with the pathological states of the hemispheres which we either observed casually or produced ourselves purposely.

The first case of this type was observed under the following circumstances. As was pointed out in one of the earlier lectures, we were able to elaborate a conditioned food reflex to very strong electric current applied to the dog's skin. Instead of the inborn defensive reaction the animal responded to it with a food reaction: it turned to the side whence the food was served, licked its lips and secreted abundant saliva (Yerofeyeva's experiments). Elaboration of the reflex began with a very weak current which was then gradually boosted to extraordinary intensity. This reflex persisted for many months; moreover, the electric current was sometimes replaced by cauterisation or mechanical destruction of the skin with the same result. The dog always remained perfectly normal, and within several months this peculiar conditioned stimulus, like all the other conditioned stimuli, slowly began to change to an inhibitory stimulus, precisely the salivary reflex beginning to be delayed from the moment the stimulus was applied. Formerly we sometimes also tried other points, besides the one point at which this reflex was initially elaborated, and then decided systematically to use our electrodes at new points. For some time the food reflex persisted without the least interference by the defensive reaction. But at a certain point everything sharply and immediately changed. Not a trace of the food reaction was left, there was only a very strong defensive reaction. Even when we used an extraordinarily weak current which was ineffective before the elaboration of the conditioned reflex, we now had the same very strong defensive reaction at the very first point on the skin as well. The same thing was repeated on two more dogs. In one of them this explosion of excitation occurred at the ninth point, while in the other it did not take place even at the thirteenth point. But, when this electric stimulation was repeated in the same experiment at many of these points, and not at one as was done before, the same thing occurred. Nothing could be done immediately after this to restore the food reflex to the current in any of these dogs. The animals became highly excitable and uneasy, as they had never been before. In one dog after a three-month intermission in the experiments we could resume elaboration of the same reflex, by elaborating it with greater caution than the first time and, finally, restore it. In other animals even the intermission did not help. The afore-mentioned procedure apparently reduced the nervous system to a chronic pathological state. Regrettably, we have not preserved any information concerning the types of nervous system of these dogs.

The afore-described fact did not attract our particularly active interest perhaps because it occurred under exceptional conditions. But some time later we observed the same thing under more usual experimental conditions. Here is this observation.

We were studying the analysing activity as regards the extent of discriminating forms of objects with the eyes (Shenger-Krestovnikova's experiments). A light form of a circle was projected on a screen before the dog and the animal was simultaneously fed. When the reflex was formed, we started differentiating from the circle an ellipse of the same lighting and the same size of area with a

2:1 ratio of the semi-axes, i.e., the appearance of the circle was followed by feeding, while no food was given at the appearance of the ellipse. A complete and constant differentiation was obtained quite soon. Then by stages (3:2, 4:3 ratios of the semi-axes, etc.) we began to approximate the ellipse to the circle continuing to elaborate differentiations to these consecutive ellipses. The elaboration proceeded with variations (at first increasingly more rapidly and then slowing down again) smoothly up to the ellipse with a 9:8 ratio of the semi-axes. Now considerable, although incomplete discrimination was attained. During the three weeks that this differentiation was applied the state of affairs did not improve but, on the contrary, changed sharply for the worse: the discrimination between the circle and this ellipse completely disappeared. At the same time the dog's behaviour markedly changed. Formerly calm, the dog now squealed in the stand, fidgeted, tore off the pieces of apparatus fastened to it or bit through the rubber tubes running from them to the experimenter, something that had never happened before. When brought into the experimental room the dog barked, which was also unusual. When the easier differentiations were tested, it was found that they had also suffered, even the very first one with the 2:1 ratio of the semi-axes. This latter had to be restored to its former precision much more slowly (more than twice as slowly) than was the case during its first elaboration. During the second elaboration of the easy differentiation the animal gradually grew calmer and, finally, completely returned to its normal state. The transition to finer differentiations occurred even more rapidly than the first time. During the first application of the ellipse with a 9:8 ratio of the semi-axes a complete discrimination from the circle resulted, but not a trace remained from this discrimination when the ellipse was used for the second time, and the dog again returned to an intensely excited state with all the former consequences. At this point all the experiments with the dog were discontinued.

Here are several actual experiments from the aforesaid work.

Experiment Conducted on August 4, 1914

Time	Conditioned stimulus applied for 30 seconds	Salivation (in drops) in 30 seconds
4:10 P.M.	Circle	4
4:22 "	"	6
4:37 "	Ellipse (4:3 ratio of the semi-axes)	0
4:55 "	Circle	4

Experiment Conducted on September 2, 1914

1:10 "	Circle	2
1:27 "	"	8
2:06 "	"	10
2:16 "	Ellipse (9:8 ratio of the semi-axes)	1
2:30 "	Circle	6
2:48 "	"	8

Experiment Conducted on September 17, 1914

3:20 "	Circle	4
3:31 "	"	7
3:54 "	Ellipse (9:8 ratio of the semi-axes)	8
4:09 "	Circle	9

Experiment Conducted on September 25, 1914

2:17 "	Circle	9
2:47 "	Ellipse (2:1 ratio of the semi-axes)	3
3:08 "	Circle	8
3:22 "	"	8
3:46 "	Ellipse (2:1 ratio of the semi-axes)	3

Experiment Conducted on November 13, 1914

10:55 A.M.	Circle	10
11:05 "	"	7
11:30 "	Ellipse (2:1 ratio of the semi-axes)	0
11:44 "	Circle	5

In the first experiment the ellipse with the 4:3 ratio of the semi-axes produced a zero effect. In the second experiment the ellipse with the 9:8 ratio produced only one drop of saliva during the first period of elaboration of a differentiation to it, but after its application for two weeks equalled in its positive effect the circle in the third experiment. After this even the ellipse with a 2:1 ratio in the fourth experiment was no longer completely differentiated and, only in the fifth experiment after constant application for six weeks, became zero again.

After this work the foregoing fact concentrated our attention on itself and we started to elaborate it purposely. It was clear that under certain conditions the meeting of the excitatory and inhibitory processes led to a disturbance of the usual balance between them and created in greater or lesser measure and for a longer or shorter period an abnormal state of the nervous system. In the first case, during the formation of a food stimulus from strong electric current, the inborn defensive reflex had to be inhibited, and in the second case, during differentiation, as we already know from an earlier lecture, inhibition also had to come into play. Up to a certain point the opposite processes were balanced, but under certain conditions of their relative intensity or spatial delimitation the normal balance between them became impossible and everything ended in the predominance of one of them (as we shall see later), i.e., a pathological state.

For our subsequent experiments we intentionally chose dogs with different types of nervous system to see how each of them was affected by the pathological state of their nervous activity produced by our functional (not surgical) influences. The first such experiments (Petrova) were performed on two dogs with, judging by their general behaviour, antagonistic properties of the nervous system. These were the same dogs which were mentioned in the lecture on sleep and in which the sleepy state produced at first was then eliminated by application of many conditioned reflexes (six) rapidly following each other and, moreover, with a five-second interval between the beginning of the conditioned stimulation and the addition to it of an unconditioned stimulus. During these experiments, in addition to eliminating sleep, we obtained vivid and precise proof of the great difference in the characters of the nervous systems of both dogs which completely confirmed the initial diagnosis of these characters made on the basis of usual observation. This proof was furnished by the process which transformed in the dogs their almost coinciding conditioned reflexes into greatly delayed ones, when the unconditioned stimulus was added to the conditioned stimulus only three minutes after application of the latter. The transformation occurred gradually: each day the unconditioned stimulus was moved five seconds from the application of the conditioned stimulus. Of course, in keeping with this, the, what we call, latent period, i.e., the space of time after which salivation begins following application of the conditioned stimulus, gradually increased. This delay was developed simultaneously to all the stimuli. While one dog with predominance of the inhibitory process, according to our preliminary diagnosis, coped with the task of delay at once and more or less calmly, the other one, with predominance of the excitatory process, reacted to the same task quite differently. When the delay reached two minutes, the dog became excited and with the subsequent delay to the marginal value of three minutes, it actually became furious: it incessantly moved all parts of its body, squealed and barked intolerably, salivated continuously, the salivation extraordinarily increasing during the action of the conditioned stimuli; not even a trace of the delay was left. Apparently, the preliminary inhibition of many conditioned stimuli required by the conditions of the experiment was greater than the dog could cope with, was too great a task for the excitable nervous system of this dog and was manifested in a natural struggle against this torture. It must be added that this difficulty of balancing the two antagonistic processes was observed by us in many dogs in the form of excitement, but this excitement had never yet reached such an extent. But, to be sure, this time the problem was also much more serious, because the two processes had to be balanced simultaneously at many points of the hemispheres. There was nothing else we could do but discontinue the experiment in that state. It is very interesting that the task which had at first proved impossible was later, nevertheless, satisfactorily accomplished by the given nervous system. For this, it was at first necessary to confine ourselves only to one conditoned stimulus. The dog grew calm and even began to sleep during the experiment not only in the stand but also on the floor outside the stand during the experiments. Then all the conditioned stimuli were applied again but only with their five-second action before the addition of the unconditioned stimulus. Later this isolated action was again gradually prolonged to three minutes. This time a good delayed reflex calmly formed as I mentioned it in the lecture on sleep. The dog was sleepy for 1.5-2 minutes from the beginning of the action of the conditioned stimulus, but at the end of the second minute, or in the very begining of the third, it quickly came out of the sleepy-passive position and a sharp food reaction, both motor and secretory, occurred. Thus, owing to rest, gradualness and repetition, we attained the balance of both processes which we had been unable to do the first time.

Since the difference in the nervous systems of the dogs became clearly defined, we turned to the main aim of our experiments, but decided to proceed to it in a manner somewhat differing from that in the afore-described casual observations. In the greatly delayed reflexes, i.e., with the long preliminary inhibitory process, we applied other types of inhibition: differentiating, conditioned and extinguishing. We had the idea that perhaps with such complex system of inhibitions we would obtain the same disturbance in the normal balance between the two nervous processes that we had in those observations. We were wrong, no disturbance occurred. But during all these additional cases of inhibition the difference between our two dogs was always in evidence. The excitable dog temporarily accompanied the elaboration of each new inhibition by considerable excitement, while the other dog barely displayed any signs of difficulty. With this state of affairs we made use of our tested method. We began to elaborate a conditioned food reflex to electric current applied to the skin. The reflex was elaborated and practised with some interruptions for a considerable length of time. Now a chronic change in the nervous systems of both dogs occurred even without continuously transferring the electrodes to new points, as had been the case in Yerofeyeva's experiments. It must be assumed that here it was the influence of the aforesaid preliminary complication of inhibitory activity. But the important and new thing was that the disturbance in the normal work of the nervous systems of both dogs was manifested in exactly opposite manners: the negative, inhibitory reflexes chronically suffered in one dog, while the positive and, only later, successively, the inhibitory reflexes suffered in the other dog.

Here is the detailed course of the experiments.

The excitable dog reacted to the following conditioned stimuli: metronome beats, bell, gurgling and mechanical stimulus applied to the skin on the thigh, and negative stimuli: hissing together with metronome beats (hissing preceded the metronome beats by five seconds) and mechanical stimulation of the skin on the shoulder. All the conditioned stimuli were continued for three minutes before the dog was given food.

Experiment Conducted on March 15, 1923
(Before Formation of the Conditioned Reflex to Electric Current)

Time	Conditioned stimulus applied for 3 minutes	Salivation (in drops) by the minute
3:00 P.M.	Metronome beats	0 5 16
3:25 "	Hissing + metronome beats	0 0 0
3:45 "	Gurgling	0 1 14
3:54 "	Bell	3 0 17*
4:00 "	Mechanical stimulation of the skin on the thigh	0 2 12
4:13 "	Same on the shoulder	0 0 0

* In the excitable dogs, especially during stronger stimulation, the beginning of the stimulation almost always evokes a short investigating reflex (orienting reaction) and in the delayed reflexes an initial rather short disinhibition of the inhibitory phase therefore takes place.

Formation of a conditioned reflex to electric current began at the end of March. It was formed in April. As long as the current used was not very strong, all types of inhibition were more or less retained. In August the current was greatly boosted. Now the delay was disturbed for the first time and the conditioned inhibition ceased to be complete. To relieve the situation all the conditioned stimuli, except the bell, were continued isolated for thirty seconds instead of three minutes before feeding the dog. Nevertheless, the inhibitory process increasingly weakened despite the fact that application of the current had been suspended. The delay disappeared altogether. The hissing which preceded the metronome beats in the inhibitory combination by 5 seconds had itself acquired a constant positive effect, i.e., it had become a conditioned stimulus of the second order, and even the differentiation to mechanical stimulation was in considerable measure disinhibited.

Concluding Experiment (November 29, 1923) of This Period

Time	Conditioned stimulus	Salivation (in drops)
3:15 P.M.	Gurgling for 30 sec.	5
3:26 "	Mechanical stimulation of the skin on the thigh for 30 sec.	8
3:40 "	Same on the shoulder for 30 sec. (differentiation)	3
4:00 "	Metronome beats for 30 sec.	6
4:12 "	Hissing +metronome beats for 30 sec.(conditioned inhibitor)	10
4:35 "	Bell for 3 min.	16 12 13
4:46 "	Mechanical stimulation of the skin on the thigh for 30 sec.	8
5:00 "	Same on the shoulder for 30 sec. (differentiation)	3

The calm dog had the same conditioned stimuli as did the excitable dog.

Experiment Conducted on March 21, 1923
(Before Formation of the Conditioned Reflex to Electric Current)

Time	Conditioned stimulus applied for 3 minutes	Salivation (in drops) by the minute
3:18 P.M.	Gurgling	0 2 6
3:54 "	Bell	0 0 12
4:13 "	Metronome beats	1 5· 15
4:35 "	Hissing + metronome beats (conditioned inhibitor)	1 0 0
4:42 "	Bell	0 6 14
4:55 "	Hissing + metronome beats (conditioned inhibitor)	0 0 0
5:03 "	Mechanical stimulation of the skin on the thigh	0 3 9
5:15 "	Same on the shoulder	0 0 0

Formation of a conditioned reflex to electric current was begun at the end of March. This reflex easily and rapidly attained the value of seven drops in thirty seconds. During subsequent boosting of the current the defensive reaction returned, but then disappeared, completely yielding to the food reaction. However, during repetition of the elaborated reflex to the current the salivary effect of the reflex soon began to diminish and the reflexes to other conditioned stimuli tested at that time almost disappeared, being manifested only feebly in the beginning of the experiment.

The following experiment performed May 30, 1923 demonstrates this state of affairs.

Time	Conditioned stimulus applied for 3 minutes	Salivation (in drops) by the minute
3:25 P.M.	Bell	0 0 2
3:35 "	Metronome beats	0 0 5
3:47 "	Bell	0 0 0
4:03 "	Mechanical stimulation of the skin on the thigh	0 0 0
4:20 "	Same on the shoulder	0 0 0
4:25 "	Gurgling	0 0 0
4:37 "	Metronome beats	0 0 0
4:48 "	Bell	0 0 0

Since the dog began to lose weight and became sluggish, all experiments were discontinued for a considerable time and the dog was given additional food, including cod liver oil. The dog regained its former weight and cheerfulness. After the interruption all the usual conditioned reflexes, except the reflex to the bell, were re-elaborated from reflexes delayed for three minutes to ones delayed for thirty seconds, but this did not essentially alter the result: the reflexes were restored only to a negligible extent. Electric current applied at this time produced a considerable salivary effect, but when the current was boosted its effect weakened again and, finally, disappeared altogether, like the effect of all the other reflexes. More than that. This time all types of internal inhibition also gradually began to disappear, i.e., the negative conditioned stimuli, formerly zero stimuli, sometimes began to be accompanied by rather considerable salivation.

The following is an experiment performed December 6, 1923; this experiment shows the positive effect of the conditioned stimulus only during the inhibitory phase of the delayed reflex.

Time	Conditioned stimulus	Salivation (in drops)
0:48 P.M.	Mechanical stimulation of the skin on the thigh for 30 sec.	0
1:00 "	Same on the shoulder for 30 sec.	0
1:07 "	Gurgling for 30 sec.	1
1:20 "	Metronome beats for 30 sec.	0
1:40 "	Bell for 3 min.	3 2 0
1:51 "	Mechanical stimulation of the skin on the thigh for 30 sec.	0
2:00 "	Same on the shoulder for 30 sec.	0
2:11 "	Metronome beats for 30 sec.	0
2:42 "	Hissing + metronome beats for 30 sec. (conditioned inhibitor)	0
2:53 "	Metronome beats for 30 sec.	0

It must be justly assumed that the positive effect of the conditioned inhibitory stimuli did not mean a weakening of the inhibitory process, but attested further affection of the excitatory process, being the ultraparadoxical phase of the state of the formerly normally irritable cells.

At that time the general condition of the dog was quite satisfactory. Thus in two dogs with different types of nervous system, under the influence of absolutely the same harmful conditions, a chronic deviation from normal nervous activity, but in different directions, developed. In one of them, the excitable dog, the process of inhibition in the cells of the cerebral cortex extraordinarily weakened and almost completely disappeared, whereas in the other, calm, usually well-inhibited dog the process of excitation in the same cells extraordinarily weakened and almost disappeared. In other words, we were dealing with two different neuroses.

The neuroses produced by us proved very stubborn and protracted. During the suspension of the experiments they displayed no tendency to recovery. Then, for the purpose of investigation, we decided to administer to the excitable dog the tested therapeutic agent—bromides, especially, since in our early experiments (P. Nikiforovsky and V. Deryabin's experiments) we sometimes observed a favourable effect produced by bromides in intensifying inhibition in cases of its insufficiency. After several months of existence of the neuroses, daily administration of 100 cm^3 of a two per cent KBr solution per rectum was started. All types of internal inhibition rapidly began to be restored in a definite sequence: differentiation was the first to become complete and stable; it was followed by conditioned inhibition and, lastly, by the delay. Towards the tenth day all the reflexes were quite normal.

Experiment Conducted on March 5, 1924

Time	Conditioned stimulus	Salivation (in drops)
3:00 P.M.	Metronome beats for 30 sec.	5
3:12 "	Hissing + metronome beats (conditioned inhibitor) for 30 sec.	0
3:28 "	Gurgling for 30 sec.	8
3:37 "	Bell for 3 min.	2 12 16
3:44 "	Metronome beats for 30 sec.	8
3:55 "	Metronome beats (differentiation) for 30 sec.	0
4:10 "	Gurgling for 30 sec.	7
4:16 "	Bell for 3 min.	2 1 9
4:25 "	Same	0 8 21

It should be noted that no diminution of the positive reflexes was observed during this experiment. The thing that particularly attracted our attention was the great constancy of these reflexes. Thus, according to our experiments, bromides do not depress nervous excitation, but, on the contrary, regulate it.

Bromides were administered only for 11 days. But this time the neurosis was radically cured, since the reflexes remained quite normal even 2.5 months later.

The neurosis of the calm dog was not amenable either to the influence of bromides or the other measures taken by us. The dog was left without experiments for a very long time during which it was not under our observation. After this interval it proved quite normal, beyond all our expectations. We shall deal with this dog once more in the following lecture.

PATHOLOGICAL STATES OF THE CEREBRAL HEMISPHERES AS A RESULT OF FUNCTIONAL INFLUENCES EXERTED ON THEM[37]

In the present lecture I am continuing the description of our experiments with and observations of the pathological states of the cerebral cortex. In our hands and before our eyes this theme is growing increasingly broader and deeper not only because we have intentionally concentrated our attention on it but also owing to some fortuities. At the same time we constantly see how the normal is by imperceptible transitions transformed into the pathological under harmful, destructive influences, and how the pathological often opens before us, breaking up and simplifying, what is hidden from us, blended and complicated in the physiological norm. In the lecture on normal hypnotic states we reported that the particularly interesting states (from the point of view of their application to man, as we shall show in the last lecture) became a subject of our investigation only since they had clearly appeared before us in a pathological case. You remember that a few positive and negative conditioned reflexes, which the dog in that case had, included a positive reflex in response to mechanical stimulation of the skin by twenty-four rhythmic contacts with the skin for a period of thirty seconds and a negative reflex to twelve contacts during the same period. The positive reflexes normally showed a distinct gradation as to the salivary effect in accordance with the strength of the conditioned stimuli. When a positive mechanical stimulus of the skin was applied in one experiment directly after a negative mechanical stimulus of the skin without the slightest interval between them, i.e., one frequency of contacts was replaced with another, a pathological state of the cortex resulted. Soon afterwards it was manifested in disappearance of all the positive conditioned reflexes and then for a period of many days in variously departing from the norm, but definitely alternating relations of the emerged salivary effect to the strength of the conditioned stimuli. This pathological state lasted five and a half weeks. This case must apparently be ranked with the ones described in the preceding lecture. What was manifested in the case of the last dog as a very strong symptom, disappearance of all positive conditioned reflexes, the symptom that persisted for many months, here terminated towards the thirty-sixth day by passing through phases approaching the norm.

At the same time it is clear that the basic mechanism of the origin of the pathological state is the same in all the heretofore cited cases. It is a difficult encounter, a collision of the processes of excitation and inhibition.

In addition to the afore-described cases of the pathological state of the cerebral cortex, we have other cases which are of no lesser, if not greater, interest as regards some peculiarities of the pathological state, as well as the somewhat different mechanism of its origin.

I shall first dwell on a case particularly carefully observed day in and day out for several months (Rikman's experiment). Owing to its exceptional interest I shall reproduce it in particular detail and with special documents. In this case we are dealing with a dog which was very inhibitable and which formerly served for many experiments and observations. This dog had a number of positive conditioned food reflexes and one negative reflex to 60 metronome beats per minute, while 120 beats per minute were a positive stimulus. The positive conditioned reflexes were distinctly arranged, according to the salivary effect corresponding to the strength of the external agents used for conditioned action. Since the negative conditioned stimulus had been repeated 266 times by the beginning of the present experiment, it was quite precise, constant and sufficiently concentrated, i.e., its successive inhibitory effect on the positive reflexes was limited to a short time.

Here is an example of a normal experiment performed December 1, 1925.

Time	Conditioned stimulus applied for 20 seconds	Salivation (in drops) in 20 seconds	Motor reaction and general behaviour
10:37 A.M.	Metronome 120	8	Lively food reaction
10:45 "	Flashing of bulb	4	" "
10 49 "	Loud tone	6	" "
10:56 "	Metronome 60	0	Remains motionless
11:00 "	Bell	9	Lively food reaction
11:05 "	Mild tone	3.5	" "

Since the dogs of this type are, as it were, specialists in inhibition, and all types of internal inhibition are easily produced in them and persist, it was decided to perform a special test of the stability of the inhibitory process on this dog. For this purpose its negative stimulus had to be changed into a positive stimulus. To do this we used the method which usually quickly brings results, i.e., a continuous, uninterrupted application of a positive stimulus, a combination of a negative stimulus with an unconditioned stimulus. May I, please, ask you to recall what I said about this in the lecture on negative induction. Despite this, the inhibitory process was eliminated slowly. Although the old negative stimulus was accompanied by feeding for three days, from four to seven times each day, the first hint of elimination of the inhibitory process was detected only during the seventeenth repetition of this procedure and only in the form of a slight secretion, but without the motor food reaction. By the twenty-seventh repetition the salivary reaction to "Metronome 60" reached a considerable value. At that time no marked disturbance of the other positive reflexes could be observed, although the strong and weak conditioned stimuli may have drawn closer to each other as to their salivary effect.

The following is an experiment performed at that time (December 14, 1925).

Time	Conditioned stimulus applied for 20 seconds	Salivation (in drops) in 20 seconds	Motor reaction and general behaviour
10:56 A.M.	Metronome 60	5.5	Orienting rather than food reaction
11:03 "	Flashing of bulb	5	
11:10 "	Metronome 120	5	
11:17 "	Bell	8	Food reaction
11:24 "	Mild tone	5	
11:31 "	Metronome 120	5.5	
11:38 "	Bell	7	

But the value of the salivary effect of "Metronome 60" just attained did not remain constant. Despite the fact that it was accompanied by feeding it immediately began to diminish and by the thirtieth repetition equalled zero. At the same time, immediately after application of "Metronome 60", almost all the other reflexes also equalled zero.

The following experiment performed December 18, 1925 illustrates it.

Time	Conditioned stimulus applied for 20 seconds	Salivation (in drops) in 20 seconds	Motor reaction and general behaviour
0:04 A.M.	Flashing of bulb	4.5	Food reaction, eats greedily
0:09 "	Metronome 60	1	Orienting reaction
0:14 "	Loud tone	0	Turned away but took the food
0:23 "	Bell	0	Turned away, did not take the food
0:30 "	Flashing of bulb	0	Did not at once take the food
0:38 "	Mild tone	0	Food reaction, did not eat at once

Outwardly the dog looked quite healthy and outside the stand ate the food as greedily as it did in the stand in this experiment during application of the first conditioned stimulus, before application of "Metronome 60".

Subsequently, although the positive effect of "Metronome 60" was somewhat restored, its strong delaying action on the other conditioned reflexes continued. However, as soon as the experiment was performed without the metronome, these reflexes proved quite normal and perhaps only the weak stimuli diminished somewhat more than usual towards the end of the experiment.

Here is an experiment, performed December 24, 1925, that proves it.

Time	Conditioned stimulus applied for 20 seconds	Salivation (in drops) in 20 seconds	Motor reaction and general behaviour
11:02 A.M.	Bell	9	Lively food reaction
11:10 "	Flashing of bulb	5.5	
11:15 "	Loud tone	7	
11:20 "	Mild tone	5	
11:28 "	Bell	6.5	
11:32 "	Flashing of bulb	3	
11:39 "	Loud tone	6	
11:44 "	Mild tone	3.5	

I am intentionally citing several experiments with normal reflexes to show how long and persistently the norm is preserved despite the recurring disturbing action of the metronome reflexes. The same situation remains. During the experiment in which they are used both metronome rhythms with the constant variations of their positive effect from 0.5 to 7.5 invariably disturb all the following conditioned stimuli, in that they completely inhibit them, and produce various transitional phases to inhibition. It is interesting that in this case "Metronome 120" often causes a deeper disturbance than does "Metronome 60".

The following are several examples from this period.

Experiment Conducted on December 28, 1925
(Equalisation phase)

Time	Conditioned stimulus applied for 20 seconds	Salivation (in drops) in 20 seconds	Motor reaction and general behaviour
10:56 A.M.	Bell	10	Food reaction
11:07 "	Flashing of bulb	6	" "
11:13 "	Metronome 60	2	" "
11:20 "	Mild tone	5	" "
11:28 "	Metronome 120	4.5	Feeble food reaction
11:33 "	Loud tone	5	Food reaction
11:40 "	Bell	4.5	" "
11:47 "	Flashing of bulb	5.5	" "

Experiment Conducted on January 5, 1926
(Narcotic phase)

0:53 P.M.	Metronome 60	6	Retarded food reaction
1:00 "	Flashing of bulb	3.5	Food reaction
1:05 "	Loud tone	6	" "
1:10 "	Metronome 120	3	" "
1:18 "	Mild tone	0	Feeble food reaction
1:25 "	Bell	4.5	Food reaction
1:30 "	Flashing of bulb	0	Turns away does not take food
1:35 "	Bell	6	Distinct food reaction, does not eat at once

Experiment Conducted on January 20, 1926
(Paradoxical phase)

10:44 A.M.	Loud tone	8	Food reaction
10:49 "	Flashing of bulb	3	" "
10:57 "	Metronome 60	0.5	Orienting reaction
11:02 "	Mild tone	5	Lively food reaction
11:07 "	Bell	4.5	Feeble food reaction
11:14 "	Mild tone	5	Lively food reaction
11:21 "	Bell	2.5	Feeble food reaction
11:26 "	Flashing of bulb	3.5	Lively food reaction
11:31 "	Loud tone	1	Food reaction

Experiment Conducted on January 21, 1926
(Complete inhibition)

11:09 A.M.	Loud tone	6	Food reaction		
11:14 "	Flashing of bulb	4.5	" "		
11:22 "	Metronome 120	3.5	" "		
11:27 "	Mild tone	0	" "		Motionless
11:32 "	Bell	3	" "		during in-
11:39 "	Mild tone	0	" "		tervals
11:47 "	Bell	0	" "		
11:52 "	Flashing of bulb	0	Feeble food reaction		
11:57 "	Loud tone	0	" "		

Experiment Conducted on January 26, 1926
(Without metronome stimulation)

11:18 A.M.	Flashing of bulb	6	Lively	Food reaction	
11:28 "	Loud tone	6.5	"	" "	
11:33 "	Bell	7.5	"	" "	
11:40 "	Mild tone	4.5	"	" "	
11:48 "	Bell	6	"	" "	
11:53 "	Flashing of bulb	2	Feeble	" "	
0:02 P.M.	Loud tone	3.5	"	" "	

Since the last experiment showed that in the experiments without metronome stimulation the reflexes began to diminish towards the end of the experiments, although the conditioned stimuli retained their normal interrelations, we used coinciding stimuli for several days and no metronome stimulation at all. After that, isolated conditioned stimulation (i.e., until the addition of the unconditioned stimulus) continued in all reflexes only for 15 seconds, and not 20 as before. Besides, during that period we added a new conditioned stimulus—gurgling (a sound produced by air bubbles passing through water) belonging to the group of strong stimuli. The reflexes became stronger and did not weaken to the end of the experiment. Then, after an eleven-day interval, metronome stimulation, and precisely with 120 beats per minute, was reintroduced into the experiment.

Here is this experiment performed March 2, 1926.

Time	Conditioned stimulus applied for 15 seconds	Salivation (in drops) in 15 seconds	Motor reaction and general behaviour
10:44 A.M.	Gurgling	6.5	Food reaction
10:54 "	Mild tone	5.5	" "
11:02 "	Metronome 120	6	At first orienting, then food reaction
11:07 "	Flashing of bulb	4.5	Food reaction
11:15 "	Bell	4.5	" "
11:23 "	Gurgling	3.5	" "
11:31 "	Mild tone	5.5	Lively food reaction
11:33 "	Bell	4.5	Food reaction

We see that introduction of "Metronome 120" (please, remember that this was an old positive stimulus) into the experiment immediately entailed disturbance of all the other conditioned reflexes again. The equalisation phase immediately emerged and passed into the paradoxical. But this is not all. The next day, and for a long time afterwards, the cortical cells were reduced to such a state that they could not endure strong stimulation without passing into a completely inhibited state. In experiments with pathological nervous states we very often observed that a deeper disturbance of nervous activity did not occur at once, but a day and more after the harmful influence.

Here is the experiment performed the next day (March 3, 1926).

Time	Conditioned stimulus applied for 15 seconds	Salivation (in drops) in 15 seconds	Motor reaction and general behaviour
3:41 P.M.	Bell	5	Feeble food reaction
3:46 "	Flashing of bulb	0.5	Delayed food reaction
3:55 "	Loud tone	0	Does not take food
4:02 "	Mild tone	0.5	Food reaction, took food
4:07 "	Bell	0	Does not take food
4:10 "	Food given without conditioned stimuli		Takes food at once

The dog looked generally healthy. This state of affairs persisted for eleven days. Then we adopted the following measure. We gave up the loud tone altogether and considerably dampened the bell and the gurgling.
Here is such an experiment performed March 15, 1926.

Time	Conditioned stimulus applied for 15 seconds	Salivation (in drops) in 15 seconds	Motor reaction and general behaviour
10:20 A.M.	Flashing of bulb	6.5	
10:27 "	Mild tone	5	
10.32 "	Soft gurgling	3.5	
10:40 "	Soft bell	6.5	Food reaction
10:48 "	Mild tone	4.5	
10:56 "	Soft gurgling	4.5	
11:04 "	Soft bell	5	
11:12 "	Flashing of bulb	4	

The experiments were continued in exactly the same manner for nine days. Strong stimuli were used again and here is the result.

Experiment Conducted on March 27, 1926

Time	Conditioned stimulus applied for 15 seconds	Salivation (in drops) in 15 seconds	Motor reaction and general behaviour
4:02 P.M.	Loud bell	4	Food reaction
4:09 "	Flashing of bulb	0.5	" "
4:16 "	Loud gurgling	0	Turns away, does not take food
4:23 "	Mild tone	0	Takes food sluggishly
4:30 "	Bell	0	Is uneasy, takes food sluggishly
4:37 "	Flashing of bulb	1.5	Did not take food at once

175

Outside the laboratory the dog behaved perfectly normally and ate the food greedily. Two days later only weak stimuli were used and all the reflexes were on hand.

Time	Conditioned stimulus applied for 15 seconds	Salivation (in drops) in 15 seconds	Motor reaction and g-neral behaviour
3:57 P.M.	Mild tone	6.5	
4:05 "	Soft gurgling	6	
4:10 "	Flashing of bulb	4.5	
4:19 "	Soft bell	6	Food reaction
4:26 "	Soft gurgling	6.5	
4:31 "	Flashing of bulb	3	
4:40 "	Soft bell	5	

The outstanding pithiness and importance of these experiments must justify the, perhaps excessive, recording of the protocol material.

In a word, what do we have in this material? Transformation of one inhibitory point into an excitable point in the sound analyser proceeded slowly and imperfectly, and, what is most important, made this point abnormal so that action on this point with a corresponding stimulus immediately reduces the entire cortex to a pathological state which is manifested in that it cannot be stimulated by strong stimuli without passing into various phases of the inhibitory state, to the point of total inhibition. At first, this state of the cortex returns to normal quite soon after stimulation of the abnormal point is discontinued and, finally, if repeated, becomes stationary. Since the other acoustic stimuli themselves act quite normally, it must be assumed that in the given case there is a partial, narrowly localised disturbance of the sound analyser, its, so to speak, chronic functional ulcer, contact with which by an adequate stimulus harmfully affects the entire cortex and, in the long run, produces a protracted pathological state in it.

In this fact it is impossible not to see vivid, tangible proof of the mosaic structure of the cortex which we discussed before.

The afore-described final disturbance of the activity of the entire cortex can be conceived as produced by two mechanisms. Either the stimulus by evoking the excitatory process at the abnormal point thereby deepens the inhibitory process at it and for some time makes it stationary there, and the inhibition, irradiating, draws the other cortical cells into the same state, or the stimulus acts as a destructive agent on this point and then this point, like any point of the body undergoing destruction, involves inhibition of the other parts of the hemispheres by virtue of the mechanism of external inhibition. The formation of the abnormal point is, apparently, a result of the clash of the processes of excitation and inhibition.

Today, in addition to the cases cited in this and the last lectures, we have many more cases in which during the difficult encounter of the antagonistic nervous processes a rather protracted deviation from the normal activity of the cortex, frequently unamenable to any of our measures, occurred now in the direction of predominance of the excitatory and now of the inhibitory process. This also occurred either during elaboration of difficult differentiations, especially during differentiations of consecutive complex stimuli (A. Ivanov-Smolensky, M. Yurman and A. Zimkina's experiments), or now during direct and now during rapid replacement of the inhibitory stimulus with a positive stimulus in the skin analyser, especially, during replacement of one frequency of mechanical stimulations of the skin by another at the same site (when they were made stimulators of antagonistic processes). In the last case with a very excitable and even aggressive type (L. Fyodorov's experiment) the excitement of the dog reached a state in which it was no longer possible to work with it. And only constant administration of calcium bromide and exclusion of even the positive mechanical stimulus of the skin from the experiment brought the dog back to the normal condition as regards the other conditioned stimuli. In the dog of a more inhibited type (Petrova's experiment), it could be assumed that a narrowly localised abnormal point was similarly formed in the skin analyser, as in the afore-cited experiments (Rikman's), and the positive stimulation of this point evoked each time, in the current experiment and sometimes even in the experiments on the days immediately following, diffuse inhibition of the entire cortex. Regrettably, further analysis of this case was interrupted by the dog's serious illness (nephritis).

In the field of pathological states of the cortex under consideration I still have to describe several cases with a different mechanism producing these states. In these cases the pathological merges with the normal particularly imperceptibly or, rather, it is in them a constant property of a weak inborn nervous system. But before discussing them it would do well, at least briefly, to dwell for the sake of clarity on the question of external stimuli which act as direct inhibitors on the cells of the cerebral cortex. There are three types of stimuli: weak, monotonously recurring, very strong and, lastly, unusual stimuli generally represented either by new phenomena or a new connection, new sequence of old phenomena.

Our life and the life of animals is so full of cases of such action of these stimuli that there is no need giving examples of them here. The biological significance of this fact is more or less clear. If stimuli of considerable strength and, what is more important, constantly changing stimuli condition and must condition the active state of the cortex to maintain a fine balance of the organism with the environment, it is natural that weak and monotonous stimuli which do not require any activity from the organism must dispose to inhibition and rest, to give the cortical cells time for recovery after work. The inhibitory action of strong stimuli is, apparently, a special passive-defensive reflex, as, for example, in so-called animal hypnosis (properly speaking, real hypnosis), since, on the one hand, the animal's immobility makes it less noticeable to the enemy and, on the other hand, eliminates or moderates the aggressive reaction of a strong rival. Lastly, a generally unusual situation must limit the former energy of the animal's movements, because with the new state of affairs the former mode of action, as perhaps unsuitable in the given situation, may result in some harm to the animal. Thus, with a new, even negligible, variation in the environment two reflexes usually take place: a positive investigating reflex and an inhibitory reflex, a reflex of, so to speak, restraint and caution. The following interesting question remains: are these two reflexes independent or is the second reflex the effect of the first one by virtue of the mechanism of external inhibition? At first sight an affirmative answer to the latter part of the question seems the more probable. The physiological mechanism of the inhibitory action of all three types of stimuli will be the subject of discussion in one of the last lectures.

An unusual natural calamity, namely, a very big flood which occurred in Leningrad September 23, 1924 gave us an opportunity to observe and study a chronic pathological state of the nervous system of our dogs conditioned by this event as by an extraordinarily strong external stimulus. The building for animals which stood on the ground a quarter of a kilometre away from the laboratory building began to be flooded. In the dreadful storm with large incoming waves striking against the buildings, the roar and rumble of broken and falling trees, we had to move our animals hastily by swimming in groups to the second floor of the laboratory and leave them there in unusual company. All this, apparently, extraordinarily inhibited all animals without exception, because during that time we did not observe any of the usual fighting among them. After this event some of the dogs, returned to their former place, remained the same as they had been before; others, especially those of the inhibited type, developed nervous diseases (and for a very long time at that) of which we convinced ourselves in our experiments with their conditioned reflexes. These are the experiments I shall now discuss.

The first dog (Speransky's experiments), already mentioned before, was a strong and healthy, but very inhibitable animal. All the conditioned reflexes of this dog were substantial, particularly constant and precise, but only on condition that the experimental situation remained strictly customary. I shall remind you that it had ten (food) reflexes of which six were positive and four—negative (differentiations); of the positive reflexes three were acoustic and three—optic; of the acoustic reflexes the strongest one—bell—evoked the greatest salivation; the optic reflexes were equal to each other in this effect and, lastly, the positive acoustic reflexes exceeded the optic ones in salivation by one-third and more. One week after the flood the dog placed in the stand was unusually fidgety, scarcely had any conditioned reflexes and, while generally very greedy, took no food and even turned away from it. It was thus for three days. The dog was left without food for another three days, but this did not alter the results. After eliminating other causes and on the basis of our observations of the dog we concluded that it was the continuing effect of the flood and took the following measure. The experimenter who usually conducted the experiment outside the room in which the dog was alone, now stayed with the dog in the room, while I conducted the experiment from the outside. The reflexes immediately appeared and the dog greedily ate the food it was given. But no sooner did the experimenter leave the dog alone than the same thing recurred. To restore the reflexes it was necessary systematically now to stay in the room and now to leave it for some time. On the eleventh day of the experiment we applied for the first time the stimulus that had until then remained unused, i.e., the bell, the most efficient, as to the conditioned effect, and at the same time the strongest physically. After this all the other reflexes immediately diminished and the dog ceased to take the food; at the same time, it became greatly excited, looked about uneasily and especially persistently looked from the stand at the floor. Application of a social stimulus, i.e., the presence of the experimenter near the dog, gradually restored the reflexes, but the bell, repeated five days later, evoked the same reaction. Then we began to use the bell only when the experimenter was in the room with the dog. The normal relations were slowly restored. The equalisation phase was frequently observed in the reflexes, during the bell the dog sometimes stopped eating and after the bell the other reflexes frequently diminished. Finally, on the forty-seventh day of the experiments, almost two months after the flood, the experiment turned out quite normal. During this experiment we employed the following procedure. We let a quiet stream of water trickle from under the door into the dog's room, the water forming a small puddle near the table on which the dog was standing in the stand.

Here is this experiment (November 17, 1924) conducted normally without the experimenter in the dog's room.

Time	Conditioned stimulus applied for 30 seconds	Salivation (in drops) in 30 seconds	Notes
10:15 A.M.	Metronome 120	15,5	
10:24 "	Strong lighting of the room	9	
10:36 "	Bell	17	
10:46 "	Appearance of a circle before the dog	9	
10:59 "	Whistle	15	Eats greedily
11:11 "	Metronome 80 (differentiation)	0	
11:20 "	Metronome 120	12.5	
11:30 "	Square before the dog (differentiation)	0	
11:41 "	Circle before the dog	9	
11:50 "	Bell	17	

Then, at 11:59 A.M., we let water trickle into the dog's room.

0:02 P.M.	Strong lighting of the room	0	The dog quickly jumped to its feet, uneasily looked at the floor, tossed in the stand. Developed dyspnoea. The stimuli only intensified this reaction. The dog did not touch the food.
0:07 "	Metronome 120	0	
0:15 "	Whistle	0	
0:25 "	Bell	0	
0:32 "	Circle before the dog	0	

Many months later, when the reflexes were on hand and the bell had been intentionally unused for a long time, its application at first produced the usual effect exceeding all the other reflexes. But repeated for a few days and only once a day the bell gradually lost its effect, dropped to zero and greatly reduced all the other reflexes. It is interesting that at that time not only the experimenter himself but also his clothes placed near the dog and unseen by it, consequently their odour, acted on the reflexes restoratively.

Thus, under the influence of an extraordinary stimulus, the cortical cells, even formerly greatly inclined toward inhibition, became chronically still more inhibitable. The stimuli which had long since become indifferent (situation of the experiment), as well as the strong agents, which had formerly already been strong, positively acting conditioned stimuli (the bell), now sharply inhibited these weakened cells. The negligible energy components of that extraordinary stimulus (flood) were enough to evoke the original reaction.

The second dog (Rikman's experiments) was the one the experiments with which were described at length in the beginning of this lecture. The state of the dog now described belongs to an earlier period. The effect of the flood on this dog was manifested in a somewhat different

pathological form but with the same basic mechanism, i.e., in the form of extraordinary inhibition.
Here is the experiment performed on the eve of the flood, September 22, 1924.

Time	Conditioned stimulus applied for 30 seconds	Salivation (in drops) in 30 seconds
0:53 P.M.	Metronome 120	6
0:58 ″	Mechanical stimulation of the skin	3.5
1:03 ″	Metronome 60 (differentiation)	0
1:13 ″	Flashing of bulb	4
1:23 ″	Loud tone	7.5

On the third day after the flood, September 26, 1924, the experiment proceeded as follows:

Time	Conditioned stimulus applied for 30 seconds	Salivation (in drops) in 30 seconds
2:42 P.M.	Metronome 120	2.5
2:50 ″	Mechanical stimulation of the skin	2
2:55 ″	Metronome 60	3.5
3:02 ″	Metronome 120	1.5
3:06 ″	Mechanical stimulation of the skin	0
3:16 ″	Metronome 120	2.5

The dog took the food, but the positive reflexes were greatly weakened and the negative stimulus produced the most positive effect (ultraparadoxical phase).
Then the following situation persisted for a long time. As long as the negative stimulus (metronome 60) was not used, the positive stimuli were satisfactory and often attained normal value. But even a single application of this

stimulus reduced all conditioned reflexes to zero or greatly diminished them for the remainder of the experiment and for many days to come. Here are two examples.

Experiment Conducted on October 6, 1924

Time	Conditioned stimulus applied for 30 seconds	Salivation (in drops) in 30 seconds
0:03 P.M.	Metronome 120	5
0:10 "	Loud tone	5
0:20 "	Mechanical stimulation of the skin	2
0:25 "	Loud tone	4
0:33 "	Metronome 60	0
0:36 "	Metronome 120	0
0:43 "	Mechanical stimulation of the skin	0

Experiment Conducted on October 20, 1924

11:41 A.M.	Mild tone	6
11:46 "	Metronome 120	7.5
11:51 "	Metronome 60	0
11:56 "	Loud tone	0
0:01 P.M.	Bell	3
0:06 "	Flashing of bulb	0
0:11 "	Metronome 120	1.5

All the transitional phases between total inhibition and the norm were observed during the period of restoration of the reflexes when the negative stimulus was excluded. At first the restoration was facilitated by our most effective methods—suspension of the experiments for a few days and shortening of the isolated action of the conditioned stimuli; but, at last, these also proved inadequate. Only one or two reflexes in the beginning of the experiment had a slight effect, while all the others were reduced to zero. The dog grew motionless and stubbornly refused the food. We had to resort to the last measure. The experiment was performed not in the stand but on the floor with the dog released, whereby a certain inhibitory effect produced by the stand was partly eliminated for such dogs and several stimulatory impulses coming from the motor apparatus were partly added to the hemispheres. This helped. The reflexes began to return and grow. Now the dog took the food. At last the norm was attained. The negative stimulus applied again now resulted in disappearance of all reflexes till the end of the experiment only for the first seven days, but did not extend its inhibitory effect to the following days. Then, for a period of two weeks, this influence was also gradually eliminated. After that we began cautiously to practise inhibition. The differentiating inhibition was repeated in the same experiment, was concentrated soon afterwards by application of a positive stimulus and was finally refined. Only after two months of experiments on the floor, eight months after the flood, was it possible to return to the experiments under the usual conditions in the stand.

Thus, the flood had conditioned such inhibitability of the cortical cells that the insignificant inhibition added by us in the form of a negative stimulus for a long time rendered the existence of the positive conditioned reflexes in our usual experimental situation impossible.

According to our experiments and observations, a chronic pathological state of the cerebral hemispheres may be produced by two factors: difficult encounter, clash of the processes of stimulation and inhibition, and strong extraordinary stimuli.

But I must also report about another dog (A. Vishnevsky's experiments) of which I cannot, as a matter of regret, definitely say whether its present state is inborn, has been effected by the general conditions of life, age, parturition, etc., or is also, as in the two preceding cases, a special result of the influence of the flood. This dog was described in the last lecture as an extreme representative of the extreme inhibitory type. It had long been unobserved before the flood and became the subject of investigation only three or four months after the flood. I have already mentioned that many even very valuable experiments with conditioned reflexes had been performed on this dog long before the flood. Now, despite all the measures we have taken, this dog is unfit for the experiments with our usual themes. We can only analyse its state. Whether the flood or something else have produced this state is still a question. The period of the dog's normal life, which is also typical of other dogs, at least under laboratory conditions, has been greatly reduced. In the laboratory it almost always either displays the passive-defensive reflex, i.e., responds with an orienting reaction to the most negligible variations in the environment and immediately inhibits all its movements, to the point of refusing food, or, as an exception to its type, sleeps. Only two procedures return it to the state customary for the other dogs. It is a very rapid transition one or two seconds after the beginning of the conditioned stimulus to feeding or performance of the experiment on the floor on the condition that the experimenter walks about the room, the dog following in his footsteps, and also provided the conditioned stimulus is soon followed by feeding. Both circumstances alter the state of the dog in that the dog ceases to react to the slight variations in the environment, as it did before, and can eat the food it is given, ceasing to eat only in response to considerable external stimuli. Now conditioned reflexes also begin to appear. But no sooner is the food delayed even 5-10 seconds from the beginning of the conditioned stimulus than the dog becomes sleepy and may even fall asleep over the feeding box during the feeding. We consider this absolutely exceptional state of the nervous system, apparently of the cortical cells, to be a state of extreme exhaustion of the cells, as the highest manifestation of their so-called excitatory weakness. I am adding the word "apparently" because only the cerebral hemispheres are capable of this fine reactivity of the nervous system, particularly of all its analysers. We are now studying this case in great detail.

APPLICATION TO MAN OF EXPERIMENTAL DATA OBTAINED ON ANIMALS[38]

If the information obtained on the higher animals, regarding the functions of the heart, stomach and other organs which are so similar to human organs, can be applied to man only with caution, with a constant check-up on the actual similarity in the activity of these organs in man and animals, think of the great restraint we must exercise in transferring the precise natural-science information of higher nervous activity of animals, now being obtained for the first time, to the higher activity of man. Indeed, it is precisely this activity that so amazingly sharply distinguishes man from the animals, places man so immeasurably high above the whole animal world. It would be extremely light-minded to regard the first steps in the physiology of the cerebral hemispheres, complete only in programme and, of course, not in content, as some solution of the great problem of the higher mechanism of human nature. Any narrow restriction of our work on this subject at the present moment would therefore only denote extraordinary narrow-mindedness. But, on the other hand, temporarily, of course, the extraordinarily simplified treatment of the subject on the part of natural science must not be received with hostility, which, regrettably, is also not infrequently the case. Science grasps the complex only in parts and in fragments, but it gradually embraces it more and more. Hence, let us hope and patiently anticipate that the exact and complete knowledge of our higher organ—the brain—will become our real property and at the same time the main basis of lasting human happiness.

After all that has been cited in the preceding lectures it can hardly be contested that the most general bases of higher nervous activity relating to the cerebral hemispheres are the same in the higher animals and man and that the elementary phenomena of this activity must therefore be the same in normal, as well as in pathological cases. I shall cite but a few normal cases, since they are obvious, and shall now occupy your attention mainly with pathological cases.

Our education, training and all forms of disciplining, as well as our various habits, are apparently long series of conditioned reflexes. Is there anyone who does not know how the established, acquired connections of certain conditions, i.e., definite stimulations, with our actions are persistently reproduced by themselves often even despite the intentional counteraction on our part? This equally applies to the performance of particular actions and their elaborated inhibition, i.e., both positive and negative reflexes. Furthermore, we all know how difficult it is sometimes to develop the necessary inhibition in individual superfluous movements in games, in manipulations in the various arts, and in actions. Practice has similarly long since taught us that difficult tasks are accomplished only when approached gradually and cautiously. Everybody knows how extra stimulations inhibit and disturb the well-arranged customary activity and how a change in the once established order of movements, actions and the entire mode of life upsets us and makes things difficult for us. It is also generally known that weak and monotonous stimuli make people sluggish and sleepy and even put some people to sleep. We are all likewise familiar with different cases of partial waking during usual sleep, for example, the case of a sleeping mother at the bedside of a sick child, etc. All these are facts which we encountered in these lectures on our animals before.

Now I shall treat of pathological cases.

Modern medicine distinguishes nervous and mental diseases, neuroses and psychoses. But these distinctions are, of course, entirely conventional. Nobody could draw a clear line between them because there is really no such line. How could we conceive of a mental disorder without disturbance of the brain tissue, if not structurally, then functionally? The difference between a nervous and mental disease is a difference either in complexity or fineness of the disturbance of nervous activity. The experiments on our animals also incline us to this idea. As long as we deal with animals in which our different functional procedures or extraordinary conditions of life (please, remember the case of the flood) or, lastly, minor operations on the hemispheres disturb their nervous activity, we can understand more or less satisfactorily the mechanism of these disturbances in terms of neural physiology. But as soon as we have destroyed large sections of the hemispheres or this is done by growing cicatricial tissue we find it always difficult to conceive fully and clearly the mechanism of the developing disorders in nervous activity and we resort to assumptions which require proof of their correspondence with reality. The difference in our position regarding the subject in either case is apparently based on the greater complexity of the disturbances in the latter case and the inadequacy of the present-day physiological analysis for them. Observing both groups of animals many physicians and psychologists would most probably say that the animals in the first group were affected nervously and those of the second group mentally. We, on the other hand, refusing to pry into the imaginary inner world of our dogs, would say that we have before us deranged activity of the cerebral hemispheres, lesser and simpler derangement in the former case, and greater and more complex in the latter case.

Now let us compare the different nervous disorders in our animals and in man.

On dogs we have acquainted ourselves with two conditions which functionally produce nervous disorders. These are: a difficult encounter, a clash between the excitatory and inhibitory processes, and strong, extraordinary stimulations. They are also the usual causes of nervous and mental diseases in man. Life situations which arouse us to the greatest extent, for example, in cases of cruel insults or great misfortune, and which at the same time obligate us to restrain and suppress our natural reactions to them, frequently lead to a deep and long disturbance of the nervous and mental balance. On the other hand, people likewise frequently become nervously and mentally ill by being exposed to extraordinary dangers which threaten them as well as their near and dear ones, or by merely witnessing terrible events which do not directly concern either them or their dear ones. In such cases, it is, as a rule, noted that the same circumstances fail to produce the same effect on other people who, as we say, are not disposed to the disease, i.e., they have a stronger nervous system. Exactly the same thing was observed in our dogs. As regards such diseases, individual animals differ very greatly. We had dogs in which one of the most effective methods of disturbing nervous equilibrium, namely, direct replacement of the inhibitory rhythm of mechanical stimulation of the skin at the same site with a positive stimulation repeated daily for a long period of time did not in any way harmfully affect the animal. In other animals the nervous disorder appeared only after numerous repetitions. In still others, the nervous state emerged after the very first application of the method. Similarly, as was mentioned before, the extraordinary flood provoked the disease, apparently analogous to traumatic shock in people, only in a few dogs, particularly the very inhibitable ones.

Furthermore, this method, as was reported before, conditions different forms of the disease, according to the different types of nervous system, either towards predominance of the process of excitation, as in the dogs with a stronger nervous system, or towards predominance of the process of inhibition, as in dogs with a weaker nervous system. As far as we can judge, mainly on the basis of our ordinary observations, it seems to me that these two variations of the disturbance of nervous activity in animals correspond to the two neurotic forms in man, namely, neurasthenia and hysteria, if we characterise the former by a predominance of the excitatory process and weakness of the inhibitory process, and the latter, on the contrary, by a predominance of the inhibitory and weakness of the excitatory process. There are practical reasons to regard neurasthenics, at least some of them, as strong people even capable of very hard work, whereas hysteriacs are, of course, absolutely unviable subjects, total invalids. The fact that neurastheniacs at the same time have periods of impotence, temporary unfitness, is understandable as long as they are so protractedly excitable and productive at other times: nervous dissipation must be compensated. We may say that they represent another periodicity in the alternation of work and rest, longer than the usual, and therefore, compared with ordinary balanced people, their periods of excitation and inhibition are so exaggerated. The fact that hysteriacs, on the other hand, have attacks of excitement, does not, of course, in any way denote any strength of their nervous system. This excitement is purposeless, futile and, so to speak, coarsely mechanical. Our observations of the dogs contain, it seems to me, some indications of the origin and character of this excitement. We had a dog (described by Frolov) of a very inhibitable type, in common parlance, an extremely cowardly and obedient animal. This dog served for experiments with gastric secretion and had to remain in the stand for many hours. In this case, we observed that the dog never slept but stood in an alert posture, surprisingly calm, barely moving, and but rarely cautiously shifting from one leg to another. This was not torpor, however. The dog reacted when called by name. But when it was taken off the stand and released from the straps, it became absolutely incredibly excited: it squealed and strove to get free with such force as to almost overturn the stand. This excitement could not be repressed by any means, either loud shouting or whipping; the dog became entirely unrecognisable. A few minutes of walking in the yard and the dog became itself again: it went to the experimental room by itself, jumped into the stand, and again stood motionless. The urinary and defecation reflexes played no essential part in this fact. A similar fact was also sometimes observed in other dogs, but it was never manifested in such extremely marked form. It can be very simply understood as a temporary positive induction, an explosion of excitation after prolonged and strenuous inhibition. This could be one of the reasons for the attacks of excitement in hysteriacs during their frequent and deep manifestations of inhibition. But there may have been also another reason, which was demonstrated by one of our other dogs (described by Podkopayev). This calm, balanced and not very active animal never jumps into the stand by itself, remains motionless in the stand, but does not sleep, however, and its positive and negative conditioned reflexes are very constant and precise. Some pieces of apparatus for mechanical stimulation of the skin are attached to one half of the dog's body, from the shin across the body to the carpus. A positive food stimulus was elaborated from the stimulation of the shin and negative stimuli—from the stimulation of all the other places. The latter were elaborated quickly and were constant. The dog remained calm during all skin stimulations, making absolutely no local movements, and even the motor food reaction was absent during conditioned stimulation; the dog took the food deliberately. Elaboration of the negative reflexes was begun by stimulation of the carpus as the point farthest removed from the point of the positive reflex. This situation obtained for some time. Then the stimulation of the carpus suddenly began to be accompanied by a motor reaction, namely, an abrupt jerking away of the stimulated limb. Sometimes these jerks coincided with the rhythm of the mechanical stimulations. Then, similar local reactions began to appear successively at the inhibited points approaching more and more the point of the positive stimulation, while the motor reactions became increasingly broader and were manifested in the shifting of all limbs. The head and neck remained motionless, indifferent, so to speak, to all that occurred in the posterior part of the body; nor did the dog salivate. When the stimulation on the thigh, the closest point to the positive stimulation, was also made positive, the afore-described motor reaction to it completely disappeared. The same thing likewise occurred with the other points, when their stimuli were also made positive, except the two most remote points which, upon stimulation, continued, together with the complete salivary effect, to manifest a local defensive reaction, even if in a weakened form. The course of development of this phenomenon (not from the beginning of the experiments with each stimulus, but only after elaboration of the differentiation) and its local character warrant the assumption that these are cerebrospinal reflexes which appeared because of a functional and partial disconnection of the cortical skin analyser. The same thing could be assumed in some cases with hysterical subjects during their cortical inhibitions.

Our material also contains other cases which likewise correspond to rather well-known pathological states of the human nervous system. May I request that you recall the dog (Rikman's) which was reduced to such a state that it endured absolutely no conditioned stimuli from among physically strong agents and infallibly at once lapsed into an inhibited state so that its conditioned reflex activity could continue only in response to weak stimuli. I will hardly stretch the point if I draw an analogy between this case not completely, of course, but only as regards its mechanism, and cases of protracted human sleep lasting for many years, as was described by Pierre Janet concerning a young girl and as was observed in an adult male in one of the Petersburg psychiatric hospitals. There were cases of patients who seemed to be immersed in continuous sleep. They did not move, did not speak, and had to be fed and kept clean artificially. Only at night, when the daily life with its various and strong stimuli died down, were they sometimes able to engage in any activity. Janet's patient sometimes ate and even wrote at night. The Petersburg patient was also reported to get up from time to time at night. When, almost after twenty years' sleep, this patient, now an old man (sixty years old), began to shake off his sleep and could speak, he declared that formerly he had also frequently seen and heard what had happened around him but had been unable to do or say anything about it. In both these cases there was clearly an extremely weakened nervous system and especially weakened cerebral hemispheres which by strong external stimuli were rapidly reduced to a continuous inhibited state, to sleep.

On the same dog we acquainted ourselves with another pathological symptom of nervous activity which, in our opinion, is also not infrequently reproduced by the neuropathological casuistry of man. This dog had a chronic, narrowly localised functional affection of the auditory analyser in the cortex, contact with which by appropriate stimulation successively evoked an inhibited state of the entire mass of the hemispheres. There are many various cases of a morbid nervous state in people, when their normal activity is more or less maintained only until they are affected by components, even if very negligible, even if in the form of verbal hints, of those strong and complex stimuli which originally provoked the nervous disease.

Lastly, we must recall the case mentioned in one of our earlier lectures; I am referring to the case in which we periodically produced visual illusions in one of our dogs. These illusions were, in all probability, based on a complication of the external stimulation of the cortex by an internal stimulation resulting from the action of a growing cicatrix. We can similarly understand in some cases the illusions of people under particular internal stimulations of the cortex.

This is from the field of pathology. The same similarity between our experimental animals and us is also observed as regards treatment of nervous disorders, besides the identical effect of pharmaceutical agents. As was already reported before, rest, suspension of the experiments in general, often helped in restoring normalcy. Certain details are observed in this case and I deem it useful to cite one of them here. One of our dogs was driven to an extraordinarily excited state by the method of colliding the inhibitory and excitatory processes (Petrova's experiments). All forms of internal inhibition were disturbed, i.e., all its negative conditioned reflexes were transformed into positive reflexes. All the conditioned stimuli, formerly positive, as well as formerly negative, gave rise to dyspnoea as the usual symptom of strong excitement. Suspension of the negative conditioned reflexes did not alter the state of affairs. Dyspnoea continued, and the positive reflexes remained greatly intensified compared with normal. Then we decided to use only the physically weak positive conditioned stimuli, i.e., optic and mechanical skin stimuli, suspending the acoustic ones which were usually physically the stronger stimuli in our experiments. A favourable result was noted immediately. The animal calmed down. Dyspnoea disappeared. The normal salivary effect was restored. Some time later, it was possible gradually to introduce the strong positive stimuli without disturbing the result of the treatment. Moreover, several days later, differentiation of the skin stimulation, according to site, as a lighter form of internal inhibition was on hand without provoking any excitement of the animal. Regrettably, the experiment was discontinued at this point because the experimenter had no more time. It is an interesting case showing how diminished external energy reaching the cerebral hemispheres in the form of conditioned stimuli decreased the pathologically intense positive tone of the hemispheres. Of course, human nervous therapy makes wide use, in the form of various vital recipes, of limitation of external stimuli falling on the morbidly stimulated hemispheres.

I take the liberty of describing in detail one more case which, to my mind, is very instructive from the point of view of therapy. It is a case of a dog with an absolutely unusual, apparently abnormal reaction to mechanical stimulation of the skin, a reaction manifested in some strong excitation of the cerebral hemispheres (Prorokov's observations and experiments). In response to our usual mechanical stimulation of the skin on the thigh the dog immediately begins to wiggle its hind quarters, shifts all its limbs, tosses its head in some strange manner, squeals and sometimes yawns. This reaction ceases, when the dog is given food and begins to eat. Beyond all our expectations, this peculiar reaction did not in any way hinder the formation of a conditioned reflex to stimulation of the skin, which is usually performed by local motor reflexes (jerking away the corresponding limb, local play under the site of stimulation, *platysma myoides*) encountered in other dogs. Here, on the contrary, the reflex was formed rapidly and, what is absolutely exceptional, in the overwhelming majority of cases, this conditioned mechanical skin reflex was, according to its salivary effect, greater than in response to the strongest acoustic stimuli. Similarly, the food motor reaction, which usually replaced the peculiar afore-described reaction at half the period of each isolated conditioned mechanical stimulation of the skin, was sharply intensified compared with what it was in response to other stimuli. Usually continuing for some time after cessation of feeding, the food excitement of the animal was in this case also longer and stronger. Besides, when the skin stimulation was used in the experiments, the dog became generally very excitable. It reacted with a complex of the same special movements to the slightest sound coming from behind the door where the experimenter was. All this warranted the conclusion that in this dog the skin stimulation evoked strong diffuse excitation of the cerebral hemispheres. We are still unclear as to the nature of this excitation. The absence of an erection denoted that this excitement was not of a sexual character. We wondered if it was not analogous to the effect of tickling. At any rate, it was an unusual, abnormal nervous phenomenon and we decided to eliminate it. To do this, we used the procedure of developing internal inhibition in the form of a differentiation of the skin stimulation at a particular point. Stimulation of the shoulder at first evoked a special and a conditioned reaction by virtue of the initial generalisation of the conditioned stimulation. But with its repetition unaccompanied by feeding the basic food reaction soon disappeared, the motor as well as the secretory (by the eighth time), and then the special motor reaction (by the fortieth time). But stimulation of the thigh produced the former picture of both the special and food motor reactions which alternated with each other. Then we added skin stimulation closer to the thigh, on the side, also differentiated. Exactly the same thing that happened during stimulation of the shoulder recurred, and the special reaction on the thigh remained without diminishing. Finally, we elaborated a differentiation on the hind leg. This time, during stimulation of the thigh the special motor reaction began to weaken and, finally, disappeared altogether. Thus, the development of extensive inhibition in the cortical end of the skin analyser eliminated the peculiar extraneous skin reflex, retaining and making normal (from increased) the conditioned skin food reflex. This case, as well as certain other observations, gave us the idea of using the method of gradual development of inhibition in the hemispheres for the purpose of restoring the generally disturbed balance in them. We tried it on a dog which had a narrowly localised pathological point in the auditory analyser described in one of the earlier lectures. Since this point was specially connected with metronome beats, while the other acoustic stimuli acted on the healthy points of the analyser, we developed differentiated inhibition expecting that its irradiation to the pathological metronome point may favourably affect it, restoring it to normal excitability and activity. The experiment is still being conducted. I do not know but that something similar may be used in human nervous therapy, not considering the different sedative procedures in the form of lukewarm baths, etc.

Now I shall occupy your attention with such states of the nervous activity of our dogs, partly normal and partly pathological, which, if we were to apply them to man, would have to be called psychic. In dogs these are the hypnotic phases, transitional between waking and sleep, and the passive-defensive reflex.

In one of the earlier lectures we saw that the transition of the animal from the waking to sleep was based on the development of the inhibitory process in the brain, beginning in the hemispheres under the influence of certain stimuli and representing various degrees of extensiveness and intensity in the different phases of the emerging sleepy state. Today, we can hardly doubt that there is quite enough of these facts in the animal for a physiological interpretation of the basic phenomena of human hypnotism.

First of all, it is a question of the conditions evoking the hypnotic states. In animals, as we already know, they emerge rather slowly under weak and moderate monotonously and protractedly recurring stimuli (ordinary case in our experiments), and rapidly under strong stimuli (case of old hypnosis of animals). Moreover, the directly acting stimuli, both weak and strong, may be signalled by other stimuli which are conditioned in relation to the former. Please, recall the special method of forming conditioned negative reflexes described at the end of one of our lectures (Volborth's experiments) when the indifferent stimuli repeated several times simultaneously with inhibitory stimuli elaborated earlier also became inhibitory. The procedure of hypnotising man completely reproduces the conditions described in animals. The early classical method of hypnotising consisted of so-called passes, i.e., weak, monotonously repeated stimulations of the skin, as in our experiments. The method constantly used today consists of repeated words (uttered in a minor, monotonous tone) describing the physiological acts of the sleepy state. These words are, of course, conditioned stimuli firmly connected in all of us with the sleepy state and therefore evoking it. On this basis everything that coincided with the sleepy state several times in the past can and does hypnotise. All these are analogues of the chain negative reflexes (Volborth's) similar to the chain conditioned positive reflexes, i.e., reflexes of different orders described in one of the earlier lectures. Lastly, hysteriacs are hypnotised, according to Charcot, by strong sudden stimuli as in the old method of hypnotising animals. Of course, physically weak stimuli may also act at the same time, if they signal the strong stimuli, i.e., if they, by virtue of coinciding in time, have become conditioned in relation to the strong stimuli. In animals, as well as in man, most of the hypnotic methods reach the goal the sooner and with greater certainty, the more often they are used.

The loss of voluntary movements and catalepsy, i.e., retention of the position of parts of the body imparted to them by an external force, is one of the first manifestations of hypnosis. Of course, this is a result of isolated inhibition of the motor analyser (motor area of the cortex) which has not descended to the motor centres underlying the hemispheres. At the same time, the other parts of the hemispheres may function properly. The hypnotised subject may understand what we say to him, may know from us the distorted posture which we imparted to him, may wish to alter it and still be unable to do it. All this is also observed during the hypnotic state in animals. In the lecture on hypnotic states, we already mentioned that some dogs completely retained an active pose, but lost all conditioned reflexes. This is a case of inhibition of the whole mass of the hemispheres without the inhibition descending below the hemispheres. Other dogs react to all the conditioned stimuli with activity of the salivary glands, but do not take the food. This is a case of inhibition of only the motor analyser. Lastly, in the animals hypnotised by the old method, the body and limbs remained motionless, while the eyes watched what was going on nearby and the animals could sometimes even eat the food they were offered. This is a case of a still more partial inhibition so that, in addition to the entire remaining mass of the hemispheres, even the motor analyser was not completely inhibited. Of course, the tonic local reflexes in response to suitable external stimuli are quite understandable, during total inhibition of this analyser in animals, as well as in man.

It stands to reason, that in more complex forms of the hypnotic state it is difficult and now even impossible, for several reasons, to draw a parallel between the animal and man. Perhaps we are not yet cognisant of all the phases of the hypnotic state, especially concerning the degree of its intensity and do not, as was mentioned before, exactly know their order and succession. We are probably unfamiliar with all the forms of its manifestation in animals, since we have not observed the animals in their usual life, both individual and social, but only in the limited situation of the laboratory experiment, i.e., abstracted, as it were, from their total behaviour. In other words, we are either as yet unable to perform all the necessary varieties of experiments or perhaps sometimes cannot properly note and understand all the phenomena belonging here, whereas in man we know them under more diverse conditions of life, reproduce and investigate them by using the great system of speech signals. Of course, we must also bear in mind that with the extraordinary difference in the complexity of behaviour of man and animals the latter may not at all have some of the forms of manifestations of the hypnotic state. We, therefore, have to use the elementary data obtained from the animals only for some tentative physiological understanding of the various manifestations of the hypnotic state in man.

Let us take the automatism of hypnotised persons when they stereotypically reproduce what the hypnotiser does before them or when they correctly perform the movements (walk) along a complex, intricate and difficult path. Here we are apparently dealing with the well-known inhibition of certain parts of the hemispheres, which excludes the normal rather complex activity directed by the new or even old, but constantly again combining stimuli of the given moment. However, this inhibition admits or even improves, outside of complex influences, the old firmly and long practised connection of certain stimuli with definite activity, definite movements. Thus, the imitative reflex is vividly reproduced under hypnosis, the reflex by means of which complex individual and social behaviour is elaborated in all of us during childhood. Similarly, the succession of objects with their peculiarities which formerly repeatedly evoked corresponding movements and actions, by successively stimulating certain analysers of the person in a definite stage of hypnosis unerringly guides him stereotypically amid this succession. Is it not the usual thing that, while occupied mainly with one matter, one thought, we can simultaneously do something else, something which we are very much accustomed to, i.e., work with the parts of the hemispheres which are in a certain degree of inhibition, according to the mechanism of external inhibition, because the point of the hemisphere connected with our main occupation is, of course, then greatly excited? I am becoming personally convinced that this understanding of the matter corresponds to the fact, now that in my old age the reactivity of my brain has diminished (poor memory of current events). As time goes on I am becoming increasingly less capable, while doing one thing, properly to do something else. The concentrated stimulation of a certain point with general diminution of the excitability of the hemispheres apparently induces such inhibition of the other parts of the hemispheres that the conditioned stimuli of the old, firmly fixed reflexes now prove below the threshold of excitation.

Perhaps we could draw an analogy between the aforedescribed state of hypnotised subjects and the hypnotic stage in dogs, which we call narcotic, when the strong and old reflexes persist, while the weak and young ones disappear.

Of the hypnotic phenomena in man so-called *suggestion* justly attracts special attention. How should it be understood physiologically? Of course, for man the word is as real a conditioned stimulus as all the other stimuli which man has in common with animals, but at the same time it is also more all-inclusive than any others and in this respect cannot in any way be either quantitatively or qualitatively compared with the conditioned stimuli of animals. Owing to the entire preceding life of the adult human being, the word is connected with all the external and internal stimuli reaching the cerebral hemispheres, signals them all, replaces them all, and can therefore evoke all the actions, reactions of the organism, which those stimuli condition. Thus, suggestion is man's most simplified and most typical conditioned reflex. The word of the person who begins hypnotising the given subject with a certain degree of inhibition developing in the cerebral cortex, concentrating the stimulation in a definite narrow region, according to the general law, at the same time evokes naturally deep external inhibition (as in my own case which I have just pointed out) throughout the remaining mass of the hemispheres and thus excludes all competing influence of all the other present and old traces of stimulations. Hence, the great, almost irresistible power of suggestion as a stimulus during hypnosis and after it. And later, after hypnosis, the word retains its effect, remaining independent of the other stimuli and immune to them as it was at the moment of its initial application to the cortex which was not connected with them. The all-embracing nature of the word makes intelligible the fact that by suggestion it is possible to evoke in the hypnotised subject so many various actions directed at the external as well as the inner world. We may wonder whence comes this power of suggestion compared with dreams which are for the most part forgotten and only rarely are of some vital significance. But a dream is a trace stimulation and at the same time for the most part an old stimulation, whereas suggestion is a present stimulation. Furthermore, hypnosis represents a lower degree of inhibition than does sleep and, consequently, suggestion has twice the stimulatory power than does a dream. Lastly, suggestion as stimulation is brief, isolated and integral, and is therefore strong; a dream usually represents a chain of various and contrary trace stimulations. The fact that the hypnotised subject may be suggested anything that is contrary to reality and a reaction diametrically opposed to the real stimulations—a sweet taste instead of a bitter taste, an unusual visual stimulation instead of a commonplace stimulation, etc., may be evoked—can be understood, without stretching the point, as the paradoxical phase in the state of the nervous system, when weak stimuli produce a greater stimulatory effect than do strong stimuli. The real stimulation, for example, from a sweet substance, proceeding directly to the corresponding nerve cell is, it must be assumed, greater than the stimulation with the word "bitter" which passes from a corresponding auditory cell into the cell which corresponds to the real stimulation with bitter, as a conditioned stimulus of the first order is always stronger than a conditioned stimulus of the second order. Even now in pathological cases the paradoxical phase may be of greater significance than we indicated before. It may be assumed that it makes itself felt also in those normal people who yield to the influence of words more than they do to the facts of surrounding reality.

Some time, we may possibly learn to make suggestions to animals under hypnosis.

The fact that certain phases of the hypnotic state remain more or less stationary in man also occurs in dogs. In man, just as in animals, under certain external conditions and depending on the individuality of the nervous system, the hypnotic state rather quickly changes to complete sleep.

The passive-defensive reflex is in a certain manner connected with the hypnotic state. As was already mentioned, the old form of animal hypnosis may justly be regarded as the passive-defensive reflex consisting, during encounter with extraordinary or strong external stimuli, in greater or lesser immobilisation of the animal by inhibition (developing primarily in the cerebral cortex) of the skeletal and motor system. This reflex was repeatedly discovered in our experimental animals in different degrees of intensity and in somewhat different forms, invariably retaining its basic inhibitory character. Its variations consisted in greater or lesser restriction of the animal's movements, as well as in weakening and disappearance of conditioned reflexes. The passive-defensive reflex was usually evoked by extraordinary and strong external stimuli. But the extraordinary character and strength of external stimuli are, of course, entirely relative values. The extraordinary character of the stimulation is determined by what the animal was subjected to before, while the strength of the action of the external stimulus depends on the state of the given nervous system: its inborn properties, health or disease, and lastly, different stages of healthy existence. We observed all this on our dogs. The dogs, earlier exhibited many times before a large audience, in the long run remained perfectly normal, while those which appeared before that audience for the first time sank into an intensely inhibited state.

The afore-described exceptional dog, named "Smarty", reacted to the slightest variations in its environment as to strong stimuli and was extraordinarily inhibited by them. Some dogs, strongly influenced by the great flood and apparently made chronically ill were inhibited by strong conditioned stimuli which had formerly never affected them that way. Lastly, some dogs are in such an inhibited state only under certain degrees of hypnosis. The latter case produces an extraordinary impression on the observer. Here is a dog which formerly always remained awake in the experimental situation and quickly and greedily ate the food it was given after application of conditioned stimuli. By frequent and continuous application of weak conditioned stimuli we induced a certain constant hypnotic state in this dog in the experimental situation and almost immobilised it. Then we observed the following strange state of affairs. We applied strong conditioned stimuli in response to which the dog turned repeatedly to the place where the food was served, then sharply turned away and did not touch the food. Anyone observing the dog would infallibly say that the dog was afraid of something. No sooner did we apply a weak conditioned stimulus than the dog walked over to the feeding box and calmly ate. As soon as we dispelled, eliminated the hypnotic state, all the conditioned stimuli evoked the normal effect. It is clear that in the special state of the animal the former usual stimuli acted as very strong ones and produced an inhibitory reflex. And, contrariwise, as soon as we were able to raise the excitatory tone in the hemispheres of our exceptionally inhibited dog "Smarty", we could immediately observe a considerable weakening of its almost constant passive-defensive reflex.

In all the aforesaid cases it is the characteristic passive-defensive poses of the animal that always strike the eye. When you see all these experiments you cannot but conclude—and this conclusion must be recognised as correct at least in many cases—that what we psychologically call fear, cowardice and timidity has as its physiological substrate the inhibitory state of the cerebral hemispheres and represents various degrees of the passive-defensive reflex. Of course, after this we are quite justified in regarding the delusion of persecution and the phobias as a natural inhibitory symptom of the pathologically weakened nervous system.

There are such forms of fear and cowardice as panic flight and special slavish poses which apparently contradict the aforesaid conclusion that they are based on the inhibitory process. It must be assumed that these are unconditioned reflexes issuing from the centres directly underlying the cerebral hemispheres and becoming active precisely during inhibition of the cerebral hemispheres. The latter is proved by the disappearance at this time of the conditioned reflexes.

Now a few words about our experiments described at the end of the preceding lecture. If they find complete confirmation during repetitions and variations, they will probably throw some light on the obscure phenomena of our subjective world concerning the relations between the conscious and the unconscious. These experiments would indicate that so important a cortical act as synthesis can take place in the parts of the hemispheres, which are in a certain degree of inhibition, under the influence of the strong excitation prevailing in the cortex at the given moment. Even if there is no awareness of this act at that time, it has taken place just the same and under favourable conditions it may appear in the consciousness ready-made and seem to have emerged in an unknown manner.

In conclusion to all these lectures I repeat that I regard all our experiments, like the similar experiments conducted by other authors, aimed at a purely physiological analysis of higher nervous activity, as the first trial which, according to my profound conviction, however, has quite justified itself. We have won the incontestable right to say that the investigations of this extraordinarily complex subject are now on the right track, on the way to complete, although, of course, not early, success. As for ourselves, we can say that we are now faced with many more questions than ever before. Formerly we artificially simplified, schematised the subject in virtue of necessity, whereas today with some knowledge of its general principles, we are beset or overwhelmed, to be exact, by a mass of particulars which require determination.

PHYSIOLOGICAL TEACHING ON TYPES OF NERVOUS SYSTEM OR TEMPERAMENTS[39]

At the present meeting, dedicated to the memory of the great Russian physician, I have been given permission, as a token of my admiration of the talents, scientific contributions and life of Nikolai Ivanovich Pirogov,[40] to report on the experimental work which I have carried out together with my associates and which, although not specially surgical, is, nevertheless, of a physiological and medical character.

Temperament forms a most important part of the constitution, and, since the constitution now uncommonly occupies the attention of the medical world, my report to physicians will thus be justified.

The physiological teaching on temperaments is a result of a new study of higher nervous activity conducted by a new method. Since this study has not yet become common knowledge, has not become part of textbooks on physiology, whence we derive the basic information on the animal organism, I must, in order to be understood, willy-nilly, touch upon certain general propositions from this study and only then pass to the special subject of my report.

The most general characteristic of a living being consists in the fact that it responds with its definite specific activity not only to the external stimuli, the connections with which exist ready-made since the day of birth, but also to many other stimuli the connections with which develop in the course of individual existence, in other words, that a living being possesses the ability of adaptation.

For greater clarity of the subject I shall begin with the higher animals. The specific reactions of the higher animals are, as is well known, called reflexes, and by these reflexes the animals establish constant relations with the environment. Of course, these relations are a necessity because, if the organism did not establish suitable, definite relations with the environment, it could not exist. The reflexes are always of two kinds: constant reflexes to definite stimuli existing in each animal from the day of birth, and temporary, variable reflexes to most diverse stimuli which each animal encounters during its lifetime. As for the higher animals, for example, dogs, with which all our investigations deal, these two kinds of reflexes even appertain to different parts of the central nervous system. The constant reflexes, i.e., what we have always called reflexes, are connected with all parts of the central nervous system, including the cerebral hemispheres, while the hemispheres are the special place, the organ of temporary connections, temporary relations of the animal with its environment, temporary reflexes.

You know very well that until recently, until the end of last century, these temporary relations, temporary connections of the animal organism with its environment were not even considered physiological, and another phrase—"psychic relations"—was used to designate them. Current studies have shown that there are no reasons whatsoever to exclude them from the field of physiological research.

From these general words I shall now proceed to a number of particular facts. Take harmful conditions, harmful influences, which the animal, of course, immediately avoids, for example, fire which burns the animal, if it finds itself in the sphere of its action, comes in contact with it. This is, of course, an ordinary inborn reflex, the function of the lower divisions of the central nervous system. But if the animal avoids the red colour and the pattern characteristic of fire at a distance, this reaction is one the animal has obtained during its lifetime, it is a temporary connection, a temporary, acquired reflex, which one animal may have and another, which has not yet been in contact with fire, will not have at all. Take another field of stimulation, for example, the food reflex, i.e., taking food. This is primarily a constant reflex: a child, as well as a newborn animal, immediately performs certain movements and introduces food into its mouth. But when an animal runs after this food from a distance attracted either by the sight of this food or by a sound produced, for example, by a small animal which serves as food for the former animal, it is also a food reflex, but this reflex has formed during the animal's lifetime by means of the cerebral hemispheres. This is a temporary reflex, and, from a general point of view, it could be called a signalling reflex. In this case the stimulus signals the real object, the real aim of the simple inborn reflex.

We have now made great progress in the studies of these reflexes. Here is an ordinary example which we always have before our eyes. You give or show food to the dog. This food evokes a reaction: the dog reaches for the food, takes it into its mouth, salivates, etc. To evoke the same reaction, motor and secretory, we can replace this food with anything we wish, any casual stimulus, but before we do this we must connect it with food in time. If you ring or whistle, or raise your hand, or scratch the dog, or do anything you please and then immediately give the dog food and repeat it several times, all these stimuli will elicit the same food reaction: the animal will reach for the stimulus, will lick its lips, will salivate, etc., i.e., you will have the same reflex as you did before, when you showed it the food.

It stands to reason, that it is extremely important for the animal under the conditions of its life to be physiologically connected so remotely and so diversely with the favourable conditions which it needs for existence or with the harmful conditions which menace its existence. If, for example, some danger is signalled by sound from afar, the animal will have time to take measures against it, etc. It is clear that the highest adaptation of animals, the highest equilibrium with the environment, is infallibly connected with this kind of temporarily forming reflexes. These two kinds of reflexes we usually designate by two special adjectives: the inborn, constant reflexes we call unconditioned reflexes, whereas those that attach themselves to the inborn reflexes during the animal's lifetime we call conditioned reflexes.

If we daily and repeatedly connect and disconnect our lamp and telephone, it would be an incredible incongruity for the vast conducting nervous system which connects the organism with the endless surrounding world to deviate from this technical principle and for this not to be its usual physiological procedure. It follows that there are no reasons for theoretical thought to object to this, whereas physiologically this has been quite confirmed. Under certain circumstances conditioned reflexes regularly form and exist like any other nervous phenomena.

We shall consider one more fact concerning conditioned reflexes. Let a tone, for example, of 1,000 vibrations per second be made a conditioned food stimulus by the usual procedure, i.e., simultaneous application of the tone and feeding. This is a reflex in which the conditioned stimulus evokes in the cortex the process of excitation, a positive food reaction.

Such a reflex we call a positive conditioned reflex. But, in addition to these conditioned positive reflexes, there are also negative reflexes, i.e., such reflexes as evoke in the central nervous system not the process of excitation, but the process of inhibition. If, after the foregoing reflex to a tone of 1,000 vibrations per second has formed, I try other tones, marginal ones, say, 10-15 tones in either direction, they will also act, but less intensely the further they are located from my tone to which I have elaborated the reflex.

Now, if I constantly accompany my tone, the initial one, as formerly with food, while I do not accompany with food the tones which began to act by themselves, in this case the latter will gradually and entirely lose their conditioned food effect.

Have they become indifferent, then? No, they have not. Instead of a positive effect they have acquired inhibitory action; they stimulate in the central nervous system the process of inhibition. The proof of this is perfectly simple. You try a tone of 1,000 vibrations per second. It elicits, as always, a positive reflex, a food reaction. Now you apply one of the tones which have ceased to act. Immediately following this, the tone of 1,000 vibrations will also temporarily lose its effect. Consequently, the marginal tone has produced inhibition in the central nervous system and it requires some time to eliminate this inhibition from the nervous system. Thus you see that with these temporary agents it is possible to produce in the central nervous system processes of excitation as well as inhibition. You understand, of course, that this is of tremendous importance in the life of animals, as well as our own life, since our life boils down to the fact that under certain conditions and at a certain moment we must act in a certain manner, while under other circumstances and at another moment we must inhibit our activity.

This underlies the highest vital orientation. The normal life of man and animals thus consists of constant and correct balancing of these two processes. We must bear in mind that these two antagonistic processes are equally important, equally essential in nervous activity.

I think I can limit my preliminary explanations to this and turn to the main subject.

During elaboration of conditioned reflexes, now positive and now negative, we observe in the dogs an enormous difference as to how rapidly these reflexes are elaborated, how stable they are and to what extent they reach the absolute. In some animals it is very easy to elaborate a positive reflex and the latter is very stable under most diverse conditions; but it is very difficult to obtain inhibitory reflexes in these animals; in some animals it is impossible to elaborate them with complete precision, since they infallibly contain a certain element of positive action. This characterises some animals. On the other hand, at the opposite end there are animals in which positive conditioned reflexes are elaborated with great difficulty, they are constantly very unstable, and are inhibited from the slightest change in the surroundings, i.e., they lose their positive effect; contrariwise, the inhibitory reflexes develop rapidly and are always very stable.

Between these extremes there is a central kind of dog or a central type of nervous system. This is a type of dog which easily develops both kinds of reflexes and which well inhibits and well forms positive reflexes, a type in which both kinds of reflexes remain stable and may be perfectly precise. It follows that the entire mass of dogs can be divided into three main groups: the excitable group, inhibitable group (extreme groups) and the central group in which the processes of excitation and inhibition are balanced. Since the cerebral hemispheres are the seat of the conditioned reflexes, in the three aforesaid groups it is a question of three types of character and, correspondingly, activity of the cerebral hemispheres.

But we have still more convincing proof of the existence of these three types of nervous system.

If we produce a very difficult encounter between the excitatory and inhibitory processes, we observe entirely different reactions of the three types of central nervous system to this procedure. I shall describe for you in somewhat greater detail the method which we constantly use and which is, so to speak, the highest test of adaptation or strength of the nervous system. We place a piece of apparatus on the skin; with this apparatus we mechanically stimulate the skin in a definite rhythm, say, every second, and this becomes a conditioned stimulus. This stimulus can be differentiated, i.e., the nervous system may be made to react differently to the different frequency of mechanical stimulation. Let us assume that, besides the 30 stimulations in 30 seconds that I used before, I shall also use 15, and that I can produce a situation in which the dog will manifest a positive food reaction when I use 30 stimulations, and this reaction will be inhibited when I use 15. Of course, this is done so that the 30 stimulations are accompanied by feeding and the 15 stimulations are not.

Thus two stimulations which differ from each other but little evoke two antagonistic processes in the nervous system. Now, if we bring these two processes together, make them directly follow one another, collide them, as it were, with one another, we obtain a very interesting result. Let us assume that I begin with 15 stimulations and the dog manifests no food reaction. If I immediately replace the 15 stimulations with 30, this will be a test of the nervous system which will very obviously distinguish the three afore-mentioned types. If the experiment is performed on a dog of one pole, say, the excitable, in which excitation predominates and inhibition is weak, the following takes place: either immediately or after several repetitions of this procedure the dog becomes sick. It retains only the excitatory process and almost completely loses the inhibitory process. In the laboratory we call this state *neurasthenia*, and this disease may last in the dog for months. If I apply the same procedure to dogs of the opposite pole, it is, contrariwise, the excitatory process that weakens in them, while inhibition remains extraordinarily predominating. We call such dogs *hysteriacs*. In both these cases the normal correlation between inhibition and excitation has disappeared. We call this a derangement. We are apparently dealing with neuroses; two true neuroses: one with predominance of excitation and the other of inhibition. These are serious diseases; they last for months and the dogs have to be treated for them. Our main treatment is suspension of all experiments, but sometimes we also resort to other means. As for the diseases of the inhibitory type we have found no other means save discontinuing the experiments with the dog, sometimes for six months and even longer. Bromides and calcium salts have proved good agents for the other neurosis. The sick animal becomes normal within a week or ten days.

Hence, it cannot be doubted that these are entirely different dogs, since they contract different diseases under the influence of the very same pathogenic procedure.

But, in addition to these extreme types, there is also the central type. The same procedure has no effect on animals of the central type; they remain well, they do not fall ill. It becomes perfectly clear that there are three different types of nervous system: central—*balanced,* and two extreme types—*excitable* and *inhibitable.* It means that the two extreme types work, if I may say so, mainly with one half of the nervous system. We may call them half-and-half types. Between them stands the integral type in which both processes work constantly and evenly.

Now the following is of some interest. The central type is available in two forms externally greatly differing from one another, although in relation to our main criterion the difference between these two forms is very slight. One form very easily balances the antagonistic nervous processes, while the other one does so with some difficulty, and that is all. It never goes as far as a pathological state.

Now if we attend to the general external behaviour of all our dogs, we observe approximately the following. The excitable type in its highest manifestation is for the most part an aggressive animal. For example, if the master, whom these animals know very well and to whom they are quite obedient, should suddenly mistreat them, say, whip them, they may bite him, may not restrain themselves. The extreme inhibitable type shows itself in that, if you shout at it or raise your hand against it, it will put the tail between its legs, crouch and even urinate. This is what we call a cowardly animal. As for the central type, the latter is represented by two forms: scarcely mobile, quiet animals which seem entirely to ignore everything in their environment (we usually call them sedate) and, on the contrary, animals who, when awake, are very lively, extraordinarily mobile, examining everything and sniffing at everything. But at the same time these animals are very peculiar in that they are strangely inclined towards sleep. As soon as they are brought into our atmosphere, are left in a separate room alone, are put in a stand and their environment ceases greatly to vary, they immediately begin to drowse and fall asleep. This is actually an amazing combination of mobility and sleepiness.

Thus all our animals are divided into four definite groups: two extreme groups of excitable and inhibitable animals and two central groups of balanced but different animals: some very quiet and others extraordinarily lively. We have to consider this a precise fact.

Can we apply this to man? And why not? I do not think it should prove offensive to man if man and dogs have the same main characters of nervous system. Today we are already so educated biologically that nobody can object to this comparison. We can attribute to man with full justification the types of nervous system established in the dog (and these types are so precisely characterised). These types are apparently what we call temperaments in man. A temperament is the most general characteristic of each individual person, the most basic characteristic of his nervous system, and the latter leaves a particular imprint on the entire activity of each individual.

In the question of temperaments, general human empiricism with Hippocrates, the brilliant observer of human beings at the head has apparently come closest to truth. It is the ancient classification of temperaments: *choleric, melancholic, sanguine* and *phlegmatic*. To be sure, this classification is now being extraordinarily altered. Some say there are only two temperaments, others establish three, still others—six, etc. However, for the past two thousand years the majority has clearly inclined towards the four types. It may be assumed that this ancient view contains the greatest amount of truth. I can show you the extent to which some of the latest authors are muddled in this question by the example of one Russian psychiatrist. He decided to recognise six temperaments: three normal and three pathological. The normal temperaments include the merry, clear and phlegmatic, while the pathological ones include the choleric, melancholic and sanguine. It is strange that, for example, the sanguine temperament is ascribed to the pathological group only because all sanguine persons are presumably light-minded. In other words, light-mindedness is a symptom of pathology.

If we take the ancient classification of the four temperaments, we shall at once see the agreement between the results of our experiments on dogs and this classification. Our *excitable* type is the *choleric*, while the *melancholic* is the *inhibitable* type. The *phlegmatic* and *sanguine* temperaments would correspond to the two forms of the *central* type. The melancholic temperament is clearly the inhibitable type of nervous system. For the melancholiac everything in life apparently becomes an inhibitory agent, since he does not believe in anything, does not hope for anything, sees only evil and danger in everything and expects only evil and danger from everything. The choleric type is clearly a militant type, with verve, easily and quickly excitable. The golden mean is represented by the phlegmatic and sanguine temperaments, balanced and, therefore, healthy, stable and truly vital nervous types, as different or even opposite the representatives of this type may appear externally. The phlegmatic person is always calm, balanced, persistent and hard-working. The sanguine person is hot-headed, and very productive, but only when he has a lot of interesting things to do, i.e., has constant stimulation. When he has no such things, however, he becomes bored and sluggish, exactly like our sanguine dogs (this is what we usually call them) which are extremely lively and business-like, when the situation excites them, and immediately begin to drowse and sleep when there are no such stimuli.

We took the liberty of assuming and thinking somewhat further by touching upon the clinical aspects of nervous and mental diseases, although our information does not go beyond that contained in textbooks. It occurred to us that among human beings the main suppliers of these clinics are also probably the extreme, unstable types or temperaments, whereas both forms of the central type remain more or less unaffected by the trials and tribulations of life. We thought it justifiable to connect neurasthenia, as the corresponding morbid form, with the excitable choleric type and hysteria, as the predominantly inhibitory form, inhibitory disease, with the inhibitable melancholic type. And, furthermore, when the disease appears as the so-called psychic forms, can we not assume that the two main groups of constitutional endogenous psychoses—cyclothymia and schizophrenia—represent by their physiological mechanism the highest stage of the same diseases?

On the one hand, the neurasthenic can develop extraordinary activity, perform enormous work. Many prominent people were neurasthenics. But, along with periods of strenuous work, the neurasthenic infallibly experiences periods of deep impotence.

And what about the cyclothymic type? The same thing. Now he is excited well beyond normal, up to attacks of frenzy, and now he sinks into a deep depressive, melancholic state.

On the other hand, our laboratory hysterical dogs apparently have very weak cortical cells which easily lapse into various degrees of the chronic inhibitory state. But the basic general feature of human hysteria is apparently the same cortical weakness. Simulation of illness, suggestibility and emotiveness (I am taking this psychic characteristic of hysteria from the pamphlet on *Hysteria and Its Pathogenesis* by Professor L. V. Blumenau[41]) are all vivid manifestations of this weakness. A healthy person will not hide behind illness, will not try to elicit lenience, compassion or interest to himself, as to a sick, i.e., weak person. Suggestibility is, of course, based on an easy transition of the cortical cells to an inhibitory state, whereas emotiveness is a predominance, a violence of the most complex unconditioned reflexes (aggressive, passive-defensive and other reflexes—functions of the subcortical centres) with weakened cortical control.

There are also reasons to regard schizophrenia as an extreme weakness of the cortex, as the highest stage of hysteria. The basic mechanism of suggestibility is a dissociation of the normal, more or less unified work of the entire cortex. Definite suggestion is irresistible precisely because it takes place in the absence of the usual influences on it from the other parts of the cortex. And if this is so, schizophrenia is the highest manifestation of the same mechanism. Let us imagine extreme general weakness of the cortex, its, so to speak, pathological, abnormal fragility. As it is possible to obtain entirely isolated invalid points and foci in the cortex of our inhibitable hysterical dogs by applying functional difficulties, in schizophrenics, under the influence of rather strong life's impressions, probably on the basis of an organic disease, increasingly more such impotent points and foci constantly and gradually appear, an ever greater dissociation of the cerebral cortex and a splitting of their normal integrated work takes place.

After all the aforesaid, it seems to me that it can hardly be disputed that in the thousand-year-old question of temperaments a weighty word belongs to the *laboratory* because of the elementary and relatively simple character of its experimental objects.

SOME PROBLEMS OF THE PHYSIOLOGY OF THE CEREBRAL HEMISPHERES[42]

Our last question will be the question of types of nervous system. The experimental material collected by us on dogs with which we performed all our experiments has grown so much that we can justly speak of main types of nervous system. In our animals the difference with regard to formation and nature of positive and inhibitory conditioned reflexes comes to the fore perfectly clearly. There is a group of dogs in which positive conditioned reflexes are formed very easily, soon reach their utmost intensity and stably persist on this level despite the frequent different inhibitory phenomena, i.e., despite the interference of irrelevant reflexes. You may even try by frequent and continuous repetition of these reflexes to decrease their effect in response to strong, as well as weak conditioned stimuli, a method which usually easily reduces the intensity of the conditioned reflexes. And yet they remain stable. But all inhibitory reflexes are acquired by these animals with great difficulty. The animals greatly resist them, struggle against them. A lot of time has to be wasted to achieve their full elaboration, if it is at all possible in them. In some of them it is entirely impossible to produce full inhibitory reflexes, for example, absolute differentiations.

In others they may be developed, but they cannot be repeated in the course of one experiment or even every day at least once in every experiment, or else they cease to be full again. Besides, they are easily disinhibited by irrelevant stimuli. At the opposite end there is the type in which, on the contrary, the positive conditioned reflexes under our conditions are formed very slowly, do not soon reach maximum intensity and are extraordinarily liable to diminish and disappear for a long time under very insignificant irrelevant and new stimuli. Frequent repetition of positive reflexes similarly rapidly leads to their diminution and disappearance. But inhibitory reflexes are produced uncommonly rapidly and are very stable. Inhibitory type is a legitimate designation for this type of animal. Concerning the cortical cells of these two groups of dogs we can say that in the excitable type the cells are strong and richly endowed with excitable substance, whereas in the inhibitory type the cells are weak and contain very little of this substance. In accordance with this, the usual strength of stimuli proves supermaximal for these latter cells and quickly brings them into a state of inhibition.

Between these extreme types there is a central type. Both positive and inhibitory reflexes are easily formed by this type and once formed they become stable. Since normal nervous activity consists in constant balancing of the two antagonistic nervous processes, and in the latter type this balancing occurs more or less uneventfully, this type has the right to be called a balanced type. So far we have used several varieties of experiments, i.e., several criteria for comparing various animals as regards their conditioned reflex activity, and the foregoing classification has always justified itself. Of course, there are also certain gradations between these basic types. This classification is also confirmed by the fact that, when faced with difficult nervous tasks or under the influence of excessively strong stimuli, or during a severe collision of the antagonistic nervous processes, when a protracted deviation from the usual state of their nervous system occurs in some of the animals (true neuroses), the afore-described types differ even more from each other. While the balanced type rather quickly, at any rate without any consequences, overcomes these difficult tasks, the extreme types clearly develop nervous diseases and different ones at that: the excitable type almost completely loses its inhibitory ability and becomes permanently and strongly excited under our conditions, as also in general; the inhibitory type, on the contrary, almost completely loses all our positive conditioned reflexes and lapses into a hypnotic state with its different phases. In this case both types require for restoration of normalcy the following treatment: prolonged rest, suspension of the experiments, or pharmaceutical agents, or both. It is interesting that the balanced type defined by our criteria is represented by two forms greatly differing in their external behaviour: some animals, which are always extremely calm, somehow strangely indifferent to everything that goes on around them, but always awake, and others, which are uncommonly mobile and lively under the usual circumstances and constantly interested in everything that happens around them, but which in a monotonous atmosphere (for example if they are left in the experimental room alone) amazingly quickly sink into a sleepy state. Although these dogs, like the calm ones, cope with their difficult nervous tasks without diseases, they do so with some difficulty.

Our types of nervous system are apparently what is usually designated by the term "temperament". A temperament is the most general characteristic of each individual person, as also each animal, the basic characteristic of the nervous system which lends a definite colouring to the entire activity of each individual. If this is so, we cannot fail to see that our types would very much correspond to the ancient classification of temperaments. The choleric and melancholic temperaments would be our extreme types—the excitable and inhibitable; the phlegmatic and sanguine types would very well coincide with the two forms of the balanced central type—calm and lively. I think that our classification of temperaments, as one based on the most general properties of the central nervous system, on the characteristics and relations of both halves of nervous activity—excitation and inhibition, may also be considered the simplest and most fundamental. The following could also be added to the aforesaid. We must assume that a temperament is determined mainly by the property precisely of the cerebral hemispheres, since in our experiments with conditioned reflexes we always deal only with cortical cells. That the essential thing in the given case is not the special most complex unconditioned reflexes, usually referred to as instincts or drives, is revealed, for example, by the fact that the food reflex is often very intense in extraordinarily inhibited animals. The conception of the predominant importance of the properties of the cortex for the temperaments will also have to be accepted for man. Considering that the subcortical centres closest to the hemispheres are centres of the special most complex unconditioned reflexes—food, active- and passive-defensive and others—and that their activity constitutes the physiological basis of the elementary emotions, the aggregate of vital functions will be determined by the character of the cerebral cortex which sends downward now mainly excitation and now inhibition, or both in their due balance.

Having finished the report of our new factual material and of a number of newly arising problems of physiology of the cerebral hemispheres and the brain in general I should like to draw two general conclusions: one purely physiological and the other one applied, of general importance to life.

If we divide the whole central nervous system only in two halves—an afferent and efferent, I think that the cerebral cortex is an isolated afferent division. In this division alone the higher analysis and synthesis of the excitation reaching it take place and from here the ready combinations of excitations and inhibitions are directed into the efferent division. In other words, only the afferent division is active and, so to speak, creative, while the efferent division is only passive and executive. Since the afferent and efferent divisions come into close contact in the spinal cord, the physiologist, during his investigations, is constantly under the impression of the combined activity of both these divisions, and, it seems to me, is deprived of the chance of establishing the, in many respects, special and full characteristic of the afferent part; for example, the constant and one-way course of an integral reflex act and special experiments on it uncommonly strengthen the idea of an always one-way conduction of the nervous process. But is this idea applicable to the purely afferent division? In the cerebral cortex we constantly happen to see the motion of both the excitatory and inhibitory processes in the two opposite directions. How are we to understand it? Is it really a two-way conduction along the selfsame paths or must we assume here special, very complex structures for the purpose of preserving the principle of one-way conduction?

As for my applied conclusion, I am drawing it under the lasting impressions of our work carried on over these many years. All of our, now very numerous, experiments with the activity of the cerebral hemispheres surprise us with the plastic character of this activity. Many nervous tasks which may at first appear entirely unaccomplishable for the given cerebral hemispheres, in the long run, with caution and gradually, are satisfactorily accomplished. And another thing. Just think of the extent to which we must take into consideration the type of nervous system of each animal in the solution of different problems! It will scarcely be light-minded on my part, if I express the hope that the experiments with the higher nervous activity of animals will also furnish not a few guiding points for the education and self-education of man. By observing these experiments I have elucidated many things at least for myself about myself and other people.

AN ATTEMPT OF A PHYSIOLOGIST TO DIGRESS INTO THE DOMAIN OF PSYCHIATRY[43]

In the course of the past thirty years I, together with my numerous colleagues, have been predominantly engaged in studying the activity of the higher parts of the brain, mainly the cerebral hemispheres; this study has been carried out on the basis of a strictly objective method, the method of the so-called conditioned reflexes. We have collected very considerable material relating not only to the normal activity of the above-mentioned parts of the brain, but to a certain degree also to their pathology and therapy. We are now in a position to produce obvious experimental neuroses in our experimental animals (dogs) and to treat them; and it is not impossible, in our opinion, to produce in the same animals states somewhat analogous to the human psychoses. It was this that induced me to make closer acquaintance with psychiatry, of which almost no traces have remained in my memory since my student days in the medical faculty. Thanks to the kindness of my medical colleagues, and especially of Prof. P. A. Ostankov and Dr. I. O. Narbutovich, I am now able systematically to observe different forms of mental disorders. Schizophrenia was the first disorder observed and studied by me. Here my attention was attracted, on the one hand, by the symptoms of apathy, torpor, inactivity, stereotypic movements, and on the other hand, by playfulness, exaggerated familiarity, childish behaviour in general, which had not been peculiar to these patients before the onset of the disease (hebephrenia and catatonia).

How can this be explained from the physiological point of view? Is it possible physiologically to generalise these phenomena and to find their common mechanism?

For this purpose it is necessary first of all to consider the facts obtained by the method of conditioned reflexes. This study has provided us with abundant data, particularly relating to the inhibitory process and its physiological and pathological significance.

Inhibition, which together with excitation constantly takes part in the diverse activity of the animal in its wakeful state, also guards the extremely reactive cells of the organism, the cells of the cerebral cortex; it protects them from highly strenuous work under the action of very strong stimuli, or even under the prolonged repetition of weak stimuli; it also ensures the necessary rest for the cells in the form of sleep after their daily normal work.

We have established the indubitable fact that sleep is inhibition, which irradiates over the hemispheres and descends along the brain to a certain level. Besides, we have been in a position to study on our animals also the intermediate phases between wakefulness and complete sleep—the hypnotic phases. These phases have been regarded by us, on the one hand, as different degrees of extensity of inhibition, i.e., of a larger or smaller extent of its irradiation over various areas of the hemispheres, as well as over various parts of the brain, and, on the other hand, as different degrees of intensity of inhibition in the form of different depth of inhibition in one and the same point. It is clear that owing to the tremendous complexity of the human brain, the diversity of separate hypnotic phenomena in man is much greater than in animals. It is possible, however, that some hypnotic phenomena are for one reason or another more manifest in animals than in man, especially since even the manifestations of human hypnosis vary considerably, depending on the peculiar features of the individual and the method of hypnotisation. And so, taking into consideration the full complex of symptoms of hypnosis, I shall further deal with hypnotic phenomena observed both in man and in our animals.

Observing the above-mentioned schizophrenic symptoms I have come to the conclusion that they are an expression of a chronic hypnotic state which I shall try to substantiate in my further exposition. Of course, apathy, dullness, inactivity, etc., are not in themselves proof of the hypnotic state of the patients, but at the same time they will not conflict in any way with this conclusion, provided my thesis is confirmed by a further comparison of more specific symptoms.

I shall first of all cite the following fact. Apathy and torpor are usually ascertained in a patient when he does not react to the questions addressed to him and gives the impression of being absolutely indifferent to them. However, if the same questions are asked not in a loud voice and not with the usual intensity, but in a low voice and in quiet surroundings, the patient reacts immediately with proper answers. This is a highly characteristic hypnotic phenomenon, to which, in my opinion, constant and proper attention is not being paid. And it is to be regretted that up to now the clinic, as far as I know, has no special term to designate this essential and important symptom as has been done with other symptoms. In our animals this symptom is one of the most frequent and persistent signs of the onset of hypnosis. In our experiments we constantly meet with the so-called paradoxical phase, when in the course of the given experiment or in one of its phases strong conditioned stimuli lose their usual action, while weak stimuli evoke in the animal a perfectly normal effect. In the well-known case of a five-year sleep, or properly speaking, hypnosis, described by Pierre Janet, the author made intellectual contact with his patient solely on the basis of this phenomenon. The patient herself emerged from the hypnotic state only at night, when all the daytime stimulations ceased.

Further phenomena of so-called negativism were observed in the analysed patients. Similarly, in our experimental animals negativism is usually in evidence at the onset of a hypnotic state. In the case of a food reflex when the conditioned stimulus is brought into action, and the food receptacle is placed before the dog, the latter persistently turns away from it. Not without interest is the following detail very clearly observed in a definite phase: when you begin to move the food receptacle away, the dog, on the contrary, reaches for it. And this is repeated several times in succession. But the moment the state of hypnosis is dissipated, the same dog devours the just rejected food. I shall analyse the mechanism of this, as well as other hypnotic symptoms, at another time; for the present I shall use them only as established facts constituting the hypnotic state.

Another symptom of schizophrenia in one of its variations is stereotypy—a persistent and prolonged repetition of definite movements. This, too, is an obvious hypnotic manifestation, and it is clearly observed in some of our dogs. When the dog is in a perfectly cheerful state, after being fed in the case of a conditioned food reflex, it often continues for a certain time to lick the anterior part of its body, usually the breast and the forelegs. With the onset of a hypnotic state the licking assumes an extremely prolonged character and often lasts until the next meal. Certain other movements, effected by the animal at one time or other, are repeated with similar persistence.

Among usual phenomena observed in schizophrenics are the so-called echolalia and echopraxia, i.e., repetition by the patient of the words addressed to him by his interlocutor and the reproduction of gestures made by someone who attracts his attention. As is known, this phenomenon is also usual in hypnotised normal persons, and, it seems to me, manifests itself with particular ease and most frequently in hypnosis evoked by passes. Catalepsy is a very ordinary phenomenon in schizophrenics, consisting in prolonged retention by the patient of different postures, which are easily, i.e., without any resistance of the musculature, imparted to his body by another person; naturally this relates also to those postures which the patient himself assumes under the influence of certain temporarily acting stimuli. This, too, is a symptom very easily reproduced in normal persons subjected to hypnotism.

A particularly striking, pronounced and tenacious symptom in certain schizophrenics, constituting even a special form of the disease, is catatonia, i.e., a state of rigidity of the skeletal musculature strongly resisting any change in the given disposition of different parts of the body. Catatonia is simply tonic reflexes, as a result of which a hypnotised person can become as inflexible as a solid board.

Finally, it is necessary to include in this group of different variations of central inhibition the symptom of playfulness or silly mannerisms, mostly observed in hebephrenics, as well as the outbursts of aggressive excitation, met with in other schizophrenics in addition to the already mentioned symptoms. All these phenomena closely resemble the initial state of ordinary alcoholic intoxication, and the state peculiar to children and young animals, for example, puppies, when they are waking up, and especially when they are falling asleep. There is every reason to assume that these manifestations result from a developing general inhibition of the cerebral hemispheres; due to this the adjacent subcortex is not only liberated from constant control, from constant inhibition effected by the cerebral hemispheres in an alert state, but, because of the mechanism of positive induction, is even brought to a state of chaotic excitation affecting all its centres. That is why the state of alcoholic intoxication is accompanied now by a causeless and unusual playfulness and joviality, now by excessive sensibility and tearfulness, now by anger, and, in the case of children when they fall asleep, by capriciousness. Particularly typical is a child in the middle of the first year of its life just going off to sleep. You can see on its face a truly caleidoscopic change of diverse expressions reflecting the chaotic activity of the child's primitive subcortex. Similarly the schizophrenic at definite stages and in definite variations of his disease exhibits this phenomenon now in a protracted form, now in the form of brief outbursts.

In view of what has been said, one can hardly doubt that schizophrenia, in certain of its variations and phases, is actually a chronic hypnosis. The fact that these variations and phases persist for years, cannot serve as a telling argument against this conclusion. Since there has been a case of a five-year sleep (described by Pierre Janet) and even of a twenty-year sleep (observed in Petersburg), why cannot hypnosis be of an equally lasting character, especially since the instances just mentioned must be regarded as states of hypnosis rather than sleep?

What is the reason for the chronic hypnosis of schizophrenics? What is its physiological, and especially pathological, basis? How does it develop and what are its consequences?

In the final analysis, of course, this hypnosis is profoundly based on the weak nervous system, and especially the weakness of the cortical cells. For this weakness various causes, both hereditary and acquired, may be responsible. We shall not touch here on these causes. But naturally, when such a nervous system encounters difficulties, more often in a critical physiological and social period of life, it inevitably becomes exhausted after excessive excitation. But exhaustion is one of the chief physiological impulses for the appearance of inhibition in the capacity of a protective process. Hence chronic hypnosis is inhibition in different degrees of extensity and intensity. Consequently, this state is, on the one hand, pathology, since it prevents the patient from normal activity, and, on the other hand, according to its mechanism, it is still physiology, a physiological remedy, since it protects the cortical cells from the danger of being destroyed as a result of too heavy work. In our laboratory we have now a striking example showing how prolonged inhibition restores normal activity for a time to weak cortical cells. There are reasons to assume that as long as the inhibitory process operates, the cortical cells are not gravely damaged, their full return to normal is still possible, they can recover from excessive exhaustion and their pathological process remains reversible. Using modern terminology, it is only a functional disease. That this is really the case, is proved by the following fact. According to Kraepelin, a leading psychiatrist, of all the forms of schizophrenia the hebephrenic, and especially the catatonic form—which is of a particularly pronounced hypnotic character—show the highest rate of complete recovery (catatonics—up to 15 per cent), which is not observed in other forms, especially the paranoic one.

In conclusion I take the liberty of offering therapeutic advice more of a practical than sentimental character. Although enormous progress has been made since olden times up to our day in the treatment of the mentally ill, still, I think, something remains *to be desired* in this respect. To keep patients, already possessing a certain degree of self-consciousness, together with other, irresponsible patients, who may subject them, on the one hand, to strong stimulations in the form of screams and extraordinary scenes, and, on the other hand, to direct violence, in most cases, means creating conditions which to a still greater extent enfeeble the already weak cortical cells. Moreover, the violation of the patient's human rights, of which he is already conscious and which partly consists in restriction of his freedom, and partly in the fact that the attendants and medical personnel naturally and almost inevitably regard him as an irresponsible person, cannot but strike further heavy blows at the weak cells. Consequently, it is necessary as quickly and as timely as possible to place such mentally diseased in the position of patients suffering from other illnesses which do not offend human dignity so manifestly.

PHYSIOLOGY OF THE HYPNOTIC STATE OF THE DOG[44]
(Jointly with Dr. M. K. Petrova)

Besides the usual classical method of hypnotising animals (laying the animal on its back and keeping it for some time in this unnatural position), which results in a hypnotic state manifesting itself in catalepsy, our laboratories were able, in the course of their research into the normal activity of the higher parts of the brain, to study in more detail the diverse and very delicate manifestations of the hypnotic state. As already established by us, the basic condition required for the development of this state is a prolonged action of monotonous stimuli, which finally bring the corresponding cortical cells to a state of inhibition. This inhibition, on the one hand, is of different degrees of intensity, and on the other hand, spreads to a greater or lesser extent over the cerebral cortex and further down the brain. Corresponding facts were cited in a book published by one of us. (I. P. Pavlov, *Lectures on the Work of the Cerebral Hemispheres*.[45])

But subsequent observations revealed a greater variety of symptoms of the hypnotic state, its more and more delicate gradations, which hardly differ from the wakeful state, and its ever-increasing mobility depending on the slightest changes in the surroundings, on insignificant modifications in the external stimuli acting upon the animal.

In the present article we shall deal with the phenomena

observed by us in two dogs. Previously they were used by one of us (M. K. Petrova) for studying the various conditioned reflexes, but now they constantly fall into a hypnotic state the moment they are placed in our usual experimental conditions and respectively equipped.

Long ago in the works which originated in our laboratories it was repeatedly pointed out that in the case of conditioned food reflexes there takes place a dissociation of the salivary secretion and the food motor reaction when the dog falls into a sleeping state. It usually happened that our artificial conditioned stimuli or more often the natural stimulation (which, as has been proved, is also conditioned) produced by the sight and odour of food, evoked a profuse secretion of saliva, although the animal did not take the food. It was in this state of the animal that very diverse and highly interesting variations of the food motor reaction were manifested in the course of our observations. These variations, which apparently represent different degrees of intensity of hypnosis, were now predominantly observed in one animal, now in another. One of the dogs, which was usually in a less profound hypnotic state, distinctly exhibited what in mental diseases is called negativism. After a conditioned stimulation applied during a certain period of time we put food before the dog; the latter turns away from the food receptacle. But when we begin to move the receptacle away, the dog makes a movement in its direction. We present the receptacle anew; the dog again turns away from it. We move it away, and the dog turns towards it once more. We have termed the reaction of turning away from the food receptacle negative, or the first phase of negativism, and the movement towards the food receptacle—positive, or the second phase. This negativism may recur many times until the animal at last partakes of the food, which happens in most cases. The degree of hypnosis is expressed precisely by the number of repetitions of this procedure. At the beginning of the hypnotic state the food is taken and eaten by the dog after the second offering. When the hypnotic state becomes more profound, both phases of negativism recur more and more often. When hypnosis reaches the highest degree, the dog rejects the food, no matter how many times it is offered. But as soon as the hypnotic state is dissipated in this or that way—for example, by removing the apparatus attached to the dog for the purpose of collecting the saliva, or by loosening the chain which is attached to the dog and which during the experiment is fastened to the upper crossbar of the stand, or by some other means—the dog immediately begins to devour the food.

In the other dog the food motor reaction during hypnosis assumed an even more complicated form. In one of the more pronounced cases the phenomena developed in the following sequence. Under the action of our conditioned stimuli (usually to the end of their isolated action) the dog, if it was in a sitting posture, rose to its feet, if standing, it turned its body in the direction whence the food was usually presented to it. But when food was offered, it turned its head away from it, thus exhibiting the first phase of negativism. Then the food receptacle was moved away, and the animal, on the contrary, turned the head towards it and followed it with its eyes; thus the second phase appeared. After some manifestations of this negativism the dog at last brought its mouth close to the food, but was unable to take it. As if with great difficulty it began, little by little and repeatedly, to open and to close its mouth, but to no purpose—it did not take the food (abortive movements). Afterwards, it began to move its jaws with greater ease, took the food, at first in small portions, finally opening its mouth wide and swallowing rapidly without interruption. Thus, in this hypnotic phase we must distinguish three different states in three parts of the skeletal musculature relating to the process of eating: strong inhibition, immobility of the muscles directly participating in the process of eating (the masticatory and lingual muscles); considerable mobility, but of a periodic character, in the form of a negativism of the cervical musculature; and finally, normal activity of the remaining musculature of the body. The more profound the hypnotic state, the more immobile and inhibited is the direct musculature: the tongue is put out as if paralysed, the jaws are absolutely motionless. In the cervical muscles only the first phase of negativism is manifested. Then the movements of the head cease completely, and only the trunk still turns under the influence of conditioned stimuli. Finally, when the hypnotic state becomes still more profound, this last motor reaction to the conditioned stimuli, as well as to food, also disappears. All these phenomena can be dissipated, abolished instantaneously by the same methods which have been described in the case of the first dog.

Concerning the food motor reaction in our cases, the following should be added. Any slight change in the usual appearance of the food, and even in the manner of presentation leads to conversion of the negative motor reaction into a positive one; in other words, the dog eats the food which it has just rejected. For example, we offer the dog slightly moistened and evenly spread powder of dried meat and bread in an ordinary cup. The dog refuses it. But if the same powder is presented partly in the form of a lump protruding from the cup, the dog seizes it greedily and then begins to eat the rest of the powder. A positive reaction can be also obtained if the powder is offered to the dog on a small plate or on a piece of paper. It takes the food also from the experimenter's hand instead of from the cup. Finally, sometimes, after the conditioned stimulation, it begins to lick up the powder spilled on the floor, although when offered in the cup, it refused it.

Along with these motor phenomena relating to the process of eating there were manifested in the course of our observations on the hypnotic state other specific motor reactions worth noting. Many dogs, after partaking of their small portion of food and being in an alert state, for a time lick their forepaws and breast. In the hypnotic state the licking usually assumes a protracted character; in the case of one of our dogs in question it soon passes into a peculiar form. The dog licks the forepaw and wets it with saliva, especially the flesh of the toes; then it brings the forepaw close to the apparatus attached to the salivary fistula and passes the toes over it—a gesture it repeats many times if not stopped. In the alert state the same dog did not do this. Some dogs in the alert state struggle against the apparatus only when it is first attached to them, afterwards they get used and pay no attention to it. We can rightfully suppose that our dog exhibited in the hypnotic state one of the specific defensive reflexes. When a dog has a wound on a part of the skin within reach of its tongue, it repeatedly cleans it with saliva, or, as we say, licks it (the auto-curative reflex). Apparently in this particular case the irritation evoked by the hardened cement, by means of which the apparatus is attached to the skin, is responsible for the manifestation of the reflex; and since the point of irritation is not accessible to the tongue, the latter is replaced by the toes of the forepaw.

Many of the above-described variations of the food motor reaction usually take place during one and the same experiment and rapidly supersede one another. This variability, this mobility of the hypnotic state, is also seen in other phenomena. We shall cite a few more cases illustrating the fluctuation of the hypnotic state and the modification of the effect of the conditioned stimulus, already described and reproduced by us, or noted for the first time in the course of our observations and experiments on dogs. These fluctuations and modifications are either due to causes still unknown or are related to definite conditions.

I repeat that, if the dog is susceptible to hypnotisation under experimental conditions, the hypnotic state usually develops immediately after the dog is placed in the stand, and sometimes the very moment it crosses the threshold of the experimental chamber. With the progress of the experiment this state grows continuously and gradually, provided it is not dissipated by certain new conditions.

Let us consider first of all the dissociation of the secretory and motor reactions of the food reflex.[46] This dissociation often assumes the form of, so to speak, reciprocal antagonism. In some cases the stimulation evokes a secretion of saliva in the absence of any motor reaction, i.e., the dog, as mentioned above, does not take the food. In other cases, on the contrary, the dog rapidly seizes the food and eats it with avidity, but there is no salivary secretion in response to well-elaborated conditioned stimuli.

Here is the example of one of our dogs—"Bek". The experiment took the following course during two days in succession.

April 17, 1930

Conditioned stimulus	Secretion of saliva in drops during 30 sec.	Food motor reaction
Rattle-box	15	Negativism, then takes food
Bell	15	Abortive movements; rejects food for a long time

April 18, 1930

Conditioned stimulus	Secretion of saliva in drops during 30 sec.	Food motor reaction
Rattle-box	1	Takes food at once, but eats inertly
Bell	0	Takes food at once and eats with relish

Sometimes these, as it were, antagonistic relations between the secretory and motor food reactions rapidly interchange in the course of the experiment.

This can be illustrated by an experiment performed on another dog—"John":

April 12, 1930
Beginning of the Experiment

Conditioned stimulus	Secretion of saliva in drops during 30 sec.	Food motor reaction
Rattle-box	5	Negativism
Bell	0	Takes food at once

In the early works that originated in our laboratories it was frequently stated that a well-elaborated inhibitory stimulus, usually a differential one, can modify the hypnotic state in two opposite directions—either intensifying, or weakening it. The same thing was often observed by us in the above-mentioned animals in their state of hypnosis.

Finally, it should be pointed out that among our usual conditioned strong stimuli a particularly powerful conditioned stimulus often eliminates or weakens the hypnotic state whereas stimuli of usual strength either leave it unchanged or even reinforce it.

Here is an example connected with the experiment performed on the above-mentioned "Bek", the beginning of which has been described above. When the experiment was continued and a differentiation applied, the conditioned stimuli of medium strength—the rattle-box, the gurgle of water and the bell—did not produce any secretory effect, and the dog, while making abortive masticatory movements, did not take food for a long time. A strong crackling sound which is a very powerful conditioned stimulus, evoked a secretion of saliva, and after a short period of negativism the dog took the food.

April 17, 1930

Conditioned stimulus	Secretion of saliva in drops in 30 sec.	Food motor reaction
Rattle-box	0	Does not take food for a long time
Gurgling sound	0	Same
Strong crackling sound	5	Negativism of short duration
Bell	0	Does not take food for a long time

How should the physiological mechanism of the above-mentioned phenomena be interpreted and understood? It is evident that at the present level of our knowledge in the field of the physiology of the higher parts of the brain it would be an extreme pretension, incompatible with the real state of affairs, to try to give a well-grounded and clear answer to all questions which may arise in this connection. However, we must constantly attempt to explain particular phenomena by the more general properties of the activity of the higher parts of the brain, to effect new variations of experiments that would ensure a closer approach to the comprehension of the extremely complex relations of reality which exist in the given case.

The difficulty which we meet when attempting to elucidate the mechanism of the above-mentioned phenomena observed in the hypnotic state, is that under stimulations, undoubtedly reaching the cerebral cells, we often do not know what in the ensuing nervous activity should be attributed to the cerebral hemispheres and what to the lower levels, the lower parts of the brain and even the spinal cord. In the course of the philogenic development of the central nervous system the nervous combinative systems, in the form of definite, so-called reflex centres, becoming more and more complex, steadily moved closer to the brain end; they effected an increasing analysis and synthesis of the stimulating agents due to the augmenting complexity of the organism and the growth of its relations with the external environment in ever-widening areas. Thus, along with a more or less stereotypic nervous activity, and with ready complexes of physiological functions, called forth by a limited number of elementary stimulations, there gradually developed the higher nervous activity dealing with an ever-increasing number of conditions, of complex, and besides, variable, stimulations. Then a very complicated problem arises before the investigator, the problem of the connection and of the forms of this connection between different levels of the nervous system. As to our first problem concerning the dissociation of the secretory and motor reactions of our conditioned food reflex, it is necessary to establish what in this reflex should be ascribed to the cortex and what to the adjacent subcortex, or, in ordinary terminology, what in this process is of a voluntary and what is of a reflex character. To be still more exact, it is necessary to know whether in the conditioned food reflex the secretory and motor components equally depend on the cortex, or whether there is a difference between them in this respect. Does not the motor component predominantly depend on the cortex, and the secretory component on the subcortex?

Let us turn to the well-known facts.

Proceeding from the phenomena of human hypnosis we must admit that in the cerebral cortex along with a grandiose representation of the external world effected through the afferent fibres (an indispensable condition for the highest regulation of functions) there is also a vast representation of the organism's internal world,[47] i.e., of the states and functioning of numerous organs, tissues and internal organic processes. In this respect particularly convincing are the facts pertaining to the so-called phantom, self-suggested pregnancy. Numerous processes relating to the activity of passive tissues, such as the adipose one, arise and become intensified under the influence of the cerebral hemispheres. But it is clear that these two kinds of representation differ greatly in degree. Whereas the representation of the skeletal musculature is highly delicate and detailed, perhaps being equal in these respects to the representation of such external energies as sound and light, the representation of other internal processes lags considerably. This is probably due to the slight practical significance of the representation. In any case, it is a constant physiological fact. And this, apparently, makes it possible to distinguish between the voluntary and involuntary functions of the organism, the former including only the activity of the skeletal musculature. This voluntariness signifies that the work of the skeletal musculature is, above all, determined by its cortical representation, by the motor region of the cortex (the motor analyser, in our terminology) which is directly connected with all the external analysers; in other words, in its orientations it is always determined by the analytical and synthetical work of these analysers.

Proceeding from these facts, we can present the mechanism responsible for the elaboration of our conditional food reflex in the following way. On the one hand, this is a union between the cortical points of application of the conditioned stimuli and the food reflex centre of the adjacent subcortex with all its particular functions; on the other hand, it is a closer connection of the same points with the corresponding parts of the motor analyser, i.e., those which participate in the process of eating. Then the dissociation of the secretory and motor components of the alimentary process taking place in the course of hypnotisation might be interpreted as follows. The hypnotisation evokes a state of the cortex when the motor analyser is inhibited, while all the other analysers are free. The latter evoke a reflex on the alimentary centre of the subcortex with all its functions, while the inhibition of the motor analyser, so to say, by direct communication, excludes the motor component from this reflex, thereby bringing the terminal points of movement, the cells of the anterior horns, to a state of inactivity. Thus, in the alimentary process only the secretory reaction remains manifest.

Here is the reverse case. An artificial conditioned stimulus does not produce a secretion of saliva, but a motor reaction is in evidence—the dog takes the food at once. Now this can be easily explained. This must be a weak inhibition of the entire cortex, and an artificial stimulation alone is not sufficient to dissipate it; only with the presentation of food, when the artificial conditioned stimulus is supplemented by natural stimuli (the sight and odour of food, which in themselves are even stronger than artificial stimuli), does there arise a complete reflex with both components.

But there is one more phenomenon which was observed by us in the course of other experiments in our laboratories and which manifested itself outside the hypnotic state; it would be opportune to analyse this phenomenon in the light of our present explanations. The dog eats the food, but no secretion of saliva is observed for ten or twenty seconds. This is undoubtedly due to the development of inhibition deliberately induced in the cortex by means of artificial conditioned stimuli for definite periods of time. How is this phenomenon to be interpreted? What mechanism is responsible for it? It must be assumed that an intense inhibition develops from the points of application of the artificial conditioned stimuli and spreads over the entire subcortical alimentary centre with both of its principal components—secretory and motor—as well as over the corresponding part of the cortical motor analyser. The moment food is presented, there arises at the points of application of the strongest natural conditioned stimuli, which have not participated in developing inhibition, an excitation rapidly affecting the alimentary region of the motor analyser; the latter is more labile in comparison with the subcortical centre, where the inhibition dissipates only if the motor effect of the unconditioned stimulus is more pronounced. One might draw a certain analogy between this phenomenon and the deliberate, volitional introduction of food into the mouth, its mastication and ingestion, in the absence of any trace of appetite.

However, it can, of course, be assumed (there are sufficient grounds for this) that the conditioned connection with the salivary secretion is likewise effected in the cortex through the cortical representation of the salivary glands, and if so, all the cases of dissociation of the secretory and motor reactions can be attributed to a different localisation of inhibition at the onset of the hypnotic state and in the course of its development.

Another hypnotic phenomenon whose physiological mechanism must be elucidated by us is negativism. This, obviously, is a manifestation of inhibition, since it is a phasic phenomenon which gradually ends in sleep. Likewise, there is no doubt that it is a cortical localised inhibition because the salivary reaction accompanying it reveals a conditioned, i.e., cortical character. Consequently, it is natural to conclude that this is a motor inhibition related to the motor region of the cortex, to the motor analyser. But how is this form of inhibition to be explained? Why does the negative phase of the motor action appear first and the positive one next? What causes the change? It seems to us that this can be easily explained by more general, already known facts. When the hypnotic, inhibitory state sets in, the cortical cells become, as it were, weaker and less efficient—the maximum limit of their possible excitability diminishes. This is the so-called paradoxical phase, when a strong stimulus usually turns into a super-powerful one and may evoke not excitation, but inhibition, or it may strengthen the latter. We must also assume that a movement proceeding from the motor analyser, as is generally the case, consists of two opposite innervations—positive and negative, a movement towards the object and a movement from the object, which is similar to the relations of the flexors and extensors in the limbs. The negativisim may be then explained in the following way. A conditioned stimulus, slightly inhibited or not inhibited at all, directs a stimulation from the cortex to a corresponding positive innervating point of the motor region which is in a paradoxical state due to a certain degree of hypnotisation. That is why the stimulation does not excite the above-mentioned point, but intensifies its inhibition. Then, this extraordinary local inhibition, in accordance with the law of reciprocal induction, excites the negative point which is closely associated with the positive one. Hence the first negative phase of negativism. When the stimulus is removed, the extraordinarily inhibited positive point, by virtue of internal reciprocal induction, immediately becomes excited itself; at the same time the negative point, excited by the induction, at once passes into a state of extraordinary inhibition and in its turn positively induces the positive point. Thus, after its first extraordinary inhibition the positive point undergoes, so to speak, a double excitation. In accordance with this, if the hypnotic state does not deepen, the positive phase usually takes the upper hand after a single or repeated presentation and removal of the food—the dog begins to take it. We observe, then, a highly labile state of the cellular activity which is one of the properties of the transitional phase. This is proved by the further course of developments. If the hypnotic state deepens, there remains only the negative phase; reverse induction becomes impossible, and no excitation of the motor innervating apparatus is observed at all.

Approximately in this period of the conditioned food motor reaction under hypnosis there is manifested one of the conditions for a fragmentary localisation of hypnogenous inhibition in the cortex. One of our dogs, as shown in the descriptive part of this article, exhibited a very interesting and peculiar phenomenon (already mentioned by one of us in a previous article[48]). This relates to a definite sequence of inhibition in the adjacent zones of the motor region. The sequence can be explained by the fact that the inhibition embraces first of all those regions whose activity was most intense before the onset of the hypnotic state. Since in the repeated process of eating the masticatory and lingual muscles worked most of all, then the cervical muscles, and finally the muscles of the trunk, the inhibition manifested itself in the same sequence.

The interesting phenomenon of a positive excitatory influence exerted in the course of hypnotisation by the slightest change in the appearance of the food and in the manner of its presentation, is likewise accounted for by the general property of the cortical activity already known to us. It was established in our laboratory long ago (by Dr. Y. V. Volborth) that there is a conditioned inhibition of the second order, just as there is a conditioned excitation of the second order. The phenomenon is as follows. If an indifferent stimulus repeatedly coincides in time with an elaborated inhibitory process (for example, in the course of a differentiation), then it soon becomes an inhibitory agent itself. It is then easily understood why everything acting on the cerebral hemispheres during the state of hypnosis (which in itself is a certain degree of inhibition) acquires an inhibitory character. Hence, it is sometimes sufficient to bring the dog into the experimental chamber to evoke in it a hypnotic state. Any new stimuli, even very insignificant ones, naturally do not produce this inhibitory effect, and consequently, evoke positive cortical activity.

The auto-curative reflex mentioned in the descriptive part of this article is simply one of the subcortical reflexes manifested in the state of hypnosis after short feeding. The process of eating, with all its exciting components, acts on the more or less hypnotised cortex as a strong stimulus and entails an intensification of cortical inhibition. A positive induction then proceeds from the cortex to the subcortical centres, which are now under the action of the ultra-weak stimuli or traces of former strong stimuli. The animal begins to sneeze, to scratch itself, etc., which was not observed in the alert state. Of a similar nature was the experimental case with a dog whose state resembled a wartime neurosis; this case is described and analysed in the present volume of Collected Papers.[49]

As to the effect of differentiations, i.e., of conditioned inhibitory stimuli, we have long known that their influence on diffused inhibition is of a twofold, contrasting character. In the case of a very feeble, diffused cortical inhibition, of a weak hypnotic intensity, the well-elaborated inhibitory stimulus concentrates the diffused inhibition to a greater or lesser degree and in doing so either fully abolishes the hypnotic state or weakens it. On the contrary, in the case of a strong inhibitory tonus of the cortex, the same stimulus intensifies the inhibition, as it were, by its summation with the existing inhibition. Consequently, the result is determined by the relations of intensity.

Let us, finally, consider the last experiment cited by us in the descriptive part of this article, when an extremely strong stimulus, contrary to stimuli of moderate strength and to weak stimuli, instead of intensifying the inhibition, often produced a positive action. The latter can be explained by the direct influence of the extremely strong stimulus on the subcortex; the intense subcortical excitation is communicated to the cortex, thus dissipating or weakening the inhibitory process in it. A special experimental method applied by us proves the correctness of this interpretation. When the monotonous experimental surroundings begin to have a hypnotising effect on some of our animals, we, incidentally, counteract it by increasing their alimentary excitability by means of a certain diminution of their daily food ration. And naturally this increase of alimentary excitability must be located in the subcortical alimentary centre.

ON NEUROSES IN MAN AND ANIMALS[50]

The *Journal of Nervous and Mental Disease*, vol. 70, printed Dr. P. Schilder's article entitled "The Somatic Basis of the Neurosis" in which the author admits that what I and my associates have called a neurosis in our experimental animals (dogs) studied by the conditioned reflex method "comprises all the phenomena of neuroses". This admission by a competent person is, of course, very valuable for us. But I must resolutely object to what the author goes on to say about the comparative studies of these neuroses in man and animals. The article contains the following passage: "These important experiments of Pavlov and his school (on neuroses) can be understood only if we look upon them in the light of our experiences in neuroses. We cannot interpret the neurosis by means of the conditioned reflex, but by means of the psychic mechanism we have studied in the neurosis, we can certainly very well interpret what takes place in a conditioned reflex."

What should we understand—and what does everybody usually understand—by the words "interpretation" or "understanding" of phenomena? Reduction of more complex phenomena to more elementary, simple phenomena. It follows that also in the given case of neuroses in man they must be interpreted, understood, i.e., analysed with the help of neuroses in animals as the naturally more simple, and not vice versa.

In the case of man we must first of all determine exactly what the deviations in behaviour are from the normal in the given case. Indeed, normal behaviour is also extraordinarily diverse in various people. Then we must find together with the patient or despite the patient, or even against his resistance, amid the chaos of life's relations, the conditions and circumstances which acted at once or gradually and with which the origin of the pathologic deviation, the origin of the neurosis may be justly connected. Moreover, we must understand why these conditions and circumstances produced such a result in our patient and left another person entirely unaffected. And what is more, why they have led to this pathological complex in one person and to an entirely different complex in another person. I am taking only the main, so to speak, group questions, omitting the enormous variety of more particular questions. Do we always have quite satisfactory answers to these questions?

But this is only part of the matter, if we want its complete, deep analysis. Of course, the deviations in the behaviour of our patient have come into play on his nervous apparatus. Who will now contest this? We must therefore still answer the following questions: What deviations from the normal processes in his nervous system have occurred under the aforesaid conditions, and how and why have they occurred? Are not all these demands real? Where are these demands satisfied?

And what do we have in the dog?

To begin with, we see that neuroses can be obtained without difficulty only in an animal in which there is normally no requisite balance between the elementary phenomena of nervous activity, as yet inaccessible to further physiological analysis, between the processes of excitation and inhibition. It is either in the animal in which the excitatory process greatly predominates over the inhibitory process so that the animal cannot *fully* inhibit its activity when this is required by the conditions of life (excitable type), or in another animal in which, on the contrary, the excitatory process is so weak that it is frequently inhibited out of measure and at variance with the requirements of life (inhibitable type).

Furthermore, we know on the same experimental animal precisely that this inadequate balance, characteristic of the given animals normally, is definitely disturbed under certain, elementary conditions. There are mainly three conditions, three cases. Either we apply extraordinarily strong stimuli, as conditioned stimuli, instead of weak and moderate ones, which determine the usual activity of the animal, i.e., we overstrain its excitatory process, or we require of the animal now very strong and now very protracted inhibition, i.e., we overstrain its inhibitory process, or, lastly, we collide these two processes, i.e., apply our conditioned positive and negative stimuli directly after each other. A chronic disorder of higher nervous activity —neurosis—occurs in the corresponding animals in all these cases. Our excitable type almost completely loses its ability to inhibit anything and becomes generally uncommonly excited; the inhibitable type, being hungry, refuses even to eat during application of our conditioned stimuli and becomes generally extraordinarily uneasy and at the same time passive during the slightest variations in the environment.

It can be assumed with all probability that if these sick dogs could observe themselves and could tell us what they experienced during that time, they would not have anything to add to what we would assume for them in their condition. They would all say that in all the afore-mentioned cases they experienced a difficult, distressing state. Then some of them would say that after that they were frequently unable to refrain from doing what they were not allowed to do and for what they were punished anyway, while others would say that they were either altogether unable to do what they generally had to do, or could not do it calmly.

Thus, what we obtained on our animals are elementary physiological phenomena, the limit (at the present state of our knowledge) of physiological analysis. At the same time this would be the very last, deepest basis of the human neurosis and would serve for its most appropriate interpretation, its understanding.

It follows that in the case of man with the complexity of his life's situation and multiformity of his reactions to it we are always faced, for the purpose of analysis, as well as cure, with a very difficult question: What life's circumstances were too intense for the given nervous system, where and when did the requirements of activity and requirements of inhibiting the activity collide beyond the endurance of this nervous system?

Then how, according to Dr. Schilder, could the innumerable experiences of the neurotic, considering the extraordinary complexity of human higher nervous activity, compared with that of the dog, yield anything useful for the explanation of the elementary animal neurosis, when they themselves were only different variations of the same physiological processes so vividly observed in the dog?

Of course, we still have a number of unanswered questions for further physiological analysis of the problem of neuroses and psychoses. Can neuroses also be produced in balanced nervous systems? Is the initial unbalance of the nervous system a primary phenomenon, i.e., an inborn property of the very nervous tissue, or a secondary phenomenon, depending on some inborn peculiarities of the other systems of the organism, besides the nervous system? Are there perhaps, in addition to the inborn property of the nervous system, also other factors in the organism which determine the particular degree of normal functioning of this system?

We are now studying some of these questions and already have some material with which to answer them.

It stands to reason that, in addition to these particular questions concerning the general problem of disorders of normal nervous activity, the physiologist continues to be faced with the question of the physico-chemical mechanism of the most elementary nervous processes: excitation and inhibition, their interrelations and overstrain.

EXPERIMENTAL NEUROSES[51]

I am reporting the results of the work done by me jointly with my collaborators. At the present time we have a good deal of material and now I can cite from it but very little and in general outline.

By neuroses we imply chronic (continuing for weeks, months and even years) deviations in higher nervous activity from normal. For us higher nervous activity is manifested mainly in the system of conditioned positive and negative reflexes to all manner of stimuli and, partly (to a slight extent), in the general behaviour of our animals (dogs).

Until now the neuroses were engendered in our animals by the following factors: firstly, excessively strong or excessively complex stimuli; secondly, overstrain of the inhibitory process; thirdly, a clash (direct succession) of the two antagonistic nervous processes, and lastly (fourthly), castration.

The neuroses were manifested in a weakening of both processes separately or together, in chaotic nervous activity, and in different phases of the hypnotic state. Various combinations of these symptoms represented very definite pictures of diseases.

The essential thing here was the following. Whether the disease develops or not, whether it is manifested in one form or another, depends on the type of the given animal's nervous system.

On the basis of our investigations we had to establish three main types. The central, ideal, truly normal type, in which both antagonistic nervous processes are balanced. We found this type in two variations: calm, sedate animals and, on the other hand, contrariwise, very lively mobile animals. The two others are extreme types: one is strong, in all probability too strong, but not entirely normal, however, because it has a relatively weak inhibitory process; the other is a weak type in which both processes are weak, especially, the inhibitory process. It seems to me that our classification of the types of nervous systems most fully coincides with Hippocrates' classical classification of temperaments.

For the sake of brevity and by way of example I shall cite in somewhat greater detail only our latest experiments (Dr. M. Petrova's) on castrated animals.

Under usual conditions the disease was observed after castration in animals of the central type only for a period of a month; subsequently the animal behaved normally. Only during increased excitability was it possible to establish a constantly diminishing efficiency of the cortical cells, whereas in cases of conditioned food reflexes it was easy to modify the excitability by different degrees of hunger.

In the weaker type the clearly pathological state following castration lasted for many months, up to one year and more, and improved but gradually. These animals were very intensely affected by the regular suspension of our experiments or administration of bromides, which temporarily restored the animal to normal. During the usual daily work the conditioned reflexes were chaotic. Three-day intervals between the experiments conditioned an entirely normal functioning of the reflexes. This fact made it perfectly obvious that each of our experiments was serious nervous work. Administration of bromides restored and retained normal activity also during the daily experiments.

The following circumstance was quite unexpected and very peculiar. Rather strong types usually manifested immediately after castration diminished efficiency of the nervous system: the positive conditioned reflexes diminished. The contrary was observed in the weak type. The conditioned reflexes became intensified for several weeks after castration. Extreme weakness of the cortical cells occurred later, and in this case administration of bromides did not improve the situation but made it worse. This peculiar fact can also be satisfactorily accounted for, but I am in no position to dwell on the details now.

I must finish my report.

To draw a serious analogy between the neurotic states in our dogs and the different neuroses in man, is a task we, physiologists, who are not thoroughly familiar with human neuropathology can scarcely cope with. But I am convinced, however, that the solution or an essential approximation to the solution of many important questions of the etiology, natural systematisation, mechanism, and, lastly, treatment of human neuroses are in the hands of the experimenter on animals.*

---

* Some of these points, it seems to me, have now received special clinical confirmation.

By artificially producing in our dogs a deviation in higher nervous activity from the normal, we observed in dogs of different types of nervous system two different forms of nervous disease, two different neuroses, resulting from the same procedures—difficult nervous tasks.

In an excitable (and at the same time strong) dog the neurosis consisted in an almost complete disappearance of the inhibitory reflexes, i.e., extraordinary weakening, almost to zero, of the inhibitory process. In another, inhibitable (and at the same time weak) dog all the positive conditioned reflexes disappeared and the dog was reduced to a very sluggish and, in our situation, sleepy state. At the same time the neurosis of the first dog quickly responded to bromides and was radically cured. In the other dog the same dose of bromides rather changed the state of affairs for the worse, and the dog recovered very slowly only through a very long rest, i.e., suspension of our experiments with conditioned reflexes.

The main aim of my participation in this Congress is therefore fervently to advise neuropathologists to work with normal and pathological conditioned reflexes.

Unfamiliar with the clinical aspects of neuroses we, at first erroneously, although guided by certain considerations, named the neurosis of the first dog *neurasthenia* and that of the second dog—*hysteria*. Of late we have found it more fitting to name the neurosis of the first dog *hypersthenia* and to retain the designation of *neurasthenia* for the neurosis of the second dog, assigning, perhaps more accurately the term *hysteria* to other disorders of the nervous system which we now discover in our experiments as a result of other causes.

At the International Neurological Congress, which just took place and at which this report was made, Dr. Szondi arrived at the conclusion in his report that the present clinical form of neurasthenia must be divided into two different neuroses corresponding to two opposite constitutions and very much coinciding, in my opinion, with the neuroses I have briefly described above.

ESSAY ON THE PHYSIOLOGICAL CONCEPT OF THE SYMPTOMATOLOGY OF HYSTERIA[52]

To my dear comrade Alexei Vasilyevich Martynov, in honour of his forty years of brilliant scientific, pedagogic and practical work,

The grateful author.

Leningrad, April 1932

The objective study of the higher nervous activity by the method of conditioned reflexes has made such progress and has been so widened and deepened that it no longer seems very risky to attempt a physiological interpretation and analysis of the complex, pathological picture presented by hysteria in all its manifestations, although hysteria is regarded by clinicians, fully or predominantly, as a mental disease, as a psychogenic reaction to the environment.

Thus, it is at the same time a test which enables one to judge to what degree the theory of conditioned reflexes is entitled to claim a physiological explanation of the so-called psychical phenomena.

Unfortunately, here again it is impossible to do without a physiological introduction, although a brief one. To this day conditioned reflexes are relatively little known even in the country of their origin; besides, the theory of conditioned reflexes is developing so rapidly that many of its important points have not yet been published and will be expounded by me here for the first time.

1

The conditioned reflexes continuously accumulated by human beings and animals in the course of their individual life are formed in the cerebral hemispheres, or, in general, in the higher part of the central nervous system. They represent a higher degree of complexity of ordinary unconditioned reflexes, i.e., reflexes which exist in the organisation of the central nervous system from the day of birth.

The biological meaning of the conditioned reflexes consists in the fact that the few external stimuli of unconditioned reflexes, given a definite condition (coincidence in time), establish a temporary connection with the countless phenomena of the surrounding medium—signals of those stimuli. Because of this, all the organic activities representing the effects produced by the unconditioned reflexes, establish more delicate and more precise relations with the environment in wider and wider areas. The theory of conditioned reflexes or the physiology of the higher nervous activity studies the laws governing the dynamics of these reflexes both in normal and pathological life.

The activity of the cerebral hemispheres and of the entire central nervous system with its two processes—excitation and inhibition—is subordinated, in our view, to two fundamental laws: the law of irradiation and concentration of each of these processes, and the law of their reciprocal induction. Experiments carried out on the normal activity of the cortex enable us to draw the conclusion that if the intensity of these processes is weak, they at once begin to irradiate from the point of their origin; if their intensity is strong enough, they concentrate, and if it is excessively strong they irradiate again. When the processes concentrate they induce an opposite process both at the periphery during their action, and at the precise point of action upon its termination.

The irradiation of the excitatory process over the entire nervous system gives rise to a summation reflex. In spreading out, the wave of new excitation is summated with the already existing, manifest or latent, local excitation, revealing in the latter case the latent focus of excitation. In the cerebral hemispheres, which are of a more complex structure and possess extreme reactivity and impressionability, the irradiation of the excitatory process leads to the formation of a temporary conditioned connection, a conditioned reflex, association. While the summation reflex represents a momentary, transient phenomenon, the conditioned reflex is a chronic phenomenon, gradually becoming stronger under the above-mentioned condition; it is a characteristic cortical process.

When the excitatory process concentrates in the entire central nervous system we meet with phenomena of inhibition—a manifestation of the law of induction. The point at which the excitation is concentrated is to a greater or lesser extent surrounded by an inhibitory process representing a phenomenon of negative induction. The latter makes itself felt both in the unconditioned and conditioned reflexes. The inhibition develops in full at once; it always arises and persists not only during the excitation by which it has been produced, but even for some time after it. The stronger the excitation and the lower the positive tonus of the surrounding brain mass the more profound, extensive and durable is its action. Negative induction acts both between the small points of the brain and its large parts. We call this inhibition external, passive, and, it can be added, unconditioned. Previously, this well-known phenomenon was termed the struggle of nervous centres, which emphasised the fact that at a particular time a physiological predominance, or, so to speak, priority of one nervous activity over the other takes place.

Along with the inhibition just mentioned the cerebral

hemispheres exhibit other kinds or cases of inhibition, although there are grounds to assume that the physico-chemical process in all these cases is one and the same. This is, first of all, an inhibition which constantly corrects the conditioned connection and accordingly restrains the excitatory process, when the signalling conditioned stimulus is not accompanied, in some cases temporarily, by the signalised stimulus, or when it is accompanied by the latter with a considerable delay. This inhibition becoming highly fragmentary, also delimits, differentiates the conditioned positive agents from the countless analogous and related negative agents. It arises of itself in the conditions mentioned above, gradually grows and gains in intensity; it can train and perfect itself. This inhibition can also become connected with any indifferent external stimulus, if the action of the latter coincides for a certain time with the presence of inhibition in the cortex; this stimulus then begins of itself to produce an inhibitory process in the cortex. From what has been said it is clear that this purely cortical inhibition, along with the conditioned connection, plays an important role in the adaptation to the surrounding medium, constantly and expediently analysing the stimulations coming from there. We have named this kind or case of inhibition internal, active inhibition. Generally speaking, the adjective "conditioned" could be accorded it as well. Then another, specific case of inhibition is observed in the cortex. All other conditions being equal, the effect of the conditioned stimulus is, as a rule, proportional to the intensity of the physical strength of the stimulus, but to a definite maximum level (and probably also to a certain minimum level). Beyond this maximum the effect no longer increases; it may sometimes even diminish. We then say that such a stimulus, on reaching this maximum level, begins to produce inhibition, not excitation. We interpret this phenomenon in the following way: the given cortical cell has a definite limit of functional capacity, i.e., of, so to speak, inoffensive, easily reversible functional wear, and the inhibition, which arises in connection with a super-powerful stimulation, does not permit overstepping this limit. The stronger the super-powerful stimuli, the more intense is the inhibition; in this case the effect of stimulation either remains at the maximum level, which is more often the case, or diminishes somewhat, if the stimulation is too intense. This inhibition could be called transmarginal.

The limit of functional capacity of the cortical cells is not of a constant nature; it may change abruptly, as well as in a chronic way. Inanition, hypnosis, disease and old age lead to a steady decline of this limit; at the same time in the surrounding environment more and more inhibitory stimuli appear which become super-powerful for the given cell. The following important fact must be also pointed out. When the excitability or lability of the cortical cells is augmented in a natural or artificial way, for example, by means of chemical substances, i.e., when a more rapid functional wear of the cortical cells is provoked, an ever-increasing number of stimuli which previously were below maximum or of maximum strength become super-powerful, leading to inhibition and a general decline of the conditioned reflex activity.

The following question remains unsolved: What is the relation between the two latter cases of inhibition and the first universal case of negative induction? If they are simply a modification of the first case, then what is the nature of the modification and how does it occur in relation to the peculiar properties of the cortex? It is probable that transmarginal inhibition is closer and more related to external, passive inhibition than to internal, active inhibition, since it, too, arises at once, and is not elaborated and trained as the latter.

These two kinds of cortical inhibition also move, spread over the brain mass. A very large number of diverse experiments were performed with the special object of studying the movement of the first kind of cortical inhibition—

internal inhibition. In these experiments the inhibition spread out as if before the eyes of the experimenters.

There is no doubt that inhibition, while irradiating and deepening, develops different degrees of a hypnotic state, and that spreading from the cerebral hemispheres downward to the utmost over the brain, it produces normal sleep. The diversity and multiplicity of hypnotic stages, which at first can hardly be distinguished from the waking state, strikingly manifest themselves even in our dogs. In respect of the intensity of inhibition the so-called equalisation, paradoxical and ultra-paradoxical phases are worth mentioning. Conditioned stimuli of different physical intensity, instead of producing effects in proportion to their intensity, as in the case of the waking state, now produce equal, or even inversely proportional and distorted effects. In rarer cases the distortion of the effects reaches such a degree that only the inhibitory conditioned stimuli produce a positive effect, while the positive stimuli assume an inhibitory action. In respect of the extensity of inhibition there are observed functional dissociations of the cortex, as well as of the rest of the brain, into larger and smaller parts. The motor area of the cortex is particularly often isolated from other areas, and even in this area sometimes a dissociation of functions comes to the fore.

It is a matter of sincere regret that up to the present time the impression produced by these laboratory experiments is weakened due to the rivalry of the so-called sleep centre suggested by clinicians and certain physiologists; meanwhile, the matter can be interpreted in a satisfactory and conciliatory way from the following point of view, which seems to me fully justified by the facts. One can hardly doubt that there are two mechanisms responsible for the onset of sleep, and that it is necessary to distinguish active sleep from passive sleep. Active sleep originates in the cerebral hemispheres and is based on an active process of inhibition, arising in the hemispheres and spreading from there to the lower parts of the brain. Passive sleep results from the diminution or limitation of stimulating impulses reaching the higher parts of the brain (not only the cerebral hemispheres, but also the adjacent subcortex). The stimulating impulses include, on the one hand, external stimuli, which reach the brain through the medium of the external receptors, and, on the other hand, internal stimuli, conditioned by the work of the internal organs and transmitted to the higher parts of the brain from the central nervous region regulating the organism's vegetative functions.

The first cases of passive sleep of a particularly pronounced character are Strümpell's well-known clinical case[53] and the analogical, more recent experiment carried out by Prof. A. D. Speransky and V. S. Galkin[54] when, after a peripheral destruction of three receptors—olfactory, auditory and visual—the dog falls into a profound and chronic state of sleep (lasting for weeks and months). The second cases of passive sleep are the clinical cases which lead to the recognition of what clinicians and some experimenters designate as the "centre of sleep".

The physiology of the muscular tissue offers us an example which in this respect is analogous to sleep. Owing to its specific physiological organisation, the skeletal muscle only contracts under the influence of its motor nerve, but the relaxation of the muscle is of a passive nature; as to the smooth muscle, its contraction and relaxation are actively effected under the influence of two special nerves—one positive and the other inhibitory.

Just as in the case of concentration of the excitatory process, the concentration of the inhibitory process engenders, by virtue of the law of reciprocal induction, an opposite process, which in the given case is, naturally, a process of excitation. The point of concentration of the inhibition is surrounded, to a greater or lesser extent, by a process of heightened excitability—a manifestation of positive induction. The positive induction makes itself felt in the unconditioned, as well as in the conditioned reflexes.

A heightened excitability arises either immediately or after a certain period during which the inhibition gradually concentrates; it persists not only for the duration of the inhibition, but for some time after its disappearance and in certain cases long after it. The positive induction manifests itself both between small points of the cortex and large parts of the brain.

I shall dwell now on some points of the physiology of the higher nervous activity which are of importance for physiological analysis of the symptomatology of hysteria.

The connection between the organism and the surrounding medium through conditioned signalling agents is the more perfect the more these agents are analysed and synthesised by the cerebral hemispheres in conformity with the extreme complexity and continuous fluctuations of the environment. The synthesis is effected through the process of conditioned connection. The analysis, the differentiation of positive conditioned agents from inhibitory ones is based on the process of reciprocal induction; the separation of different positive agents, i.e., of agents related to different unconditioned reflexes, is accomplished by a process of concentration (new experiments by Rikman[55]). Thus, precise analysis requires a sufficient intensity both of the inhibitory and excitatory processes.

Further, of particular significance for the physiological study of hysteria are our data relating to the types of nervous system. First of all, we distinguish very strong animals, but unequilibrated, in which the inhibitory process always lags to a certain degree and, consequently, does not conform to the excitatory process. When these animals are confronted with difficult nervous tasks calling for considerable inhibition, they almost fully lose their inhibitory function (special neurosis) and become painfully restless; in some cases this restless state is periodically superseded by depression and drowsiness. In their general behaviour animals of this category are aggressive, provocative, and lacking in self-control. We call such dogs excitable or choleric. Next comes the type of strong and at the same time equilibrated animals, in which both processes are of equal strength; because of this, it is difficult and sometimes even impossible to induce neuroses in such animals by means of complex nervous tasks. This type assumes two forms—the quiet (phlegmatic) and the very lively (sanguine) forms. Finally, there is the weak inhibitable type, in which both processes are insufficient, particularly and more often the inhibitory process. It is this type which specially furnishes experimental neuroses, reproduced in them with extreme ease. Animals of this type are cowardly; they are constantly in a state of uneasiness or display excessive fussiness and impatience. They are incapable of enduring strong external agents acting as positive conditioned stimuli, any considerable normal excitation in general (alimentary, sexual, etc.), even a slight intensity (continuation) of the inhibitory process, and still less a collision of the nervous processes, any complex system of conditioned reflexes and finally any change in the stereotype of the conditioned reflex activity. In all these cases they exhibit a weakened and chaotic conditioned reflex activity and very often fall into different phases of hypnosis. Moreover, in these animals separate, even very small, points of the cerebral hemispheres can be easily rendered pathological, and when adequate stimuli affect such points a rapid and drastic decline of the general conditioned reflex activity takes place. Although the general behaviour of these animals is such that they cannot always be described as melancholic, nevertheless there is every reason to include them in the category of melancholic animals, i.e., those in which the vital manifestations are in many cases constantly suppressed and inhibited. In our exposition of the types of nervous system we implied, when we spoke of the equilibrium between excitation and inhibition, the so-called internal inhibition. In the weak type, with its weak internal inhibition, the external inhibition (negative induction) is, on the contrary, highly predominant and, above all, determines the entire external behaviour of the animal. Hence this type is called *weak, inhibitable*.

In concluding the physiological part of this article, I must point to the following circumstance which is of particular importance for the comprehension of some of the special symptoms of hysteria. There are sufficient grounds to assume that centripetal, afferent impulses produced by each element and moment of movement reach the cerebral cortex (motor region) not only from the skeletal motor apparatus, which makes possible an exact cortical regulation of the skeletal movements, but also from other organs and even separate tissues; because of this, the cortical regulation of the latter is likewise possible. At the present time, conditioning, which must be related to the higher part of the central nervous system, assumes greater biological significance since the possibility of conditioned leucocytoses, immunity and other various organic processes, has been demonstrated, even though we do not yet know the exact nervous connections participating, directly or indirectly, in this phenomenon. But this possibility of cortical influence is deliberately utilised and is revealed by us in very rare cases under exceptional artificial or abnormal conditions. This is explained by the fact that, on the one hand, the autoregulation of the activity of other organs and tissues, apart from the skeletal motor apparatus, is chiefly effected in the lower parts of the central nervous system, and, on the other hand, is disguised by the fundamental activity of the cerebral hemispheres aimed at regulating the most complex relations with the surrounding medium.

2

Let us turn now to hysteria.

Concerning the general concepts of hysteria held by the clinicians, some of them give a fundamental general characteristic of the pathological state and some bring forward certain particularly pronounced traits or symptoms of this state. Some clinicians speak, as it were, of a return to instinctive, i.e., emotional and even reflex life; others attribute the disorder to suggestibility, explaining the entire behaviour of hysterical persons and the so-called stigmata of hysteria (analgesia, paralyses, etc.) by suggestion and autosuggestion. Certain clinicians advance to the foreground the desire to be ill, to take refuge in illness; others regard as particularly important the manifestation of fantasticism, the absence of a real perception of life; still others look on the disease as chronic hypnosis, and finally there are clinicians who ascribe it to a reduced capacity for psychical synthesis or to split personality. I believe that all these concepts taken together fully cover the entire syndrome and the entire nature of hysteria.

First of all, we must consider as a generally recognised fact that hysteria results from a weak nervous system. Pierre Janet plainly states that hysteria is one of an immense group of mental illnesses caused by weakness and cerebral inanition. If that is so, then the above characteristic—taking into account that the weakness mainly relates to the higher part of the central nervous system and especially to the cerebral hemispheres as its most reactive part—becomes comprehensible in the light of the physiology of the central nervous system and of its higher part as now presented by the theory of conditioned reflexes.

Usually the cerebral hemispheres which represent the highest organ of correlations between the organism and the surrounding medium and hence the constant controller of the executive functions of the organism, always exert influence on the adjacent parts of the brain with their instinct and reflex activity. From this it follows that the elimination or weakening of the activity of the cerebral hemispheres must necessarily lead to a more or less chaotic activity of the subcortex devoid of the right measure and of adequacy to the given surroundings. This is a well-known physiological fact which manifests itself in animals after the extirpation of the cerebral hemispheres, in adults when they are in different states of narcotisation and in children when they fall asleep. Thus, using the above-mentioned physiological terms, the alert, active state of the cerebral hemispheres, manifested in the unceasing analysis and synthesis of external stimuli, of the influences of the surrounding medium, negatively induces the subcortex, i.e., inhibits its activity as a whole, liberating in a selective way only the activity needed by conditions of place and time. On the contrary, an inhibited state of the hemispheres liberates or positively induces the subcortex, i.e., strengthens its general activity. Consequently, there are adequate physiological grounds for the occurrence of various affective outbursts and convulsive fits in hysterical persons under acute and abrupt inhibition of the cortex resulting from unendurable stimulations—and such stimulations are not infrequent in the case of a weak cortex. These outbursts and fits are sometimes expressed in more or less definite instinctive and reflex activities and sometimes in absolutely chaotic forms, depending on the varying localisation of inhibition over the cortex and the adjacent or more distant subcortex.

But this is an extreme and active expression of the pathological state. When the inhibition spreads further down the brain, we witness another extreme, but passive state of the organism of the hysterical person in the form of deep hypnosis and, in the end, of complete sleep lasting for hours and even for days (lethargy). This difference between the extreme states is probably determined not only by various degrees of weakness of the excitatory and inhibitory processes in the cortex, but also by the force correlations between the cortex and subcortex, which sometimes vary in an acute or chronic way in one and the same individual, and sometimes are also related to different individuals.

This varying chronic weakness of the cortex, apart from being the cause of the extraordinary and extreme states of the organism just described, invariably conditions also the permanent peculiar state of hysterical persons—their emotivity.

Although our life and that of animals is directed by the basic tendencies of the organism—alimentary, sexual, aggressive, investigatory, etc. (functions performed by the subcortex adjacent to the cerebral hemispheres), nevertheless, for the purpose of co-ordinating and realising all these tendencies, indispensably in connection with the general conditions of life, there is a special part of the central nervous system; this part moderates each particular tendency, harmonises them and ensures their most rational realisation in the conditions of the surrounding medium. These are, of course, the cerebral hemispheres. Thus, there are two ways of action. In the first place it is the way of rational action which is effected after, so to speak, a preliminary (though sometimes almost instantaneous) investigation of the given tendency by the cerebral hemispheres and its transformation, in the requisite measure and at the appropriate moment, into a corresponding motor act or behaviour with the help of the cortical motor region. It is, in the second place, the way of affective, passionate action, realised (perhaps even directly through the subcortical connections) under the influence of the given tendency alone, without the above-mentioned preliminary control. In hysterical persons the latter way of action predominates in most cases, and its nervous mechanism is quite clear. The tendency arises under the influence of external or internal stimulation and evokes the activity of a corresponding point or region of the cerebral hemispheres. Under the influence of emotion and due to the irradiation from the subcortex, this point becomes extremely charged. If the cortex is weak, this is sufficient to provoke a strong and greatly extended negative induction, which excludes any control, any influence of all other parts of the cerebral hemispheres. And it is precisely these parts which locate the representation of other tendencies and of the surrounding medium, the traces of previous stimulations and emotions, the acquired experience. This is joined by another mechanism. The strong excitation produced by emotion intensifies the excitability of the cortex; this rapidly leads the excitation of the cortex to the limit of its functional capacity and exceeds it. Consequently, negative induction is joined by transmarginal inhibition. Hence, a hysterical person lives to a greater or lesser degree not a rational but an emotive life, and is directed not by the cortical, but subcortical activity.

Suggestibility and auto-suggestibility are directly connected with this mechanism of hysteria. What are suggestion and auto-suggestion? They are a concentrated excitation of a definite point or region of the cerebral hemispheres in the form of a definite excitation, sensation or its trace—an idea now called forth by emotions, i.e., excited from the subcortex, now produced abruptly from the outside, now by means of internal connections, associations—an excitation which acquires a predominant, undue and irresistible significance. It exists and acts, i.e., passes over into movement, into one or another motor act, not because it is maintained by various associations, that is, connections with many present and past stimuli, sensations and ideas—this would produce resolute and sensible action, such as is usual with a normal strong cortex—but because in a weak cortex with a low, weak tone this concentrated excitation is accompanied by a strong negative induction which detaches and isolates it from all indispensable extraneous influences. This is the mechanism of hypnotic and post-hypnotic suggestion. During hypnosis we observe even in a normal and strong cortex a lowered positive tone owing to irradiated inhibition.* When the word or command of the hypnotist is directed to a definite point of such a cortex as a stimulus, the latter concentrates the excitatory process in a corresponding point and is immediately followed by negative induction, which, meeting little resistance on its way, spreads over the entire cortex; thanks to this, the word or command is completely isolated from all influences and becomes an absolute, irresistible stimulus, continuing to operate even subsequently, when the individual returns to an alert state.

Exactly the same as to its mechanism, but in lesser degree, takes place constantly and spontaneously in old age when the excitatory process in the cortex undergoes a natural decline. In a still strong brain the internal or external excitation, concentrating, even though considerably (but not excessively, as in exceptional cases), in a definite point or region of the cortex, is naturally accompanied by negative induction, which, because of the strength of the cortex, does not represent complete and widely spread inhibition. Therefore, along with the predominant excitation, some other concomitant excitations act, which evoke corresponding reflexes, especially old and fixed ones, or the so-called automatic reflexes. Usually our behaviour consists not of isolated, but complex reactions, corresponding to the constant complexity of the surroundings. The picture is altogether different in old age. When concentrating on a certain excitation, we exclude by means of negative induction the action of all other extraneous but simultaneous stimulations, and that

---

* Despite the very rich material accumulated by the physiology of the nervous system in general, and by the theory of conditioned reflexes in particular, the question of the relation between excitation and inhibition still baffles solution. Is it one and the same process interchanging under definite conditions, or a couple, strongly knit together, which, as it were, revolves under certain conditions and shows, to a greater or lesser extent, or even in full, now one of its sides, now the other?

is why we often act not in compliance with the given conditions, i.e., our reaction to the entire surroundings remains incomplete. Here is a simple illustration. I look at the object which I need, I take it in my hand but at the same time do not notice all or practically all other objects surrounding and adjoining it; as a result I knock against the other objects, derange them without any need, etc. This is described, erroneously, as senile distraction, whereas, on the contrary, it is concentration, but involuntary, passive and defective. Precisely for the same reason an old man, who thinks of something or talks to somebody while putting on his outdoor clothes, sometimes forgets to put on his hat, takes one object instead of another, etc.

As a result of constant extraneous and involuntary suggestions and auto-suggestions, the life of a hysterical person is overcharged with extraordinary and peculiar manifestations.

To begin with, let us take the case of war hysteria which was thoroughly studied during the world war. Being a permanent and serious menace of death, war, of course, is one of the most natural incentives to fear. Fear has definite physiological symptoms which in individuals with a strong nervous system either do not manifest themselves at all, being suppressed, or quickly disappear; in persons with a weak nervous system they are of a more prolonged character, with the result that such persons are no longer able to participate in military operations and thus are discharged from the obligation of exposing their life to danger. These persistent symptoms could also disappear of themselves with the lapse of time, but in a weak nervous system, precisely because of its weakness, a mechanism sets in which maintains them. The persistent symptoms of fear and the resulting temporary safety thus coincide in time and, by virtue of the law of conditioned reflexes, must become associated, interconnected. Hence, the sensation and representation of these symptoms assume a positive emotional shade and, naturally, are repeatedly reproduced. Then, on the one hand, according to the law of irradiation and summation, they, acting from the cortex, maintain and reinforce the lower centres of the reflex symptoms of fear, and, on the other hand, being emotionally charged, they are accompanied, in a weak cortex, by an intense negative induction, and thus exclude the influence of other representations which could oppose the feeling of conditioned agreeableness or desirability of these symptoms. We, therefore, have no sufficient grounds to affirm that this case represents a deliberate simulation of symptoms. In effect, it is a case of fatal physiological relations.

But a hysterical person displays a multitude of similar cases even in his everyday life. Not only the horrors of war, but many other dangers (fire, railway accidents, etc.), numerous life shocks, such as the loss of close relations or friends, unfaithful love and other deceptions encountered, the loss of property, collapse of convictions and beliefs, etc., and in general difficult conditions of life—unhappy marriage, poverty, violation of self-respect, and so forth—all these factors produce in a weak individual, at once or eventually, violent reactions accompanied by different abnormal somatic symptoms. Many of these symptoms, which appear at the moment of strong excitation, are impressed in the cortex for a long time or forever, just as are many strong stimulations in normal persons (kinesthetic stimulations included). But other symptoms, which in a normal subject can be effaced with the lapse of time—whether because of fear of their abnormality, inconvenience, direct harmfulness and merely indecency, or, the reverse, because they are advantageous or simply interesting—become more and more intense, extended (through irradiation) and stable, owing to the same mechanism as in the case of the war hysteria mentioned earlier, as well as to their emotional reinforcement. Naturally, in a weak subject, an invalid in life, unable to win by positive qualities respect, attention and favour of other people, the latter motive acts most and contributes to the prolongation and fixation of the morbid symptoms. Hence, one of the most striking features of hysteria is the desire to be ill, to take refuge in illness.

Along with positive symptoms, there are negative ones, which are produced in the central nervous system not by the process of excitation, but by the inhibition process, for instance, analgesia and paralysis. They attract special attention, and some clinicians (for example, Hoche in a recent article) regard them as specifically hysterical symptoms which seem absolutely incomprehensible. But this is an obvious misunderstanding: they do not differ in any way from positive symptoms. Do not we, normal people, constantly repress some of our movements and words, i.e., do not we send inhibitory impulses to definite points of the cerebral hemispheres? As pointed out in our physiological introduction, in the laboratory we constantly elaborate, along with conditioned positive stimuli, conditioned negative stimuli. In hypnosis by means of stimulating words we produce anaesthesia, analgesia, general immobility or inability to move certain parts of the body, functional paralysis. A hysterical person often can and must be regarded, even in normal conditions, as being in a chronic state of hypnosis to a certain degree, since owing to the weakness of his cortex, ordinary stimuli become super-powerful and are accompanied by a diffused transmarginal inhibition, just as in the paradoxical phase of hypnosis observed in our animals. Therefore, besides the fixed inhibitory symptoms, which, like the positive ones, appear at the moment of violent nervous trauma, the same inhibitory symptoms may arise in a hysterical hypnotic as a result of suggestion or auto-suggestion. Any notion of an inhibitory effect evoked either by fear, interest or advantage, repeatedly concentrates and intensifies in the cortex and, owing to the emotivity of the hysterical person, just as in hypnosis the word of the hypnotist, provokes these symptoms and fixes them for a long time, until, finally, a stronger wave of excitation effaces these inhibitory points.

The same mechanism of auto-suggestion produces in a hysterical person a multitude of other symptoms, some of which are rather ordinary and frequent and some extraordinary and highly peculiar.

Any slight sensation of pain or the slightest anomaly in any organic function engenders in a hysterical person the fear of becoming seriously ill; and this suffices not only to maintain these sensations, again by means of the above-described mechanism, but to reinforce them and bring to such a pitch of intensity as to render the subject invalid. However, this time it is not the positive aspect of the sensation that is responsible for its frequent reproduction and predominant action in the cortex, as is the case in war hysteria, but, on the contrary, its negative aspect. This, naturally, makes no difference as regards the essence of the physiological process. Unquestioned cases of phantom pregnancy accompanied by corresponding changes in the mammary glands, by an accumulation of fat in the abdominal wall, etc., are examples of peculiar manifestations of hysterical auto-suggestion. This is further confirmation of what has been said in the physiological introduction to this article concerning the cortical representation not only of the activity of all organs, but of separate tissues. At the same time this testifies to the extreme emotivity of hysterical persons. It is true that in this case the maternal instinct, powerful in itself, reproduces by auto-suggestion such a complex and specific state of the organism as pregnancy, at least certain of its components. The same mechanism is responsible for the states and stigmas of religious ecstatics. It is a historical fact that the Christian martyrs endured their tortures with patience, even with joy, and when dying, lauded those for whom they sacrificed themselves; this is striking proof of the power of auto-suggestion, i.e., of the strength of concentrated excitation in a definite cortical region, excitation accompanied by a very intense inhibition of all other parts of the cortex representing, so to speak, the fundamental interests of the entire organism, its integrity, its existence. If the power of suggestion and auto-suggestion is so great that even the destruction of the organism can take place without the slightest physiological resistance on its part, then, in view of the already proved high ability of the cortex to influence the processes of the organism, it is easy to understand from the physiological point of view the partial violation of the organism's integrity produced by suggestion and auto-suggestion by means of trophic innervation, the existence of which has been also proved.

It is, therefore, impossible not to see the erroneousness of the extreme point of view put forward by Babinski,[56] although in general he correctly appraises the fundamental mechanism of hysteria. In his view the only symptom that should be regarded as hysterical, is the one provoked or eliminated by suggestion. This conclusion overlooks the extreme intensity and incessant action of the given emotivity, which cannot be produced in a full measure deliberately by suggestion, especially since the real cause and nature of this emotivity may remain unrevealed.

Finally, it is necessary to touch on the fantasticism of hysterical persons, on their detachment from reality and frequent twilight states. It can be assumed that these symptoms are interconnected. As shown by the observations made by Bernheim[57] and others on hypnotised normal subjects, as well as by our observations on dogs mentioned in the physiological part of this article, we must distinguish in hypnotism a number of gradations, beginning with a state, which hardly differs from wakefulness and ending with complete sleep.

In order to embrace and fully understand all the degrees of hypnosis, especially in man, I think it is necessary to dwell on the following problems, which have not only been insufficiently elaborated by science, but are not even properly formulated.

Life clearly reveals two groups of human beings: artists and thinkers. There is a striking difference between them. The first group, artists of all kinds—writers, musicians, painters, etc., perceive reality as a single whole, i.e., the entire living reality without breaking it up or decomposing it. The other group, the thinkers, on the contrary, dismember it, thereby, as it were, killing it and making of it a kind of temporary skeleton; only afterwards do they gradually as if anew assemble its parts and try to revive it, but this, however, they are unable fully to accomplish. This difference is particularly manifest in the so-called eudetism of children. I recall a case which greatly amazed me forty or fifty years ago. In a family of a marked artistic disposition the parents used to entertain their two- or three-year-old child (and amuse themselves at the same time) by showing him a collection of twenty or thirty photos of different relatives, writers, actors, etc., and simultaneously pronouncing their names. The effect was that the child memorised the photos and then called all the persons represented on them by their proper names. But how great was the general surprise one day when it was discovered that the child could give the right names by looking even at the back of the photo. Apparently in this case the brain, the cerebral hemispheres, perceived the optic stimulations in exactly the same way as a photographic plate reacts to the fluctuations of the intensity of light or as a phonographic disc records the sounds. And this, perhaps, is the essential feature of any kind of artistic faculty. Generally, such an integral reproduction of reality is inaccessible to a thinker. That is why the combination in one and the same person of great artist and great thinker is an exceedingly rare phenomenon. In the overwhelming majority of cases they are represented by different individuals. Of course, in the mass there are intermediates.

I believe that there are definite physiological grounds, although as yet not very convincing, for interpreting the matter in the following way. In the artist the activity of the cerebral hemispheres, while developing throughout their entire mass, least of all involves the frontal lobes and concentrates mainly in other parts; in the thinker, on the contrary, it is most intense in the frontal lobes.

Repeating what I have just said, for the sake of systematisation, I view the higher nervous activity as a whole like this. In higher animals, including man, the first system establishing complex correlations between the organism and the external environment is represented by the subcortex adjacent to the cerebral hemispheres with its highly complex unconditioned reflexes (in our terminology), or instincts, drives, affects, emotions (in the usual diverse terminology). These reflexes are produced by a relatively limited number of unconditioned external agents, or in other words, those which act right from the day of birth. Hence, a limited capacity of orientation in relation to the surrounding world and at the same time a low degree of adaptation. The second system is represented by the cerebral hemispheres, excluding, however, the frontal lobes. It is here that a new principle of activity arises with the help of conditioned connection or association—the signalisation of a limited number of unconditioned external agents by a countless number of other agents, which at the same time are constantly subjected to analysis and synthesis and ensure very wide orientation in relation to the same medium and thereby a much higher degree of adaptation. This is the only signalling system in the animal organism and the first signalling system in man. In the latter another system of signalisation is added; it can be assumed that this system relates to the frontal lobes,[58] which in animals are much less developed than in man. It represents a signalisation of the first signalling system by means of speech and of its basis or basal component—kinesthetic stimulations of the speech organs. In this way a new principle of nervous activity arises—abstraction and at the same time generalisation of the countless signals of the first signalling system which is again accompanied by analysis and synthesis of the new generalised signals—a principle which ensures unrestricted orientation in relation to the surrounding world and the highest degree of adaptation, namely, science, both in the form of human universal empiricism and in specialised forms. This second system of signalisation and its organ, representing the latest acquisition in the process of evolution, are bound to be most fragile and susceptible to diffused inhibition when it arises in the cerebral hemispheres at the initial stages of hypnosis. Then, instead of the activity of the second signalling system, usually predominant in the alert state, the activity of the first system comes to the fore, liberated from the regulating influence of the second system; at first it takes the more stable form of reverie and fantastic imagination and subsequently the more acute form of a twilight state or light sleep (corresponding to the intermediate state between sleep and wakefulness or to the state of falling asleep). Hence the chaotic character of this activity, which no longer reckons with reality, or if it does, then only slightly, and is mainly dependent on the emotional influences of the subcortex.

From what has been said it will not be difficult to appreciate from the physiological point of view what the clinicians term disturbance of psychical synthesis in hysteria (the expression used by Pierre Janet) or the split "ego" (Raymond's expression). Instead of a co-ordinated and well-equilibrated activity of the three systems mentioned, in hysteria this activity is continually dissociated, and the natural and law-governed interdependence of the systems is deranged; meanwhile the interconnection and proper interdependence of the work of these systems constitute the foundation of a sane personality and underlie the integrity of our "ego".

In the final analysis, different combinations of the following three particular physiological phenomena are constantly manifest and make themselves felt against the fundamental background of cortical weakness in hysterical persons: quick susceptibility to varying degrees of hypnotic states due to the fact that even normal life stimuli are super-powerful and are accompanied by transmarginal diffused inhibition (the paradoxical phase); extreme fixation and concentration of the nervous processes in definite points of the cortex due to the predominance of the subcortex; and, finally, undue intensity and extensity of negative induction, i.e., of inhibition caused by low resistibility of the positive tone of other cortical parts.

In conclusion, I take the liberty of saying a few words about hysterical psychoses. A case of this kind of psychosis has been demonstrated to me; it is a case of hysterical puerilism in a woman of more than forty, who became ill as a result of severe shocks experienced in family life. She was unexpectedly deserted by her husband who some time later also deprived her of her child. After an attack of stupor and a general prolonged paresis the woman sank into dotage. At present she behaves like a child, without, however, manifesting any obvious general defects in the intellectual and moral sphere or in personal life. A closer examination of the patient shows that everything seems to be accounted for exclusively by the absence of the analytical inhibition which always accompanies our behaviour, our movements, words and thoughts and which distinguishes the adult from the child. Does not the development of our personality consist in the fact that under the influence of education and religious, social and civic requirements, we gradually learn to inhibit, to repress that which is not admitted, which is prohibited by the factors just mentioned? Is not our behaviour in the family circle or in the company of friends quite different in all respects from that under other conditions? The universal experiments of life prove this beyond all doubt. Do we not constantly encounter the fact that in fits of passion, which overcome the cortical inhibition, men speak and act in a manner which they regard as inadmissible when they are calm? And do they not bitterly regret such behaviour when the fit of passion recedes? This is particularly evident in the state of alcohol intoxication when all brakes are abruptly switched off, as aptly expressed in the Russian proverb: to the drunkard the sea seems up to his knee.

Will this patient ever return to a normal state? Well, it depends. The psychiatrists affirm that in youth such a state persists only for hours or days, although it is sometimes more protracted. In the given case it is a state of relative calm and satisfaction; it is probably determined by the previously described nervous mechanism, which makes the patient take refuge in illness in order to escape the difficulties of life and owing to which this pathological state may in the end become irremediably habitual. On the other hand, the disturbed and overstrained inhibition may weaken and disappear altogether.

Is hysteria in general a curable disease from the physiological point of view? In this respect everything depends on the type of nervous system. It is true that the predominant and encouraging impression produced by our work on conditioned reflexes in dogs is that the cerebral hemispheres offer great possibilities for their training, although naturally these possibilities are not unlimited. When dealing with an extremely weak type we can, in exceptional, so to speak, hot-house experimental conditions, obtain an improvement, a regularisation of the animal's general conditioned reflex activity, and nothing more. A durable transformation of the type is, of course, out of the question. But since certain hysterical reactions of a general physiological character can also take place in more or less strong types as a result of powerful stimulations or violent shocks, a full return to the normal is, of course, possible in this case. However, the return can occur only if the series of shocks and excessive stimulations do not overstep their limits.

While it is impossible to read without keen interest the really brilliant pamphlet by Kretschmer on hysteria, in which the author reveals a strong and almost constant tendency to interpret the hysterical symptoms physiologically, Hoche's article in *Deutsche Medizinische Wochenschrift* in its January issue this year, makes a strange impression. Is it really the case that modern physiological knowledge does not throw any light on the mechanism of hysteria, that the clinic and physiology "have halted before hysteria as they would at closed doors"? The following reasoning in Hoche's article seems quite strange. Adhering to the view that analgesiae and paralyses constitute the fundamental feature of hysteria, he addresses the supporters of the theory of the pathogenic force of motives in hysteria with the question: Why would the strong indignation felt by some of his listeners and readers in consequence of his adverse opinion of the above-mentioned theory not render them insensitive to pain, if it were caused by a faradic current of high intensity? Then he cites other analogous cases: for example, why are the patients not cured by a similar method, i.e., by a strong desire to get rid of their illness, of their neuralgiae? In this connection I recall an instance from my student days which deeply impressed me and all who witnessed it. A young woman was undergoing a plastic operation on her nose which had been dreadfully deformed by some disease. Right in the middle of the operation the woman, to everyone's surprise, suddenly made a calm remark in response to something said by the professor performing the operation. Evidently, the anaesthesia (which was general) had practically no effect. Yet the same woman attracted general attention by the fact that during the daily dressing of the post-operative wound she exhibited extreme sensitivity to pain. Clearly the strong desire to get rid of the deformity, probably intensified by sexual emotion, rendered the woman insensitive to the operation trauma and made her hope and believe that the surgical intervention would end in complete success. But after the operation, at any rate for a period immediately after it, when the coarse, strange-looking artificial nose bitterly and cruelly disappointed her, the same emotion, on the contrary, rendered her highly sensitive even to what was now carefully done to her nose.

Many cases of this kind are met in everyday life, as well as in history. When dealing with such cases, it is necessary to take into account: in strong and normal individuals the harmonious complex of strong emotions and of predominant cortical associations accompanied by an equally strong negative induction in all other parts of the cerebral hemispheres; in the weak nervous type—the hysterical mechanism described above.

PHYSIOLOGY
OF HIGHER NERVOUS ACTIVITY[59]

Since this, I suppose, is my last opportunity to address a general meeting of my colleagues, I shall take the liberty of calling your attention to the general, most systematised and summarised results of my recent work, which I have carried out jointly with my esteemed fellow-workers and which comprises a full half of my entire physiological activity; naturally, I shall repeat many of the already published facts. I pass on to you the results of our work, passionately dreaming of the majestic, ever-widening horizon opening up before our science, and of the ever-growing influence exerted by science on human nature and human destiny.

For the anatomist and histologist the cerebral hemispheres have always been as accessible and tangible as any other organ or any other tissue, i.e., that they possess similar workability and are susceptible of investigation, but, of course, commensurately with their specific properties and construction. Quite different was the position of the physiologist. Every organ of the animal body, the general role of which in the organism is known, its actual function, and the conditions and mechanism of this function, are objects of study. As to the cerebral hemispheres, their role is well known—they effect the organism's most complex relations with the environment; but the physiologist did not engage in a further study of their activity. For him the study of the cerebral hemispheres did not begin with the concrete reproduction of their activity, only after which the gradual analysis of the conditions and mechanism of this activity is possible. The physiologist possessed many facts relating to the cerebral hemispheres, but these facts were not manifestly and closely connected with their usual normal activity.

Today, after thirty years of diligent and ceaseless work jointly with my numerous collaborators, I make bold to say that the situation has radically changed, that while remaining physiologists, i.e., the same objective observers as in all other branches of physiology, we are studying at present the normal activity of the cerebral hemispheres and at the same time constantly analysing it in ever-increasing measure. The generally recognised criteria for every true scientific activity, namely, precise prevision and control over phenomena, testify to the serious character of this study, which is irrepressibly advancing, overcoming all obstacles. An ever-growing number of relations which constitute the most complex external activity of the higher animal organism, unfolds before us.

The central physiological phenomenon in the normal work of the cerebral hemispheres is that which we have termed the *conditioned reflex*. This is a temporary nervous connection between numberless agents in the animal's external environment, which are received by the receptors of the given animal, and the definite activities of the organism. This phenomenon is called by psychologists *association*. The fundamental physiological significance of this connection is as follows: in the higher animal, for example, in the dog which was the object of our investigations, the basic, most complex correlations established between the organism and the environment in order to preserve the individual and the species, are determined first of all by the activities of the subcortex which is nearest to the cerebral hemispheres; this was demonstrated long ago in Goltz's experiment with the extirpation of the cerebral hemispheres in a dog. These activities include the search for food, or the alimentary activity; the avoidance of injurious factors, or the defensive activity, etc. They are usually called instincts or inclinations; psychologists term them *emotions*, but we designate them by the physiological term *most complex unconditioned reflexes*. They exist from the very day of birth and are indispensably called forth by definite, though very limited in number, stimuli which are sufficient only in early childhood, under the conditions of parental care. It is this latter circumstance that makes an animal with extirpated cerebral hemispheres disabled, incapable of a self-dependent existence. The basic physiological function of the cerebral hemispheres throughout the subsequent individual life consists in a constant addition of numberless signalling conditioned stimuli to the limited number of the initial, inborn unconditioned stimuli, in other words, in constantly supplementing the unconditioned reflexes by conditioned ones. Thus, the objects of the instincts exert an influence on the organism in ever-widening regions of nature and by means of more and more diverse signs or signals, both simple and more complex; consequently, the instincts are more and more fully and perfectly satisfied, i.e., the organism is more reliably preserved in the surrounding nature.

The basic condition for the formation of a conditioned reflex is a single or repeated coincidence in time of indifferent stimuli with unconditioned reflexes. This is the same principle of coincidence in time, on the basis of which groups of various agents or elements of nature, both simultaneous and consecutive, are synthesised by the animal into units. In this way the *synthesis* is effected in general.

But owing to the complexity of the permanent movement and variation of the natural phenomena, the conditioned reflex must, of course, also undergo certain changes, i.e., be constantly corrected. If for some reason or other the conditioned stimulus in the given conditions is not accompanied by its unconditioned stimulus, then, when repeated, it quickly loses its effect, however, temporarily, being restored spontaneously, after a certain lapse of time. If the conditioned stimulus constantly and greatly precedes in time the moment when the unconditioned stimulus is added, then its distant part, which is, so to speak, premature and violates the principle of economy, proves ineffective. When the conditioned stimulus, connected with another indifferent one, is permanently not accompanied by an unconditioned stimulus, it remains, in this combination, ineffective. Finally, if agents closely akin to the given elaborated conditioned stimulus (for example, close tones, other spots of the skin, etc.) are usually effective immediately after the elaboration of the first one, they gradually lose their effect when repeated later on without the accompaniment of the unconditioned stimulus, or, in our usual terminology, without reinforcement. All this ensures the differentiation, the *analysis* of the surrounding world with all of its elements and moments.

In the long run, the cerebral hemispheres of the dog constantly effect in the most varying degrees both the *analysis* and *synthesis* of stimuli coming to them, and this can and must be termed *elementary, concrete thinking*. And it follows that this thinking is responsible for the perfect adaptation of the organism, for its more delicate equilibration with the environment.

This real activity of the cerebral hemispheres and of the nearest subcortex, just described in general outline, the activity which ensures normal complex relations between the organism as a whole and the external world, must be rightly considered and denoted as *higher nervous activity*, the external behaviour of the animal, instead of "psychical" as it was termed previously; it should be distinguished from the activity of other parts of the brain and of the spinal cord which are mainly in charge of the correlations and integration of separate parts of the organism; this activity should be termed the *lower nervous activity*.

Now the following questions arise: What intrinsic processes and laws govern the higher nervous activity? What has it in common with, and how does it differ from, the lower nervous activity which until now has been the predominant object of physiological study?

The basic processes of the entire central nervous activity are, obviously, always the same, namely, the excitatory and inhibitory processes. There are sufficient grounds for assuming that the fundamental laws governing these processes are also of a constant nature—irradiation and concentration of the processes and their reciprocal induction.

It seems to me that experiments with conditioned reflexes on the cerebral hemispheres, given normal conditions, permit a more complete and exact formulation of these laws than was possible on the basis of experiments performed mainly on the lower parts of the central nervous system, and which, in most cases, were acute experiments.

Concerning the cerebral hemispheres we can say that the following phenomenon is observed in them: when the excitatory and inhibitory processes are weak, then, under the action of corresponding stimuli there takes place irradiation, diffusion of the processes from the point of origin; when they are of medium strength, a concentration of the processes occurs at the point of application of the stimulus, and when they are very strong, irradiation is again in evidence.

In the entire central nervous system, on the basis of irradiation of the excitatory process, a summation reflex sets in, i.e., a summation of the spreading wave of excitation with a local manifest or latent excitation; in the latter case the latent tonus becomes revealed—a phenomenon already known for a long time. While in the cerebral hemispheres the confluence of waves irradiating from various points leads to a quick development of a temporary connection, to an association of these points, it bears a momentary, transient character in the remaining part of the central nervous system. This connection in the cerebral hemispheres probably owes its emergence to their extremely high reactivity and ability to impress, and is a permanent and inherent property of this part of the central nervous system. Moreover, in the cerebral hemispheres the irradiation of the excitatory process instantly and for a short period of time eliminates, washes off the inhibition from the inhibitory, negative points of the hemispheres, converting these points for the same period of time into positive ones. This phenomenon is called disinhibition.

Under the irradiation of the inhibitory process there is observed a decline or complete disappearance of the effect of the positive points and an increased effect of the negative points.

When the excitatory and inhibitory processes are concentrated, they induce the opposite processes (both at the periphery during their action and in the place of action upon its termination); this is the law of reciprocal induction.

In the entire central nervous system when there is a concentration of the excitatory process, we meet with phenomena of inhibition. The point of concentration of the excitation is encircled to a greater or lesser extent by the inhibitory process; this is the phenomenon of negative induction. This phenomenon manifests itself in all reflexes, develops at once and in full measure, persists for some time after the termination of excitation and exists both between the small points and the large parts of the brain. We call this external, passive, unconditioned inhibition. This phenomenon, which has also been known for a long time, was sometimes called the conflict of centres.

There are in the cerebral hemispheres also other kinds or cases of inhibition, in all probability, having one and the same physicochemical substratum. This is, in the first place, the inhibition effecting the correction of the conditioned reflexes, already mentioned and arising when the conditioned stimulus in the above-indicated conditions is not accompanied by its unconditioned stimulus; it gradually grows, becomes stronger and can be trained and perfected; this, too, is due to the exceptional reactivity of the cortical cells, and hence to the particular lability of inhibition in them. We call this inhibition internal, active, conditioned. The stimuli, which are thus converted into permanent agents of inhibition in the points of the cerebral hemispheres, are called by us inhibitory, negative. Similar inhibitory stimuli can be also obtained in another way—if we repeatedly apply indifferent stimuli during the inhibitory state of the cerebral hemispheres (experiments of Prof. Volborth[60]). As is known, the initial inhibitory reflexes are also developed in the lower parts of the brain and in the spinal cord; but here they appear at once in a finished and stereotyped form, while the same inhibitory reflexes of the cerebral hemispheres arise gradually and are always observed by us in the process of formation.

There is one more case of inhibition in the cerebral hemispheres. All other conditions being equal, the effect of conditioned stimulation, as a rule, is proportionate to the intensity of the physical strength of the stimulus, but to a certain maximum (and probably to a certain minimum, too). Beyond this limit the effect does not increase; it either remains unchanged or declines. We have grounds for assuming that beyond this margin the stimulus together with the excitatory process evoke also an inhibitory process. We interpret this fact in the following way. The cortical cell possesses a certain limit of efficiency, and beyond this point there arises inhibition which prevents an excessive functional exhaustion of the cell. The limit of efficiency is not constant; it undergoes both acute and chronic changes—in cases of inanition, hypnosis, disease and in old age. This inhibition, which can be called transmarginal, arises sometimes instantaneously and sometimes manifests itself only when the super-powerful stimuli are repeated. It can be assumed that analogical inhibition also exists in the lower parts of the central nervous system.

Peculiar internal inhibition could also be considered as transmarginal inhibition, in which case the intensity of excitation is, as it were, replaced by its long duration.

Any inhibition irradiates in the same way as excitation but the irradiation of internal inhibition is particularly distinct in the cerebral hemispheres where it is very easily observed in various forms and degrees. There is no doubt that inhibition, when spreading and deepening, calls forth different degrees of a hynotic state, and when irradiating to the utmost from the cerebral hemispheres down the brain, produces normal sleep. Particularly manifest, even in our dogs, is the diversity and multiplicity of the stages of hypnosis, which at first hardly differs from the wakeful state. In respect of intensity of inhibition the following stages are worth mentioning: the so-called equalisation, paradoxical and ultraparadoxical phases. Now conditioned stimuli of different physical strength produce either an equal, or even an inversely proportional effect; in rare cases only the inhibitory stimuli act positively, and the positive stimuli are converted into inhibitory ones. In respect of extensity of inhibition, functional dissociations in the cortex itself are observed, as well as between the cortex and the lower parts of the brain. In the cortex the motor region is particularly often isolated from other regions, and even within this region a distinct functional dissociation sometimes comes to the fore.

Unfortunately, the rivalry of what the clinicians and some experimenters designate "the centre of sleep" prevents these facts from being generally recognised and properly utilised for an understanding of the multitude of physiological and pathological phenomena. However, it is not difficult to reconcile and combine these facts. Sleep can be originated in two ways—either by irradiation of inhibition from the cortex, or by limiting the stimulations reaching the higher parts of the brain both from without and from within the organism. Strümpell[61] long ago produced sleep in a patient by means of drastic limitation of external stimulations. Recently Prof. Speransky and Galkin[62] by means of a peripheral destruction of the olfactory, auditory and visual receptors in dogs obtained a very deep and chronic sleep (lasting weeks and months). Similarly, as a result of a pathological or experimental exclusion of stimulations, constantly reaching the higher part of the brain there sets in due to the vegetative activity of the organism an exaggerated and more or less profound and chronic sleep. It can be recognised that in some of these cases too, sleep, in the final stage, is produced by similar inhibition which becomes predominant when the number of stimuli is limited.

The law of reciprocal induction begins to operate when there is a concentration of the inhibitory process, just as it does when there is a concentration of the excitatory process. The point of concentration of the inhibition is to a greater or lesser extent encircled by the process of heightened excitability; this is the phenomenon of positive induction. The heightened excitability arises either instantly or gradually and persists not only during the action of inhibition, but for some time after, and in some cases even for a quite considerable length of time. The positive induction manifests itself between the small points of the cortex, when the inhibition is fragmentary, as well as between the large parts of the brain, when it is more diffused.

The permanent operation of the above-mentioned laws helps us to understand the mechanism of the origin of the numerous separate phenomena (among which are many peculiar, at first sight enigmatic, phenomena) of the higher nervous activity; however, I cannot dwell on them here. I shall refer only to one of a series of similar cases which for a long time completely baffled comprehension. It relates to the complex influence of accessory stimuli on the delayed conditioned reflex (experiments performed a long time ago by our colleague Zavadsky).

Let us suppose that a delayed conditioned reflex is being elaborated, the conditioned stimulation constantly lasting three minutes before the unconditioned stimulus is added to it. When such a reflex has been elaborated, the conditioned stimulus does not produce any effect during the first minute. Half-way through or towards the end of the second minute the stimulus begins to produce a certain effect, and maximum effect is attained only during the third minute. Thus, the conditioned reflex consists of two external phases—ineffective and effective. Special experiments, however, have established that the first phase is not a zero phase, but an inhibitory one.

Now, if simultaneously with the conditioned stimulus there are applied accessory stimuli of different intensity calling forth only an orienting reaction, a number of changes are observed in the delayed reflex. When the stimulation is weak the ineffective phase becomes effective, that is, the special effect of the conditioned stimulus is manifested; the effect of the second phase either remains unchanged or is slightly increased.

When the stimulation is more intense the same thing occurs with the first phase, but the effect of the second phase drastically declines. Under the strongest stimulation the first phase again remains ineffective, while the effect of the second completely disappears. At present, on the basis of the latest, not yet published, experiments carried out by our colleague Rikman, we interpret all these phenomena as a result of the operation of the following four laws: 1) irradiation of the excitatory process, 2) negative induction, 3) summation, and 4) the law of maximum. Given a weak orienting reflex the spreading wave of excitation eliminates the inhibition of the first phase; this reflex, which soon all but disappears when the same stimulation is continued, either does not influence the second phase at all, or, owing to a slight summation, somewhat intensifies it. With a more considerable orienting reflex the effect persists longer; consequently, along with the disinhibition of the first phase, due to a considerable summation of the effective phase of the conditioned reflex with the irradiated wave of excitation of the orienting reflex, transmarginal inhibition takes place during the last minute of the delayed reflex. Finally, given a very strong orienting reflex there takes place a complete concentration of excitation accompanied by a strong negative induction which merges with the inhibition of the first phase and abolishes the effective phase.

Despite the fact that a multitude of particular relations between the excitatory and inhibitory processes have been studied by us, the general law of the interconnection of these processes cannot, as yet, be exactly formulated. As for the profound mechanism of both processes, many of our experimental facts incline us to the point of view that the inhibitory process is probably connected with assimilation, just as the excitatory process is naturally connected with dissimilation.

As for the so-called *voluntary volitional movements*, in this field, too, we have accumulated some material. In keeping with earlier investigations we have shown that the motor region of the cortex is first of all a receptor one, like all its other regions—visual, auditory, etc., since the animal's passive movements, i.e., the kinesthetic stimuli of this region can be transformed by us into conditioned stimuli in the same way as all external stimuli. Another ordinary phenomenon, reproduced by us also in the laboratory, is the temporary connection established between various external stimuli and passive movements which in response to certain signals evokes definite active movements of the animal. However, it is still not clear whether the connection between the kinesthetic stimulus and the corresponding motor action is of an unconditioned or of a conditioned character. Beyond this extreme point the entire *mechanism of volitional movement is a conditioned associative process* which obeys all the above-mentioned laws of the higher nervous activity.

The cerebral hemispheres are continually receiving countless stimuli both from the external world and the internal medium of the organism itself. These stimuli are conducted from the periphery along definite and numerous paths and, consequently, they first of all come to definite points and areas in the mass of the brain. Thus we have before us in the first place a highly complex structure, a mosaic. Countless and varied positive processes enter the cortex along the conductor paths, and in the cortex itself they are joined by inhibitory processes. From each of the separate states of the cortical cells (and there is an infinite number of such states) a specific conditioned stimulus may arise, as constantly observed by us in the course of our investigation of the conditioned reflexes. All these meet, collide, must come together and be systematised. Thus, in the second place, we have a vast dynamic system.[63] We observe and study in the conditioned reflexes of our normal dogs this continual systematisation of the processes, this, one may say, constant tendency towards a dynamic stereotype. Here is a most illustrative fact. If we elaborate in an animal a number of conditioned positive as well as inhibitory reflexes from stimuli of different intensity, and apply them during a certain period of time from day to day at regular intervals between the stimuli and always in a definite order, we establish thereby a stereotype of processes in the cerebral hemispheres. This can be easily demonstrated. If we now repeatedly apply throughout the experiment at equal intervals only one of the positive conditioned stimuli (better, one of the weak stimuli), it will reproduce in the proper sequence the fluctuations in the strength of the effects, as they were represented by the entire system of the various acting stimuli.

Not only the establishment, but a more or less lasting maintenance of the dynamic stereotype, is a nervous task of considerable difficulty, the degree of which depends on the complexity of the stereotype and on the individuality of the animal. There are, of course, nervous tasks the solution of which requires even from animals of the strong nervous type painful efforts. Other animals react to any simple change in the system of conditioned reflexes, such as the introduction of a new stimulus, or even to a certain transposition of the old stimuli, by complete loss of the conditioned reflex activity, sometimes lasting for a considerable period. Some animals can retain the proper system only if there are recesses in the experiments, i.e., if they are allowed certain rest. And finally, some animals show regular work only under a very simplified system of reflexes, consisting, for example, of two stimuli, both of them positive and of equal intensity.

It can be assumed that the *nervous processes in the cerebral hemispheres, when establishing and maintaining a dynamic stereotype,* are what we usually call *senses* in their two categories—positive and negative, and their extensive gradation of intensity. The processes of establishing a stereotype, of fully accomplishing it, of its maintenance and derangement are subjectively different positive and negative senses, and that has always been manifested in the motor reactions of the animals.

Our entire work gradually enabled us to establish various types of nervous system in our animals. Since the cerebral hemispheres are the most reactive and supreme part of the central nervous system, their individual properties, naturally, must determine to a great extent the principal nature of the general activity of each animal. Our systematisation of types coincides with the ancient classification of the so-called tempéraments. There is the type with a strong excitatory process, but a relatively weak inhibitory process. Animals belonging to this type are aggressive and unrestrained. We call them strong and excitable or choleric. Next comes the type of strong and at the same time equilibrated animals, in which both processes are of equal strength. This is an easily disciplined and highly practical type which is met in two variations— quiet, sedate animals and active, lively ones. We name them respectively phlegmatic and sanguine. And finally, there is the weak inhibitable type, in which both processes are weak. We call such animals weak and also inhibitable since they are highly susceptible to external inhibition. They are cowardly and fussy and can be also characterised as melancholic, since everything constantly upsets them.

That our investigation of the higher nervous activity has taken the right road, and our definition of its phenomena, as well as our analysis of its mechanism are correct, is most convincingly proved by the fact that at present we are able in many cases to produce with great exactitude its functional chronic disturbances, and at the same time subsequently to obtain a return to the normal at will. We know which type of our animals can be easily turned into neurotics, we know how to achieve this, and the kind of disorder that will set in. The strong, but unequilibrated, excitable and weak inhibitable types prove to be the best objects for the elaboration of experimental neuroses. If an excitable animal is persistently offered such tasks, the solution of which requires strong inhibition, then it loses it completely and is deprived of the ability to correct the conditioned reflexes, i.e., ceases to analyse, to distinguish the stimuli reaching it as well as the intervals of time. Stimulations produced by the strongest agents have no noxious pathological influence in this case. With equal ease the weak inhibitable type becomes ill both under slightly strained inhibition and under the action of very strong stimuli; it either fully loses its conditioned reflex activity under our experimental conditions, or manifests it in a chaotic way. As for the animals of the equilibrated type, we did not succeed in inducing nervous disorders in them even by colliding the opposite processes, which is a particularly morbific method.

Bromide proved to be the most reliable remedy against neuroses, just as it is in the human clinic; as shown by our numerous and in many respects instructive experiments, it has a special bearing on the inhibitory process, greatly tonifying it. However, very strict dosage is essential; for the weak type the dose of bromide must be from five to eight times smaller than that for the strong type. Rest, i.e., a recess in the experiments, often produces good results.

Among animals of the weak type there are frequent instances of natural neurotics.

We already have and we can even produce certain symptoms of psychotics: stereotypy, negativism and circularity.

Last year I specially acquainted myself with the clinic of human hysteria, which is regarded as being entirely or predominantly a mental disease, as a psychogenic reaction to the surroundings; as a result, I have become convinced that its symptomatology can, without any hesitation, be interpreted physiologically, from the point of view of the described physiology of the higher nervous activity, and I have expressed the conviction in the press.[64] However, some particulars of this symptomatology made us guess the existence of an addition which should be taken into consideration in order to get a general idea of the human nervous activity as well.[65] This addition relates to the speech function, which signifies a new principle in the activity of the cerebral hemispheres. If our sensations and notions caused by the surrounding world are for us the first signals of reality, concrete signals, then speech, especially and primarily the kinesthetic stimuli which proceed from the speech organs to the cortex, constitute a second set of signals, the signals of signals. They represent an abstraction from reality and make possible the forming of generalisations; this constitutes our extra, *specially human, higher mentality* creating an empiricism general to all men and then, in the end, science, the instrument of the higher orientation of man in the surrounding world and in himself. The extreme fantasticism, the twilight states of hysterical persons, and the dreams of all men, are nothing more than the vitalisation of the imaginative and concrete first signals, as well as of the emotions; the oncoming hypnotic state first of all switches off the organ of the system of the second signals—the most reactive part of the brain, which always predominantly functions in the wakeful state, and which regulates, and at the same time to a certain degree inhibits both the first signals and emotional activity.

The frontal lobes, in all probability, represent the organ of this additional purely human mentality, but it can be assumed that it is subordinated to the same general laws of the higher nervous activity.

The foregoing facts, as well as the considerations based on them, are bound to lead to the closest connection between physiology and psychology—a development particularly observed in American psychology. In the 1931 Address of Walter Hunter, President of the American Psychological Association, despite strenuous efforts on the part of the speaker—who is a psychologist-behaviourist—to detach physiology from his psychology, it is absolutely impossible to see any difference between them. But even psychologists not belonging to the camp of behaviourists admit that our experiments with the conditioned reflexes have been of great help to the association theory of the psychologists. Other facts of a like nature could be cited.

I am convinced that an important stage in the development of human thought is approaching, a stage when the physiological and the psychological, the objective and the subjective, will really merge, when the painful contradiction between our mind and our body and their contraposition will either *actually* be solved or disappear in a natural way. Indeed, when the objective study of the higher animals, for example, the dog, reaches the level when the physiologist is able to foresee with absolute exactitude the behaviour of this animal under any conditions (and this level will be reached), then what will be left to prove the independent, separate existence of the subjective state, which the animal, of course, possesses but which is as peculiar as our own? When that occurs will not the activity of any living thing, man included, be indispensably regarded by us as a single, indivisible whole?

EXAMPLE OF AN EXPERIMENTALLY PRODUCED NEUROSIS AND ITS CURE IN A WEAK TYPE OF NERVOUS SYSTEM[66]

Last year I reported to the International Neurological Congress in Bern on our experimental neuroses only in most general outlines. Today I shall cite in detail an individual example of neurosis but recently thoroughly studied by Petrova, one of my oldest and most valuable collaborators.

In questions of pure experimental neuroses we cannot fail to begin with the question of the types of nervous system of animals (in our case—dogs). We distinguish three basic types: *strong*, even very strong, but *unbalanced*, in which inhibition is weak in relation to the excitatory process; *strong* and *balanced*, i.e., with both antagonistic processes on the same level, and *weak*, i.e., with both weak processes, but sometimes with either one or the other particularly weak. Of course, there are also different degrees or variations of these types, especially, the weak type. We have a considerable number of tests by which we determine these types and their degrees. We elaborate these tests gradually and in some cases must use them all for an unmistakable diagnosis.

Until now we have been able to produce pure experimental neuroses, i.e., caused only by difficult conditions of nervous activity, difficult nervous tasks, without any organic disorders only in the animals of the extreme types.

In them we can do it easily and by several methods. I shall now describe a case of a repeated neurosis in a dog of the weak type.

This dog looks like a cross between a mongrel and a fox terrier and weighs about 12 kg. By outward behaviour, work with conditioned (food) reflexes and some tests as to type, this dog was at first taken to be even a strong and balanced animal, but two subsequent tests, incontestably characterised it as a weak type. These were increased food excitability (leaving the dog without food on the eve of the experiment) and administration of considerable doses of bromides.

With increased food excitability in animals of strong types, either the effects of all conditioned positive stimuli increase (if the effects of the strong are not marginal), or (on the contrary) only the effects of the weak ones approximate to the strong.

Even large doses of bromides administered daily for many weeks and even months produce no impression on them, whereas in the strong and unbalanced types they produce even a useful effect, strengthening their inhibitory function and thus helping to regulate their nervous activity.

In our dog both these methods resulted in diminution, disturbance of the conditioned reflex activity: the effects of the positive stimuli diminished and the negative stimuli ceased to evoke total inhibition. In this case it was found that by gradually reducing the dose of bromides it was possible to reach a dose which was not only well tolerated, but which also somewhat improved the nervous activity. Earlier we made a mistake in our conclusion at this point: without suitably dosing the bromides we thought that for weak animals bromides were never beneficial and in a larger dose were even harmful.

Thus our animal belongs to the weak type, but of a moderate degree. Under usual conditions it works quite satisfactorily, since the system of six positive stimuli of different quality and strength and one negative, inhibitory stimulus, stereotypically reproduced in the same succession and with the same intervals between the stimuli every day, constantly produces the same corresponding effects in this dog. The behaviour of the dog during the experiment is rather alert and uniform. In other words, it is an object fit for studying the conditioned reflexes. We have observed this situation for a period of 5 months.

Then we produce the neurosis.

Until now the inhibitory stimulus always acted only for a period of thirty seconds. During the next experiment we continue it for five minutes. The next day we repeat a five-minute inhibition. And this is enough radically to change everything in the dog, to make the dog acutely ill.

Not a trace has been left of the regular work with conditioned reflexes. Each day there is a new picture of the work. All the positive reflexes have uncommonly diminished and some have disappeared altogether. The inhibitory reflex has become disinhibited. Sometimes the ultraparadoxical phase comes to the fore, i.e., the positive stimulus remains ineffective, and the inhibitory stimulus differentiated from it produces a positive effect. During the experiment the dog is extraordinarily excited, sometimes it has intense dyspnoea, and is very uneasy, or falls deeply asleep and snores, or manifests the highest degree of excitatory weakness by reacting sharply to the most negligible variation in the situation. It often refuses food, which is usually offered after each positive conditioned stimulus. In a word, any systematic work with conditioned reflexes on this dog is out of question and only a constantly extremely chaotic state of nervous activity is observed. The same thing is observed in the general behaviour of the dog. It has become difficult to put the dog in the stand and make it ready for the experiment, as well as to take it out of the stand after the experiment, because it is very impatient and unrestrained. Out in the open it also behaves very unusually and even strangely: for example, sprawling on the floor it lies on one side and in this manner reaches out to somebody, etc., something it was never observed to do before. The attendants who bring the dog and take it away say that it has become rather mad.

Neither suspension of the experiments, i.e., rest, nor discontinued application of the inhibitory stimulus with its positive stimulus have exerted any favourable influence on the state of the animal. This state has not in any way improved and, rather deteriorating, has lasted for two months.

Then we have instituted treatment. Thirty or forty minutes before each experiment we give the dog 0.5 g of sodium bromide. Improvement is clearly marked on the following day and on the third day the dog becomes normal in every respect. Administration of bromides is discontinued after twelve doses. The dog is normal for another ten days.

We perform another experiment.

Among the old conditioned positive stimuli, instead of the loud, although not particularly loud, crackling, we use for 30 seconds, like all the other positive stimuli, extraordinarily loud crackling, which even our ears can barely tolerate, and then offer to the dog some food. The dog displays an intense reaction of fear, tries to get out of the stand and does not take food even after cessation of the stimulus. However, it responds with the usual reaction and takes food to the two usual stimuli that follow. Application of the extraordinary stimulus is limited to this one incident, but the following day the afore-described pathological state of the dog fully returns and, despite the additional interruptions for long periods (10-15 days) and regular rests for one or two days this state has persisted unchanged for more than a month.

The dog is given the same dose of bromides again; improvement is noted on the third day and towards the sixth-eighth day we have a quite healthy, normal animal. After ten doses administration of bromides is suspended.

We have thus ended the experiments before the beginning of our present vacations.

I think we can say without exaggeration that these experiments are, as it were, of a machine character. In the first place they show two disease-producing factors for the nervous system: overstrain of the inhibitory process and very strong external stimulation. Then, as a therapeutic factor, the great importance of restoring and strengthening the inhibitory process is clearly emphasised in both cases, since, on the basis of many of our other experiments, besides the foregoing experiment, we must ascribe to bromides a direct bearing on the inhibitory process, precisely as an agent which restores and strengthens it. And, lastly, exact doses of bromides corresponding to the types and degrees of nervous system must be considered of paramount importance.

FEELINGS OF POSSESSION
(LES SENTIMENTS D'EMPRISE)
AND THE ULTRAPARADOXICAL PHASE[67]
(Open Letter to Prof. Pierre Janet)

Would you deem it interesting to print this letter in your journal and at the same time express your views on the points made by me after careful study of the article published by you last year: "Emotions of the Persecution Delusion"?

I am a physiologist and of late, together with my colleagues, have devoted myself exclusively to study of the physiological and pathological work of the higher part of the central nervous system in higher animals (dogs), which corresponds to our higher nervous activity, usually called psychical activity. You are a neurologist, psychiatrist and psychologist. It seems that we should give proper consideration to our reciprocal work and co-operate in our research, for, after all, we are investigating the activity of one and the same organ (concerning which there can hardly be any doubt now).

The third part of your article attempts to interpret the feelings of possession. The basic phenomenon is that the patients objectivise their weakness, their imperfections, and attribute them to others. They want to be independent, but they are adamant in believing that other people regard them as slaves who are obliged to execute orders. They want to be respected, but it seems to them that they are being insulted. They want to have their own secrets, but it appears to them that their secrets are constantly being disclosed. Like everybody else, they have their own intimate thoughts, but in their imagination these thoughts are being stolen from them. They have annoying habits or painful fits, but they ascribe them to other people.

You interpret this phenomenon in the following way. Many of the ordinary circumstances of life are very difficult, unbearable and painful for these patients. For instance, the presence at the dinner table of two ladies of the patient's acquaintance, towards whom she had never been ill-disposed before. This constant difficulty and the natural frequent failures fill the patients with anxiety and fear, and inspire in them the desire to get away from it all. Like children or savages, they attribute all their troubles to the malignant actions of others, and this signifies deliberate objectification. Further, you devote attention to the following detail: in all the cases cited by you, we have to do, in your terminology, with binary social acts: to be master or slave, give or steal, strive for solitude or seek company, etc. These contrasts are confused by the patients when they are in a state of depression, the disagreeable opposite usually bearing an objective character and relating to other people. For example, the patient passionately wants to be alone, locked up in her room, and actually she remains alone, but she is tortured by the thought that some malevolent person has contrived to get into the room and is watching her.

One cannot but agree with all the foregoing, which represents an extremely interesting psychological analysis. But I take the liberty of disagreeing with you on the interpretation of the last point. You repeat more than once that, contrary to the general belief, these contrasts are not so easily distinguishable. You say: *"To tell* and *to be told* form a single whole and the one is not easily distinguished from the other, as is usually believed." And further: *"The act of insulting* and *the act of being insulted* are united by the general concept of insult; but the disorder shows that they may be confused, that one may be mistaken for the other." You explain this confusion by a rather complex combination of feelings.

Availing myself of the facts established and systematised by you, I have resolved to take another way and to interpret them physiologically.

Our general notion (category) of contraposition is one of the fundamental and indispensable general notions, which, along with all others, facilitates and controls normal thinking and even makes it possible. Our attitude towards the surrounding world, social environment included, as well as towards ourselves, would be distorted to a very great degree if there were constant confusion of opposites: I and not I; mine and yours; I am simultaneously alone and in company; I offend and I am offended, etc. Consequently, there must be a profound reason for the disappearance or weakening of this general notion, and, in my opinion, this reason can and must be sought in the fundamental laws of nervous activity. I think that in present-day physiology there are definite indications to this effect.

In the course of our study of the higher nervous activity by the method of conditioned reflexes we observed and investigated in our experimental animals the following precise facts. In different states of depression, inhibition (more often in various hypnotic states) the equalisation, paradoxical and ultraparadoxical phases are manifest. This signifies that the cortical nervous cells, instead of normally producing (within certain limits) effects proportional to the intensity of the stimulating agents, in states of various inhibition, begin to produce effects either of equal strength, or inversely proportional to the intensity of the stimulus, and even of an entirely opposite character; this means that the inhibitory stimuli produce a positive effect, and the positive stimuli a negative effect. I make so bold as to suppose that it is precisely this ultraparadoxical phase which causes the weakening of the notion of contraposition in our patients.

All the conditions necessary for the development of an ultraparadoxical state in the cortical cells of our patients, are in evidence and have been clearly established by you. When these patients, being of weak constitution, come up against a multitude of life situations, they easily fall into a state of depression, anxiety and fear; they can, however, still desire or not desire something, they have their emotionally-reinforced and possibly concentrated ideas of what is desirable or undesirable (I am the master, not the slave; I want to be alone and not in company; I want to have secrets, etc.). And in such conditions this is sufficient to evoke in a fatal way an opposite idea (I am a slave; there is always somebody near me; all my secrets are being disclosed, etc.).

The physiological explanation of this phenomenon would be as follows. Let us suppose that a definite frequency of the metronome acts as a conditioned food positive stimulus, since its application is accompanied by feeding and, because of this, evokes a food reaction. Another frequency of the metronome acts as a negative stimulus, since it is not reinforced by feeding and produces, therefore, a negative reaction: the animal turns away when it is applied. The frequencies of the metronome beats constitute a physiological pair, the components of which, being opposites, are associated and at the same time reciprocally induced, i.e., one frequency stimulates and reinforces the action of the other. This is an exact physiological fact. Further, if a positive frequency acts on a cell which for some reason or other is in a weak state (or in a hypnotic state), then this frequency, according to the law of maximum, which is also a strictly established fact, inhibits the cell. This inhibition, in conformity with the law of reciprocal induction, conditions a state of excitation instead of inhibition in the other component of the associated couple. That is why the stimulus related to the latter now provokes excitation, not inhibition.

This is the mechanism of negativisim or contralism.

If food is offered to a dog when it is in a state of inhibition (or hypnosis), i.e., when you induce it to positive activity—to the act of eating—it turns away and rejects the food. But when the food is moved away, i.e, when you give the dog a negative impulse aimed at inhibiting the corresponding activity, at discontinuing the act of eating, the dog, on the contrary, begins to reach for the food.

Evidently this law of reciprocal induction of opposite actions must also be applied to contrary ideas, which, naturally, are connected with definite (verbal) cells and also constitute an associated pair. Due to a state of depression or inhibition (in our experiments any difficulty arising in the higher nervous activity is usually reflected by inhibition), more or less intense stimulation of one idea leads to its inhibition and, by means of the same mechanism, induces the opposite idea.

It is easy to see that this explanation naturally embraces the peculiar symptom of the schizophrenics—ambivalence—which arises under a highly extended and profound ultraparadoxical state.

Many people, even scientifically-minded people, are moved almost to the point of anger by the attempts to give a physiological interpretation of psychical phenomena; they retort that such explanations are "mechanical", since they want to stress as strongly as they can the obvious inaptitude and absurdity of trying to link subjective feelings and mechanics. In my view this is an obvious misunderstanding.

At present, of course, there can be no talk of representing our psychical phenomena *mechanically, in the full sense of the word*. We are also far from being able to do this with regard to all physiological manifestations; the same thing applies, although in lesser degree, to chemical phenomena, and it applies fully to physical phenomena. A truly mechanical interpretation is still the goal of natural-science research; the study of reality as a whole, including ourselves, is advancing very slowly towards this goal, and much time will be required before it is reached. Modern natural science as a whole is but a series of many *stages of approximation* to this mechanical interpretation, stages linked throughout by the supreme principle of causality or determinism, according to which there is no action without cause.

And if possibilities are now opening up for explaining the so-called psychical phenomena physiologically, they can be regarded as a certain, slight, very slight degree of approximation towards a mechanical interpretation. It seems to me that in many cases these possibilities are opening up.

Being now at the psychological stage of your research, you are interpreting the feelings of possession, establishing the conditions under which they arise, reducing them to their elementary components and, in this way, elucidating their general structure, i.e., you are also dealing with their mechanics, with their general structure, but in your own way. I, in the physiological stage of my research, am trying to bring our common problem a bit nearer to true general mechanics, interpreting your fact concerning confusion of opposite ideas, as the specific interaction of elementary physiological phenomena—nervous excitation and inhibition. In their turn chemistry, and, finally, physics, will further disclose these phenomena and their mechanism, thus steadily approaching the solution of our problem.

ATTEMPT AT A PHYSIOLOGICAL INTERPRETATION OF COMPULSIVE NEUROSIS AND PARANOIA[68]

New laboratory facts obtained in studying conditioned reflexes on dogs served as the point of departure for a physiological interpretation of these pathological forms.

When conditioned stimuli are elaborated from various external agents (let us take, for example, conditioned food reflexes), the first reaction to the formed conditioned stimulus is usually a movement towards this stimulus, i.e., the animal turns to the location of this stimulus. When this stimulus is within our animal's reach, the latter tries to come in contact with it, especially by its mouth; for example, if the conditioned stimulus is a flashing bulb, the dog licks it, and if the conditioned stimulus is sound, the dog even catches air with its mouth (in cases of very high food excitability). Thus the conditioned stimulus really fully replaces, as it were, food for the animal. With different conditioned stimuli coming from different points in the environment the animal naturally turns to all of them.

Among other stimuli a conditioned stimulus of extraordinarily weak noise coming from under the right side of the table on which the animal stood was formed in one of our dogs (I. Filaretov's experiments). On perceiving this sound the animal stood on the very edge of the table, sometimes even placed one of its legs beyond the edge of the table and lowered its head as much as possible towards the source of the sound. The other conditioned stimuli were located in various other places, but the dog preferred to turn to the location of the noise even when the other stimuli were used.

This fact appeared particularly strange when the noise was no longer used as a conditioned stimulus during continuation of the experiments with other stimuli. The motor reaction in the direction of the former location of the noise invariably existed and still continues to exist to date, eighteen months after suspension of this stimulus. During application of all the other stimuli, wherever they may have been, there was movement only in the direction of the location of the noise until the moment the dog was given food, when it, finally, turned to the feeding box.

Towards the end of the usual interval between applications of conditioned stimuli, i.e., before the next stimulus, dogs often develop certain food excitation (reflex of time) and turn to the location of the feeding box or to the location of some other conditioned stimulus. This dog continued to turn only to the location of the old noise.

This reaction must apparently be recognised as pathological, since it made no sense at all, i.e., it was coarsely, sharply at variance with the actual relations. Regarding it as such we decided to cure it. And if we could cure it, it would, of course, be further confirmation of its undeniable pathological character. We chose a suitable dose of bromides as a therapeutic agent, since we had already had many cases in which bromides had decisively helped in our experimental neuroses and even in certain inborn defects of the nervous system in general. Our expectations were justified. The reaction sharply diminished. With other conditioned stimuli it disappeared altogether, giving way to a legitimate, appropriate motor reaction to the location of these stimuli.

The same phenomenon was later also observed on some other dogs; in one of them bromides eliminated this abnormal reaction completely.

It is clear that what we have in the afore-described

facts is a pathological disorder of the function of nerve cells, a change in the normal relations between the two aspects of their activity (excitatory and inhibitory processes), i.e., the excitatory process abnormally prevailed. This was also attested by the favourable effect of bromides as an agent which is known to intensify the inhibitory function of the cell.

Overstrain of the excitatory process must most appropriately be regarded as the cause of the pathological phenomenon in the foregoing experiment, since the exceptional weakness of the external stimulus caused extraordinary strain of the orienting motor apparatus, the general locomotor, as well as the special, i.e., adjusting apparatus of the receptor of the given stimulation.

Another analogous fact was soon added to the aforedescribed fact. In one dog of the weak type, but of a stronger variant, and in castrated dogs of various types we attempted to investigate the solution of a difficult problem by them, namely, transformation of conditioned action into its opposite—a pair of metronomes with different frequencies of beats having antagonistic conditioned significance: positive and negative, i.e., transformation of a stimulus evoking the process of stimulation in the cerebral cortex into a negative stimulus, and of a stimulus eliciting the inhibitory process into a positive stimulus (Petrova's experiments). For this purpose the metronome having a well-elaborated positive effect was now used without accompaniment with food, and, contrariwise, with the inhibitory stimulus we now gave the dog food. In one of the castrates of an exceptionally strong type the transformation was quite successful; in the other animals experimented upon it seemed to begin, but then things came to a special pass. In some animals it even seemed that the aim was quite accomplished: the use of metronomes produced results corresponding to the new conditions of the experiment several times on end, but then, gradually or at once, everything completely returned to the old relations, although the transformation procedure, already used dozens of times, was continued without interruption.

What did this mean, then? Did everything concerning the character of the excitatory and inhibitory processes now really remain unchanged in the cell despite the external similarity in the action of the metronomes at this stage of the experiments with their former action?

This had to be settled by a special investigation. The experiments we performed revealed serious disturbances of normal relations in the nerve cell. The excitatory process was now not what it had been before: it became more stable, less, so to speak, inclined to yield to the inhibitory process; or else we had to take it that the inhibitory process was very weak with the result that the excitatory process relatively predominated. Here are these experiments. When the metronome which evoked this modified excitatory process was used in the same experiment several times without reinforcement with food, i.e., it was extinguished, it diminished much less and much more slowly than the other positive stimuli under the same conditions. There was another peculiarity: after extinction of the stimulus that was being transformed we frequently scarcely noticed diminution in the usual scope of action of the other conditioned stimuli that followed it (secondary extinction). This denoted insufficient participation of the inhibitory process in the procedure of extinguishing this stimulus. On the other hand, during extinction (and even to zero) of other conditioned stimuli the stimulus we were investigating immediately after them often remained unchanged or was weakened but little, whereas the other positive stimuli diminished very much and were found to have a lesser effect even on the following day. Clear stability of the excitatory process of the cell together with weakening of the inhibitory process. At the same time our attention was further attracted by the fact that now there was a sharp difference between the other acoustic conditioned stimuli as regards the stability of the excitatory process.

The tone stimuli, farthest removed from the metronome in the character of sound, remained normal, while the stimuli with an element of knocking came closer, as regards stability, to the pathologically acting metronome.

In the experiment with transforming the effect of the metronome we, consequently, obtained the same abnormality as in the formerly described experiments; there—in the cells of the motor analyser, here—in the cells of the auditory analyser; there—during overstrain of the excitatory process, here—during collision of the antagonistic processes; both here and there bromides effected a return to the normal relations. The latter gave us one more reason to see one of the mechanisms of the new pathological phenomenon in the weakening of the inhibitory function of the cell and to understand why this phenomenon was observed on the castrated animals of the strong type. We had long since known that one of the essential effects of castration was weakening of the inhibitory function of the cell.

The aforesaid pathological phenomenon may be given several descriptive names: stagnancy, uncommon inertness, intensified concentration, and extraordinary tonicity.

From now on we shall prefer to use the term "pathological inertness".

The foregoing new facts are confirmation and extension of our old and more general fact that in the cerebral cortex it is possible to obtain experimentally by the functional method (i.e., without mechanical influence) a very limited pathological point. In our former experiments such a point represented a paradoxical or ultraparadoxical state, i.e., the stimulus related to it produced a greater effect when it diminished in strength and not contrariwise, as when it was normal, or even produced a negative instead of a positive effect. At the same time the given point could remain in such a state without affecting all the other points of the hemispheres or pass into the next stage of the pathological state in which stimulation of it with an appropriate stimulus led to disturbance in the activity of the entire cortex manifested in general inhibition of this activity. Now we also had isolated pathological points of the cerebral cortex whose pathological state represented a special phase and was manifested in that the process of excitation in them became abnormally inert.

Thus we have adequate reason to assume that under the influence of various pathogenic causes of a functional nature *sharply isolated pathological points* or *regions* may arise in the cerebral cortex; at the same time we can expect this experimental fact to take place and be of great importance in the pathology of man's higher nervous activity.

I find it possible to assume that in stereotypy, iteration and perseveration as symptoms, as well as in the essence of the compulsive neurosis and paranoia, the basic pathophysiological phenomenon is the same, namely, what came to the fore in our experiments and what we have designated by the term "pathological inertness". Stereotypy, iteration and perseveration are a pathological inertness in the motor area of the cortex (general skeletal, as well as special speech motion), while in compulsive neurosis and paranoia it is a pathological inertness in other cortical cells connected with our other sensations, feelings and ideas. These last sentences must not, of course, exclude the possibility of emergence of the same pathological state also in the underlying parts of the central nervous system.

Let us go on to the, so to speak, clinical atmosphere in the different neuroses and psychoses of this pathological phenomenon, as one of the manifestations, one of the phases of the pathological state of the nerve cells. Stereotypy and perseveration form one of the frequent symptoms, for example, of hysteria. One hysteriac complains that once she begins to comb her hair she cannot stop, cannot finish it in due time. Another hysteriac cannot, as a result of a short catatonic attack, utter a word without repeating it many times in order to finish his sentence. These phenomena are encountered still more often in schizophrenia, even characterise it, especially its catatonic form. Pathological inertness in the motor sphere is manifested now at individual points, and now embracing the entire system of skeletal muscles, as can be observed in some catatonic patients whose any group of muscles passively set in motion repeats this motion an enormous number of times.

Later we shall dwell especially on compulsive neurosis and paranoia as separate, independent diseases in which the phenomenon we are interested in is the main characteristic symptom or almost the whole disease.

To be sure, we can hardly contest the fact that, if pathological inertness is obvious and must be accepted as a fact in motor phenomena, the same thing is quite admissible, legitimate also as regards all the sensations, feelings and ideas. Who can doubt that the aforesaid phenomena are normally, of course, a manifestation of the activity of the nerve cells and, consequently, that compulsive neurosis and paranoia are a pathological state of the corresponding cells of the cerebral cortex, in the given case their pathological inertness. In compulsive neurosis and paranoia we have excessively, illegitimately fixed ideas, feelings and then actions which do not correspond to the proper natural and special social relations of man and therefore lead him into difficult, distressing, harmful conflicts with nature, as well as other men and, primarily, of course, with himself. But all this pertains only to the morbid ideas and sensations, while outside their sphere the patients think and act like quite healthy people and may even be higher than average persons.

Compulsive neurosis and paranoia are usually sharply distinguished as morbid forms clinically (the former is a neurosis and the latter—a psychosis). However this sharp distinction is not recognised by all neurologists and psychiatrists; some of them assume transitions from one form to the other, reducing their differences to degrees or phases of the pathological state and certain additional features.

The following are quotations from these authors. Pierre Janet says: "The delusion of persecution is closely related to obsessive ideas and I am surprised that they have been entirely separated from each other." Kretschmer says: "In the old disputable question of whether there are any essential differences between delusions and obsessive ideas we can arrive at the exact conclusion in a negative sense." R. Mallet says: "In delusion and obsession ... the organic damage is of the same nature."

The two pathological forms in question differ from each other in two basic features. In compulsive neurosis the patient is cognisant of the morbid nature of his pathological state and as far as possible fights it, although on the whole, unavailingly; the paranoiac does not have this critical attitude to his illness, he is in its power, in the power of persisting sensation, feeling and idea. The second difference is the chronic course and incurability of paranoia.

But these distinguishing features of the two given forms do not essentially exclude the identity of their basic symptom. This is the more true since many clinicians observed indubitable transitions, both acute and chronic, of obsession with criticism into obsession without criticism. The grounds on which the general main symptom arose and what actually evoked it in each individual case could serve as the difference between the two forms, as a basis for their clinical distinction.

A few words about the basis and causes of the disease in question, according to our laboratory material. We have long since observed on our animals that succumbing to different experimental neuroses under the influence of the same pathogenic procedures depends on the inborn type of nervous system: only representatives of the weak type and the strong but unbalanced type easily succumb to the disease. Of course, by intensifying the pathogenic procedures it was possible, in the long run, to overcome, break down also the balanced strong type, especially if some organic trauma, for example, castration, was added beforehand.

In particular, during the transformation of antagonistic conditioned reflexes as a procedure with which we produced the afore-described pathological inertness, there was an enormous variety of results, both within normal limits and with pathological deviations, depending on the individuality of the animals. In strong and entirely normal types this transformation proceeds properly to the required end, but in a very different tempo and with different variations and details of the transformation. In a giant of nervous power (even after castration), whose equal I never saw during the thirty years of my work on conditioned reflexes, this transformation began from the first time and without any variations was entirely ready by the fifth time. In others, numerous repetitions of the procedure failed to produce complete results: sometimes the new positive stimulus remained weaker than the former one, and sometimes the new inhibitory stimulus failed to come down to zero, as the former one. In one animal it was the positive stimulus that was transformed sooner, in another it was the negative. All this concerns cases of successful transformation. The same diversity was observed in pathological deviations during the solution of this problem: as already mentioned in the beginning of this article, we observed now one of these deviations and now another. The pathological inertness, as one of the morbid phasic consequences of the transformation, similarly rapidly passes into another form of the disease or remains more or less constant. In the weak type the pathological inertness usually quickly passes into another pathological state. Chronic pathological inertness is often observed in castrated animals of the strong type.

I have intentionally dwelt somewhat longer on our laboratory material in order to show how different the solution of the same life's problem must be in people, depending on the difference in the types of nervous system, and how different the pathological consequences must be when abnormal types fail to solve this problem.

So much for the basis. As for the immediate causes of the disease in question, we have seen in our present experiments (as yet not numerous) two causes producing it: in one case it is a strong and prolonged stimulation, i.e., overstrain of the process of excitation, and in another case it is a clash of the antagonistic processes.

When we deal with people, we must naturally also bear in mind different causes, as well as different bases which must, of course, lead to different degrees, as well as a different course, even if of the same basic pathological disorder.

The very first cause studied on our animals opens a long series of possible cases of the disease investigated in man. Both, an abnormal development and a temporary aggravation of one of our emotions (instincts) as well as the pathological state of some internal organ or a whole system may send to corresponding cortical cells, at a certain time or continuously, incessant or excessive stimuli and thus, at last, evoke in them a pathological inertness—an obsessive idea or sensation, when the real cause has already ceased to act. The same thing could be effected by some strong, staggering life's impressions. No fewer, if no more, cases of pathological inertness should also have been produced by our second cause, since all our life is a continuous struggle, a clash of our basic strivings, desires and tastes with the natural, as well as the special social conditions.

The aforesaid causes could concentrate the pathological inertness of the excitatory process at different points of the cerebral cortex—now in the cells directly stimulated by the external, as well as internal agents (first signalling system of reality), now in different cells (kinesthetic, auditory and visual) of the verbal system (second signalling system), and at both points with different degrees of intensity: once on the level of ideas, and the next time bringing the intensity up to a power of real sensations (hallucinations).

On our dogs we observed that sometimes, owing to pathological inertness, the effect of an appropriate stimulus sharply rose above the healthy effects of the other stimuli. As for the basis, it must naturally be the same for compulsive neurosis and paranoia, i.e., susceptibility to disease, as in our laboratory material; but this will be, however, either the weak type or the strong but unbalanced type of nervous system. And we know from our laboratory experience how essential this difference is for the immediate character of the disease. In this respect one can hardly raise any objections to the legitimacy of transferring this conclusion from animals to man. Of course, besides the inborn basis, cases of unstable, fragile nervous system engendered by unfortunate events are inevitable; these include injuries, infection, intoxication and life's great misfortunes.

Thus the difference between our two pathological forms, as regards their chronic nature and incurability, is determined by the difference in the immediate impulses to the disease, as well as the types of nervous system. The immediate impulses may be, on the one hand, temporary, transitory, and on the other, continuous and constant, till the end of life. In its turn the excitatory process is either generally relatively weak, unstable in its nature, and easily yields to the inhibitory process in the weak type, or is strong from the very beginning, stable, and generally predominates over the inhibitory process. It stands to reason, that during pathological inertness there are few or no chances at all in the latter case that this inertness may sometimes be entirely eliminated or reduced to the lowest degree which is relatively normal for the given animal. To confirm this we can cite the following fact from our laboratory material. Whereas in one of the dogs with a compulsive movement, belonging to the rather strong type, bromides have only sharply weakened, limited this compulsion, in a dog of a clearly weak type the compulsion entirely disappeared under the influence of bromides. Moreover, as was mentioned before, a more chronic pathological inertness was most frequently encountered in castrates of the strong type. In connection with this E. Bleuler's remark is of some interest; in the latest edition of his textbook he says that he would not like to regard as accidental, in the cases well studied by him, the coincidence of paranoia with sexual inadequacy.

As for the other sign of difference between the two forms in question (absence of critical attitude to the pathological symptom in paranoia and its presence in the compulsive states), it must naturally be reduced to the difference in intensity of pathological inertness. As the aforesaid indicates, the strong type must have considerable pathological inertness of the excitatory process and this will naturally be connected with greater independence and even its invulnerability to the influence of the healthy regions of the cortex, which physiologically conditions the absence of a critical attitude. Besides, it is probable that the inert excitatory process of considerable intensity must produce on the periphery, on the basis of the law of negative induction, strong and widespread inhibition, which must again lead to the same result, i.e., exclusion of the influence of the rest of the cerebral cortex on it.

We shall illustrate our general considerations by particular examples taken from life. Let us take a person of the excitable type, i.e., one in whom the excitatory process is not balanced with the inhibitory process. Let a rather frequent striving for domination prevail in his emotional (instinctive) make-up. Since childhood he has always strongly wished to advance, to be the first, to lead the others, elicit admiration, etc. But at the same time nature failed to endow him with any outstanding talents, or, if he did have them, they were unfortunately not recognised in due time, or else, the conditions of his life prevented him from making due application of them, and he concentrated his energies on activity for which he was unfit. Inexorable reality naturally prevented him from achieving his goal: he had won neither influence nor success, but, on the contrary, deserved rebuff and knocks, i.e., he never had any luck. All he could do was to submit, reconcile himself to the role of a modest worker, i.e., inhibit his aspirations. And yet there was no necessary inhibition, while this emotion constantly and imperatively demanded its satisfaction.

Hence, at first, further extraordinary but vain efforts in his hapless occupation or change to another with the same results and then, according to the property of his type (strong), a shrinking into himself with his internal satisfaction and constant vivid idea of his real or imaginary gifts and vital rights and privileges together with the additional idea of the intended hindrances and persecution on the part of those around him. This naturally results in a sufficiently conditioned phase of pathological inertness at the corresponding points of the cortex, which has destroyed the last remnant of inhibition in them. And now we see the absolute power of the idea which, not by active inhibition on the basis of other associations, other signals, witnesses of reality, but by passive inhibition, a process of negative induction, has excluded all that does not suit it and has become transformed into a fantastic idea of imaginary greatness, imaginary successes. Since the emotion lives to the end of the subject's life, the pathological idea also exists with it but remains isolated without interfering with anything that does not come in contact with it. Before us is true paranoia in Kraepelin's sense.

Now I take concrete cases from Kretschmer's[69] book *Der sensitive Beziehungswahn*. It is a question of two girls of the rather weak type, but practical, modest, and pretentious only as regards their religious, moral and social decency and not their life's rights and privileges; the pretence of the latter kind is very frequently, nearly always, combined with the strong excitable type.

A mature girl experiences normal sexual desire for a young man, but the individual, ethical and social requirements have not allowed, have always hindered her from gratifying this desire, i.e., there is a clash of nervous processes. The result is a difficult state of nervous activity and it is manifested in pathological inertness in the parts of the cortex which are connected with the struggling feelings and ideas. The girl acquires an irresistible, obsessive idea that her face shows the sexual urge in the form of coarse sensuality. In the clinic she hides her face into a pillow even from the physician. Naturally, she has already avoided going out into the street because she thought that everyone looked at her, spoke about the expression of her face and laughed. Until then, however, it had all remained within the limits of the really possible, although imaginary. Then comes a leap which is unintelligible as the work of even pathologically fixed thought. Under the influence of a chat with a girl-friend who asserted that in the Garden of Eden Eve had talked to the serpent not as to a mental, but as to a sexual seducer, our patient immediately developed an unexpected and irresistible idea and sensation that she had a serpent in her which was constantly moving and that sometimes its head reached her throat. Here we see a new inert idea. But how, by what process did it arise? Kretschmer called this phenomenon inversion, considering it a reflex inversion (*reflektorische Umschlag*).

As regards an identical phenomenon in another clinical case Kretschmer says that "it has emerged reflexly, without logical mediation, even in direct contradiction to it". But what kind of reflex is it? Where does it begin and how does it end? We have this process, we know it in the laboratory and can interpret its physiological mechanism. Moreover I deem it essential to say, to emphasise, that in this case the physiological and psychological particularly clearly overlap, merge, and, one may say, become identical.

Let us recall the two antagonistically acting metronomes, one stimulatory and the other one—inhibitory. If general inhibition develops in the cortex, for example, in the form of hypnosis, or local inhibition in the region of the metronome's action, the positively acting metronome becomes negative and the negatively acting one—positive. This is the so-called ultraparadoxical phase.

It is this physiological fact that we encounter in the afore-described leap in our patient. The girl had a strong and constant idea of her sexual purity, inviolability, considering it, under certain conditions, morally and socially shameful to have sexual desire, even though suppressed and not in the least gratified. On the basis of general inhibition, in which state our patient found herself and which in weak nervous systems usually accompanies a difficult state, this idea was irresistibly physiologically transformed into its opposite (slightly disguised), into an idea even bordering on a sensation of having the sexual seducer in her very body. This is exactly what happens in the delusion of persecution: the patient wants to be respected, and yet he is tormented by a contrary and erroneous idea of being constantly insulted, or he wants to have secrets, and yet he has the obsessive idea, the contrary thought, that all his secrets are discovered by others, etc. I have already expressed this physiological interpretation in an open letter to Professor Pierre Janet as regards the feelings of possession (*les sentiments d'emprise*).

This delusion is based on two physiological phenomena —pathological inertness and the ultraparadoxical phase, now existing separately, now appearing together, and now replacing each other.

On the whole, almost the same thing happened to the second girl. The same clash of the natural sexual desire with the practical and persistent thought of the incompatibility of ages: the object of her love was much younger. The same results, to the point of inversion; moreover, this patient was tormented by the absurd idea that she was pregnant, whereas the object of her love did not even note her dispositon for him because she was restrained in manifesting her feelings.

In this case traced by Kretschmer over a period of many years one could clearly see how the obsessive ideas and sensations sometimes reached a degree of ideas and sensations which, according to the patient herself, were very real and which, she did not know, were pathological, how they persisted in this form for some time and then were again interpreted by the patient objectively as manifestations of disease. This was connected with life's trials and tribulations and, consequently, with a change in the state of the nervous system, which now recovered and now was again depressed and weakened. Finally, as time wore on, everything naturally ended well.

I was very happy to come across the theory of the French psychiatrist Clérambault in one of the few books on neurology and psychiatry I have read. This theory considers the appearance of what he calls "mental automatism", "parasitic words and ideas", about which the delusion later systematically develops, the primary symptom of paranoia. What else can we interpret as mental automatism, but the point of a certain pathologically inert excitatory process about which all that is close, similar and related concentrates (on the basis of the law of generalisation) and from which everything that is alien is repulsed, according to the law of negative induction?

I am not a clinician (I have always been a physiologist) and now, so late, I shall, of course, have no time and shall be unable to become a clinician. For this reason in my present observations, as in my former excursions into neuropathology and psychiatry, I dare not, in discussing corresponding material, claim sufficient competence from the clinical point of view. But I shall probably not be mistaken now if I say that clinicians, neurologists and psychiatrists must, in corresponding fields, inevitably regard as fundamental the following pathophysiological facts: the complete isolation of the functionally pathological (in the etiological sense) points of the cortex, as well as the pathological inertness of the excitatory process and the ultraparadoxical phase in them.

GENERAL TYPES OF ANIMAL AND HUMAN HIGHER NERVOUS ACTIVITY[70]

The mode and standards of our own behaviour, as well as of the behaviour of the higher animals close to us and with which we are in constant vital relations (for instance, dogs), represent a great, a truly boundless variety, if behaviour is considered as a whole, in its smallest details, especially as manifested in man. But since our behaviour, as well as that of higher animals, is determined and controlled by the nervous system, it is possible to reduce the above-mentioned variety to a more or less limited number of basic properties of this system, with their combinations and gradations. This makes it possible to distinguish between the types of nervous activity, i.e., between these or other complexes of the basic properties of the nervous system.

The observation and study of a large number of dogs, using the method of conditioned reflexes, carried out in our laboratory for many years, have gradually disclosed to us these properties in their vital manifestations and combinations. These properties include: in the first place, the *strength* of the basic nervous processes—excitatory and inhibitory—which always constitute the sum total of nervous activity; in the second place, the *equilibrium* of these processes; and, finally, in the third place, their *mobility*. It is obvious that while all these properties exist and act simultaneously, they provide the highest adaptation of the animal's organism to the surrounding world, or, in other words, the complete equilibration of the organism as a whole with the external environment, i.e., they secure the organism's existence. The significance of the strength of the nervous processes is clearly shown by the fact that in the surrounding medium there arise (more or less often) unusual, extraordinary developments, powerful stimuli, and that, naturally, other external conditions of a similar and even greater force not infrequently necessitate the suppression or retardation of the effects of these stimuli. And the nervous cells must endure this extraordinary tension in their activity. From this also follows the importance of equilibrium between both processes, their equal strength. Since the organism's external environment is constantly—and often powerfully and abruptly—fluctuating, both processes must, so to speak, keep pace with these fluctuations, i.e., they must possess great mobility and be able, in compliance with the demands of the external conditions, rapidly to recede, to give preference to one stimulus, to excitation before inhibition and vice versa.

Leaving aside the gradations and considering only the extreme cases, only the limits of fluctuation, viz., strength and weakness, equality and inequality, lability and inertness in both processes, we obtain eight combinations, eight different complexes of basic properties of the nervous system, eight types of the nervous system. If we also take into account that in the absence of equilibrium the predominance may, generally speaking, be on the side now of the excitatory, now of the inhibitory process, and that in the case of mobility, inertness or lability may also become a property now of one, now of the other process, then the number of possible combinations increases to twenty-four. And finally, if we also take into consideration even the rough gradations of the three basic properties, we shall thereby again greatly augment the number of possible combinations. However, only extensive and thorough observation can establish the presence, frequency and intensity of these or other actual complexes of basic properties, of the actual types of nervous activity.

Since normally our general behaviour, as well as that of higher animals (we imply here healthy organisms), is directed by the higher part of the central nervous system—by the cerebral hemispheres and the adjacent subcortex—the study of this higher nervous activity under normal conditions by the method of conditioned reflexes is bound to lead to knowledge of the actual types of nervous activity and the basic standards of behaviour of human beings and higher animals.

It seems to me that this problem was solved—of course, only in general outline—by the Greek genius in his system of the so-called temperaments, where the basic components of the behaviour of human beings and higher animals were exactly emphasised and advanced, as we shall show in our further exposition.

But before proceeding to our factual material, I must touch on one very substantial and so far almost insurmountable difficulty connected with the definition of the type of nervous activity. Human and animal behaviour is determined not only by congenital properties of the nervous system, but also by the influences to which the organism is continuously subjected during its individual existence; in other words, it depends on constant education and training in the broadest sense of these words. This is due to the fact that along with the above-mentioned properties of the nervous system, another very important property incessantly manifests itself—its high plasticity. Consequently, since this is a question of the natural type of nervous system, we must take into account all the influences to which the organism has been exposed from the day of its birth to the present moment. With regard to our experimental material (i.e., our dogs) in the overwhelming majority of cases the fulfilment of this requirement still remains a passionate desire. We shall be able to fulfil it only when our dogs are born and reared before our eyes, under our unremitting observation. We shall soon have convincing corroboration of the importance of this requirement. So far there is only one way of overcoming the above-mentioned difficulty: it is necessary to increase and to diversify the forms of our diagnostic tests as much as possible in the hope that in this or that case we shall succeed in bringing to light the specific changes in the natural type of nervous system that were determined by the definite influences of the individual existence; in other words, by means of a comparison with all other features of the type we shall reveal both the more or less disguised natural features and the elaborated, acquired ones.

Right from the very beginning of our experiments with dogs based on the method of conditioned reflexes we (like others) were struck by the different behaviour of the bold and the cowardly dogs. The former offered no resistance when led to experimentation; they remained quiet in the new experimental conditions, both when they were placed in the stands mounted on tables, and when certain apparatuses were attached to their skin and even placed in their mouths. When food was given to them by means of an automatic device, they began to eat it at once. Such was the behaviour of bold animals. But the cowardly animals had to be accustomed gradually to the procedure—a process which required days and even weeks. Another difference was observed when we began to elaborate conditioned reflexes in these dogs. In the first case the conditioned reflexes developed rapidly, after the application of two or three combinations; they reached considerable strength and remained constant, no matter how complicated the system of reflexes. In the second case, on the contrary, the conditioned reflexes were formed very slowly, after many repetitions; their strength increased at a very low rate, and they never acquired stability, being sometimes even at zero, no matter how considerably their system was simplified. It was, therefore, natural to assume that in the first dogs the excitatory process was strong, while in the second it was weak. In the bold dogs the excitatory process, which from the biological point of view arises properly and in time, for instance, at the sight of food, constantly resists minor influences, remaining, so to speak, legitimately predominant. In the cowardly dogs the strength of the excitatory process is insufficient to overcome conditions which are less important in the given case and which produce what we term external inhibition; for this reason we say that such dogs are inhibitable. In the bold dogs even physically excessive external stimuli, when conditionally connected with physiologically important functions, continue to serve their purpose without bringing the nerve cell to a pathological state; thus they represent an exact index of the intensity of their excitatory process, of the strength (i.e., working capacity) of their nerve cells.

It is here that the specific difficulty, which I have just mentioned made itself felt. All the dogs which seemed to us cowardly, i.e., which only very slowly became accustomed to our experimental conditions and formed conditioned reflexes with difficulty (since their entire conditioned reflex activity was easily disturbed by insignificant new external influences), were regarded by us, quite groundlessly, as belonging to the weak type of nervous system. This even resulted in a blunder—at one time I regarded these dogs as experts in inhibition, i.e., as being strong in this respect. The first doubts as to the correctness of this diagnosis arose in connection with the external behaviour of these animals in their habitual surroundings. Further, it seemed strange that their conditioned reflex activity, despite its high complexity, should be of a perfectly regular character so long as the surrounding conditions remained strictly uniform. But the final solution was found thanks to a special investigation. We (Vyrzhikovsky and Mayorov) took a litter of puppies and divided it into two parts: half of the puppies, from the very day of their birth, were kept in the kennel, the others were given complete freedom. All the animals of the first group turned out to be cowardly and susceptible to inhibition given the slightest changes in the surroundings; in the animals of the second group nothing of the kind was observed. It became clear that when the puppies first appeared in the external environment they were provided with a special reflex, sometimes referred to as a panic reflex, but which I suggest should be termed an initial and temporary reflex of natural caution. The moment acquaintance with the new environment begins it is necessary to wait some time for the consequences of any new stimulation, no matter which receptor it affects, i.e., to abstain from any new movement and to repress the existing movement, since it is not known what the new phenomenon promises the organism, whether harmful, useful, or of no consequence at all. And only in the course of the gradual acquaintance with the environment is this reflex replaced, little by little, by a new, special, investigatory reflex, and, depending on its effect, by other corresponding reflexes. The puppy, which is not given the opportunity to gain this practical experience independently, retains the persisting temporary reflex for a very long time if not for life, and the reflex constantly disguises the real force of the nervous system. What a vital pedagogical fact this is! A sure sign of this unduly persisting feature, apart from the fact that in many respects it contradicts other stable inborn features, is the inhibitory action not so much of the particularly strong stimulations but of the new stimulations—no matter how weak they may be in themselves (Rozental, Petrova).

Thus, the strength of the excitatory process was regarded by us as the first property of the type of nervous system. Hence the initial division of all our dogs into strong and weak ones.

Another property of the nervous system, clearly observed by us and according to which the animals are subdivided into new groups, is the equality or inequality of the two opposite nervous processes—excitation and inhibition. We imply here the higher active cortical inhibition (or according to the terminology used in the theory of conditioned reflexes—internal inhibition), which, together with the excitatory process, continuously maintains the equilibration of the organism with the surrounding medium and helps (on the basis of the analysing function of the organism's receptors) to distinguish between the nervous activity corresponding to the given conditions and moments and that which does not (extinction, differentiation and retardation).

The significance of this property was first observed by us in dogs with a very strong excitatory process. We soon noticed that whereas in such dogs positive conditioned reflexes were formed rapidly, inhibitory reflexes, on the contrary, were elaborated very slowly, with obvious difficulty; this was often accompanied by a violent resistance on the part of the animal; it was manifested either in destructive actions and barking, or, on the contrary, in stretching out the forepaws, as if imploring the experimenter to release it from the task (the latter, however, is rarer). At the same time, these reflexes are never fully inhibited; they are often disinhibited, i.e., greatly deteriorate in comparison with the degree of inhibition obtained previously. The following phenomenon is usually observed: when we subject the cortical inhibition in such animals to severe strain by means of very delicate differentiation, or by a frequent or protracted application of difficult inhibitors, their nervous system becomes fully, or almost fully, deprived of the inhibitory function; real neuroses set in, typical and chronic nervous diseases, which must be treated either by allowing the animals a very long rest, i.e., by a complete discontinuance of the experiments, or by giving bromide. Together with such animals, there are others in which both nervous processes are at an equally high level.

Consequently, the strong animals are divided into two groups—equilibrated and unequilibrated. Unequilibrated animals belonging to the category described above are met with quite often. It might seem that there should also be unequilibrated dogs of another kind, namely, with a predominance of the inhibitory process over the excitatory. But so far we have not met with such absolutely incontestable cases, or at least we have not been able to discern them. However, we have had fairly obvious and not infrequent cases when, after a time interval and with the help of gradual and repeated exercises, the initial disequilibrium levelled out to a considerable degree. And this is just another instance when the natural type of nervous system proved to be disguised to a great measure as a result of lifetime training.

Thus, we have a perfect group of strong and equilibrated dogs. However, the animals with this type of nervous system differ greatly, even in appearance. Some are extremely reactive, mobile and lively, i.e., as it were, extremely excitable and alert. Others, on the contrary, are only slightly reactive, sluggish and self-contained, i.e., in general, so to speak, little susceptible to excitation, inert. This difference in the general behaviour must, of course, be due to a specific property of the nervous system and may be best accounted for by the mobility of the nervous processes. Like everybody else we long ago observed this external difference between animals, but we lag considerably in elucidating, on the basis of the conditioned reflex activity, its cause—the mobility of the nervous processes. Only now is this mobility being systematically investigated on two dogs—strongly pronounced representatives of the latter group. Strong and equilibrated, these animals differ greatly in external behaviour. On the one hand, we (Petrova) have an exceedingly lively and reactive animal, on the other (Yakovleva)—an extremely inert and indifferent one. The different mobility of the nervous processes in these animals is distinctly manifested in their conditioned reflex activity which, unfortunately, was not investigated in identical experiments.

The first animal ("Boy") even in the course of usual experimentation with conditioned reflexes displays an amazingly rapid transition from extreme excitation at the beginning—when being placed in the stand and equipped with the apparatus—to a state of petrifaction, to a statuesque posture, and, at the same time, to a good working state in the course of the experiment. In the intervals between the conditioned food stimuli the animal remains in a very strained posture, evincing no reaction to extraneous accidental stimuli; but under the action of conditioned stimuli a strictly recurring salivary reaction sets in immediately, and the dog gulps the food placed before it. Subsequently, this high mobility of the nervous processes, their rapid interchange, manifested themselves, so to speak, with incredible force also in the course of special experiments. In our "Boy" we long ago elaborated two opposite conditioned reflexes to a metronome; one frequency of the metronome acted as a positive conditioned food stimulus, while the other acted as a negative inhibitory one. We then began to reverse the action of the metronome. The negative stimulus was reinforced, i.e., it had to be transformed into a positive stimulus, while the positive one was no longer accompanied by feeding and had to be converted into an inhibitory stimulus. Next day we were able to observe the onset of this reversal and by the fifth day it had been fully accomplished—a rare case of such rapid transformation. One day later an error was made—the metronomes were applied in accordance with their previous significance, namely, the old positive stimulus was again reinforced, while the old inhibitory stimulus was left without reinforcement; as a result, the old relations were immediately re-established. When the error was corrected, the new relations again quickly reappeared. But this dog presented a truly wonderful, unprecedented example of the formation of a delayed reflex. Generally the elaboration of a delayed reflex, when one and the same stimulus during different periods of its action produces now an inhibitory, now an excitatory effect, is in itself a difficult task. But its elaboration after a long experience of short-delayed reflexes, and even during it, is a truly complicated task, one that cannot be accomplished by the overwhelming majority of dogs and which in successful cases requires much time, even many months. Our dog accomplished this task in the space of a few days. What an extraordinary rapid and free use of the two opposite processes!

All that has been said about this dog entitles us to state that it represents the most perfect type, since it ensures strict equilibration with all that is taking place in the external environment, no matter how strong the stimuli are—both those to which the response must be positive activity, and those the effect of which must be inhibited—and no matter how quickly these different stimuli may interchange. It should be added that these extremely difficult tests were endured by the dog after it had been castrated.

The very opposite, in relation to the property of the nervous system under consideration, is the other dog ("Zolotisty", used by Yakovleva), whose general behaviour has been characterised above. Particularly manifest in the study of the conditioned reflex activity of this dog was the impossibility of obtaining a constant and adequate salivary food reflex; it fluctuated chaotically, often falling to zero. What did this signify? If the reflex tended to be strictly related to the moment of reinforcement, i.e., of feeding, why did it fluctuate and not become constant? This could not have been caused by insufficient inhibition, since we knew that the dog could endure protracted inhibition. Besides, the absence of preliminary salivation is by no means a manifestation of perfection; on the contrary, it indicates an obvious defect. Indeed, the importance of this salivation consists in the fact that the food introduced into the mouth immediately meets with the substance it needs. That this interpretation conforms to reality is proved, in the first place, by its universality, and, in the second place, by the fact that the extent of the preliminary salivation, which is biologically indispensable and important, always strictly corresponds to the amount of food. The natural explanation for the peculiarity of our dog must be sought in the fact that the initial inhibition, which exists in each delayed conditioned reflex—the period of retardation (or the latent period, as we called it previously)—although strong, is obviously insufficiently labile to keep within the proper time, and owing to inertness, oversteps the normal limits. None of the measures aimed at obtaining a constant salivary effect was successful.

Since the excitatory and inhibitory processes were strong in the dog, it was offered a very difficu't task, one, however, that is satisfactorily solved by some other dogs. Among other elaborated conditioned stimuli, and at different moments of this system of reflexes, a new stimulus was applied four times in the course of the experiment, but it was reinforced only when applied the last time; this was a task which required all the resources of the nervous system, and above all a high mobility of the nervous processes. Our dog did its best to solve this problem in a roundabout way, holding on everything which could be a simple, ordinary signal of the fourth reinforced application of the new stimulus. First of all it made use of the noise produced by the food receptacle which was moving before its eyes; during the first three applications of the new stimulus, when no food was offered and consequently no movement of the food receptacle took place, the dog remained in sitting posture. When, during the intervals between the stimulations, empty food receptacles were placed before it in order to deprive it of the signal connected with the reinforcement, it looked into them to see whether there was any food, and only when this was the case, did it stand up (usually it was sitting). When the receptacle was placed too high so that the dog could not see whether it contained anything, it rejected the food altogether, remaining in sitting posture regardless of the stimulus applied. In the case of a positive stimulus, it was necessary to enter the chamber and show the dog that the receptacle contained food, i.e., to invite it to eat, and only then did it begin to eat. Then both the new stimulus and the presentation of empty receptacles were discontinued. Only the old stimuli were applied, of course accompanied by reinforcement. And only *gradually* did the dog begin to rise under the action of the stimuli and to eat. Again the reflex evoked by the empty receptacle was extinguished. The dog continued to rise under the action of the old conditioned stimuli but—which was the usual thing with it—did not always exhibit any preliminary secretion of saliva. Now the new stimulus was again applied four times, being reinforced only the last time; during the first three applications the food receptacle was not placed before the dog, since, as has just been mentioned, the reflex to it had been extinguished. This time, too, the problem was solved by means of a simple, but new signal, namely, a complex stimulus formed from the new stimulus plus the noise of the moving food receptacle. When the new stimulus was applied for the first three times without the addition of the last stimulation, there was no reaction. But when during these first applications the receptacle was placed before the dog, but with no food in it, i.e., when the complex stimulus was depreciated, the dog, after rising several times in vain, definitely and completely ceased to react to the new stimulus, rising only under the influence of all the other stimuli. Then it was decided to restore the extinguished reflex to the new stimulus, abolishing all other stimuli and reinforcing the new stimulus eight times in succession in the course of the experiment. The rehabilitation of the reflex proceeded *very slowly*. The new stimulus was reinforced in the course of two days, that is, sixteen times, but despite the fact that the experimenter entered the chamber more than once and during the action of the new stimulus showed the food to the dog (only after which it rose to its feet and began to eat) it never stood up by itself under the action of the new stimulus. At first the same thing was observed on the third day; only during the nineteenth application of the new stimulus, when it was prolonged after the expiration of the usual thirty seconds and when new food receptacles were placed at intervals of ten seconds, did the dog, at the fourth presentation of a food receptacle, rise and eat the food. And only later, at first with considerable omissions on the part of the animal, a motor food reflex formed; for the purpose of accelerating its full restoration the dog was more than once left without food for a space of twenty-four hours. Afterwards, on the fifteenth day, there finally developed a full reflex accompanied by a preliminary secretion of saliva, but, inconstant, as usual. On the twentieth day, in order to obtain a constant salivary reflex, the dog was given only half the usual portion of food and this reduced ration was offered for a period of ten days. But the aim was not achieved—the salivary reaction remained inconstant, and even the motor reaction manifested itself either at the end of the action of the conditioned stimulus or only after the presentation of the food receptacle. What striking inertness of the *inhibitory* process! After this, for a period of fourteen days, the dog was given only a quarter of the normal quantity of food, but this, too, hardly changed the picture as far as the reflexes were concerned.

Against this background we began once again to elaborate a new and extremely simplified differentiation: in strict alternation the new stimulus was now reinforced, now not; it was necessary to elaborate reflexes to a single rhythm. In a period of eight days we failed to observe even the slightest trace of a reflex. What striking inertness of the *excitatory* process! Thinking that this phenomenon was partly due to excessive alimentary excitability we increased the quantity of food to half the usual ration. As a result, the difference in the extent of the salivary reaction under reinforced and non-reinforced stimuli now began gradually to manifest itself, and finally a stage was reached when, in the case of reinforced stimuli, the reaction became very considerable, while in the case of non-reinforced stimuli it fell to zero. However, the motor reaction persisted in all cases, although under positive stimuli it appeared quicker. When the experiments were prolonged in order to obtain a complete differentiation also of the motor reaction, the dog began to whine, at first before the experiment and then in the course of it, and tried all the time to escape from the stand. The motor reaction under a non-reinforced stimulus was fully differentiated in some experiments only when it came first in the experiment. The more time passed, the more difficult became the state of the dog; it no longer entered the experimental chamber of its own accord and when taken forcibly would turn back and run away. While in the chamber it kept on howling and barking. Under the action of stimuli the howling and barking became louder. This general behaviour was in striking contrast with the previous behaviour of the animal over a period of three years. In order to help the dog to attain complete differentiation, it was given a full daily ration of food; it gradually calmed down, went to the stand willingly, stopped howling and barking. At the same time a secretion of saliva was observed also under the action of a non-reinforced stimulus; then the salivary secretion induced by the action of the two kinds of stimuli began steadily to diminish until it reached zero. Finally, the motor reaction to a repeated stimulus also fully disappeared. The dog refused to perform its task and lay quietly throughout the experiment, searching for fleas or licking its body. After the experiment it devoured its food with avidity.

Thus, during the long period of the elaboration of a differentiation (the latter being at first difficult, and then quite simple), we observed the extreme inertness both of the excitatory and inhibitory processes. Particularly interesting and clear as to its mechanism was the last period— when a simple differentiation was being elaborated. Owing to a considerably heightened alimentary excitability this differentiation was at last almost completely worked out, but it was accompanied by extreme excitement on the part of the animal; this testified to the difficult state of its nervous system. But when the alimentary excitability declined to the level usually displayed by all the dogs during the experiments, our previous success in keeping the opposite nervous processes within the time limits required by the external conditions was reduced to naught. It proved more difficult for the dog to interchange the excitatory and inhibitory processes at intervals of five minutes, i.e., to maintain the almost elaborated procedure, the already formed nervous stereotype, than to repress the rather strong alimentary excitation, under which all our dogs worked quite satisfactorily during the experiments; this excitation was also in evidence in our dog, as proved by the fact that it eagerly devoured the food placed before it after the experiments. This fact strikingly testifies to the great importance of the normal mobility of the nervous processes, as well as to its obvious and considerable insufficiency in our dog, whose nervous processes, however, possessed great strength.

It is now possible clearly to see how the Greek genius, personified (individually or collectively) by Hippocrates, succeeded in discerning the fundamental features in the multitudinous variations of human behaviour. The singling out of melancholics from the mass of people signified the division of the entire mass of human beings in two groups —the strong and the weak, since the complexity of life must, naturally, tell with particular force on individuals with weak nervous processes and darken their existence. Thus, the paramount *principle of strength* was clearly stressed. In the group of strong individuals the choleric is distinguished by his impetuousness, i.e., inability to repress his temper, to keep it within the proper limits; in other words, he is distinguished by a predominance of the excitatory process over the inhibitory. This, consequently, established the *principle of equilibrium* between opposite processes. Finally, by means of a comparison between phlegmatic and sanguine types the *principle of the mobility* of the nervous processes was established.

There remains the question whether the number of basic variations of human and animal behaviour is confined to the classical figure "four". After years of observations, and as a result of numerous investigations on dogs, we acknowledge at any rate, for the time being, that this number conforms to reality; at the same time we admit that there are minor variations in the basic types of nervous system, especially in the weak type. In the strong unequilibrated type, for example, the animals with a particularly weak inhibitory process and, at the same time, quite a strong excitatory process, stand out. In the weak type the variations are, above all, based on the same properties which underlie the subdivision of the strong type into equilibrated and unequilibrated, active and inert animals. But in the weak type the feebleness of the excitatory process, so to speak, depreciates the significance of these other properties and actually makes this type, to a greater or lesser degree, an invalid one.

Now I shall dwell in more detail on the methods, on the more or less definite forms of experimentation already mentioned and which clearly disclose the basic properties of the types; I shall also touch on other, less manifest, forms, which are capable of demonstrating the same properties, though not so distinctly, and at the same time reveal to a greater degree the complexity of the type, even its entire outline. It should be added, however, that many forms of our experiments have not yet assumed definite importance in the solution of the problem of types. Of course, were our knowledge of the subject complete, everything observed by us in our animals, everything recorded by us, would find its proper place in this problem. But this is still far from being the case.

We have already mentioned a definite method of ascertaining the strength of the excitatory process, believing that this strength is most inherent in the strong type. It is a physically most powerful external agent which the animal is able to endure and to turn, along with other less powerful stimuli, into a certain signal, a conditioned stimulus, which remains active for a long period. For this purpose we usually apply very strong sounds produced by a special rattle which our ear endures with difficulty. In some dogs this stimulus, when reinforced, could be developed, equally with all others, into a real conditioned stimulus, and even take first place among them by virtue of the law of proportionality between the extent of the effect and the intensity of the external stimulus. In other dogs, in accordance with the law of maximum, its effect declined compared with the other strong conditioned stimuli, however, without interfering with the action of the other stimuli. In still other dogs, when applied, it led to the inhibition of the entire conditioned reflex activity, without becoming a conditioned stimulus. And finally, there were dogs in which one or two applications of this stimulus immediately evoked a chronic nervous disorder—a neurosis which did not disappear of itself and had to be treated.

The second method employed in the case of conditioned food reflexes consists in augmenting alimentary excitability by means of a more or less protracted state of hunger. As a result, in dogs with a strong excitatory process the effects of the strong stimuli, in some cases, are increased; however, there also takes place a relatively greater increase of the effects of weak stimuli, so that they fully or almost fully approximate to the effects of the strong stimuli. In other cases the effects of the strong stimuli remain unchanged, since they have reached their limit and have even somewhat overstepped it; and only the effects of weak stimuli increase, to the degree that they may even exceed the effects of strong stimuli. But in dogs with a weak excitatory process, a heightened alimentary excitability usually leads to a decline in the effects of all stimuli.

The two methods make it possible to determine directly

the maximum possible tension of the nerve cell, the limit of working capacity, either directly by the application of extremely strong external stimuli or through the action of stimuli of average strength, provided there is heightened reactivity of the cell, that its state is labile, which is essentially the same thing.

The third method consists in administration of caffeine. In the strong type a definite dose of caffeine increases the effect of the excitatory process; in the weak type it diminishes this effect, causing the cell to overstep the limits of its working capacity.

The weakness of the excitatory process is manifested with particular distinctness, perhaps, in the following experiment; it relates to the course of the excitatory process during the period of the isolated action of the conditioned stimulus; the ascertainment of the effect is facilitated by dividing this period into smaller time units. Three cases are possible: the effect of stimulation may increase regularly and progressively until it is joined by the unconditioned stimulus; it may, on the contrary, be considerable at the beginning and then gradually diminish; and finally, fluctuations of the effect may be observed—now increasing and now declining during the above-indicated period. This fact can be interpreted in the following way. The first case might indicate the presence of a strong excitatory process developing irresistibly under the unceasing action of the external stimulus. The second case, on the contrary, can be interpreted as the manifestation of a weak process for the following reason. In particular cases, for example, after local extirpations of the cerebral cortex, when under usual conditions the effect of the corresponding stimulus disappears, it is still possible to re-establish it in a very weak form in the course of the following experiment. At first the corresponding stimulus is applied several times, being reinforced each time almost immediately after the beginning of its action (in one or two seconds); then, when there is a considerable delay (twenty to thirty seconds), a positive effect is observed immediately after the beginning of the stimulation, which, however, declines rapidly, falling even to zero by the end of the isolated action of the stimulus. This is an obvious manifestation of the weakness of the excitatory process. Finally, the third case which is simply a struggle of opposite processes; the isolated action of the conditioned stimuli leads first to the development of inhibition, since each of our conditioned reflexes is a delayed reflex, i.e., one in which the excitatory process, being premature, must, for a longer or shorter period, be preceded by an inhibitory process and temporarily eliminated.

An absolute, and not relative, determination of the strength of the inhibitory process can be effected, above all, by testing its duration, i.e., by finding out how long the nerve cell can endure a state of continuous inhibition. As mentioned above, the main principle underlying this distinction is as follows. The strong, but unequilibrated, animals, as well as the weak ones, cannot endure a protracted inhibition, with the result that the entire system of conditioned reflexes is temporarily disturbed, or a chronic nervous disorder—neurosis—sets in. The strong animals cannot endure this, since they possess a very strong excitatory process to which the inhibitory process, being sufficient in itself, does not correspond as far as intensity is concerned; this is a case of relative weakness of the inhibitory process. In weak animals both the excitatory and inhibitory processes may be weak—this would be a case of absolute weakness. When the inhibitory process is strong (specially differentiated) its instantaneous or chronic prolongation to a period of five to ten minutes may not evoke any disturbance at all, or cause only a very slight one. But when the inhibitory process is weak, its chronic prolongation, for example, to thirty seconds instead of fifteen, often cannot be effected without causing serious consequences; a prolongation to five minutes, even if effected once, is sufficient to cause a failure of the entire conditioned reflex activity in the form of a persistent neurosis.

The second essential index of the strength of the inhibitory process is its ability rapidly and exactly to concentrate. Usually when an inhibitory process begins to develop at a definite point, it invariably first irradiates and produces a prolonged, successive inhibition. But as soon as the animal possesses a strong inhibition, the latter inevitably begins to concentrate to an ever-increasing degree and, finally, the successive inhibition wholly or almost wholly disappears. When the inhibition is weak, it may remain forever in a more or less pronounced form. The concentration of a strong inhibition entails an acute positive induction, i.e., one which appears immediately or after a short period of time; it is manifested in heightened excitability both in relation to the stimulus closest in time, and to the positive stimulus at the point of inhibition (on its termination).

Another index of the strength or weakness of the inhibitory process is the duration of the development of the inhibitory conditioned reflexes; the delay in elaborating an inhibitory reflex may be due to the very great strength of the excitatory process and, consequently, to the relative weakness of the inhibitory process, as well as to an absolute weakness of inhibition. But the end of the elaboration is still more instructive. No matter how long the elaboration of an inhibitory process may last, it remains incomplete forever; more often this takes place when the excitatory process is strong, when there is a relative weakness of the inhibitory process. In some cases the inhibitory process is obviously insufficient and reveals constant fluctuations, even to the extent of complete disappearance; this usually occurs in weak animals with an absolutely weak inhibitory process.

The weakness of the inhibitory process is also expressed in the fact that an almost complete inhibitory conditioned reflex can be obtained only when in the course of the experiment it is evoked first, before any of the positive conditioned reflexes; but if it is evoked in between the latter, it becomes considerably or almost completely disinhibited.

Finally, the absolute weakness of the inhibitory process may also be seen from the animal's attitude towards bromide. In weak dogs only very small daily doses of bromide, not more than a few centigrammes, or even milligrammes, and at most amounting to several decigrammes, prove to be efficient and useful, i.e., maintain a considerable conditioned reflex activity. This fact is explained as follows: since bromide undoubtedly bears a relation to the inhibitory process, in the sense that it strengthens it, only a slight intensification of this process under the influence of bromide can be endured when there is an inborn weakness of the inhibitory process.

Probably the following phenomenon, too, should be taken into consideration when determining the strength or weakness of the inhibitory process. When a differentiation is elaborated along with a positive stimulus, two contrary consequences are usually observed: either the effect of the positive stimulus increases, or, on the contrary, there is a decline of the effect compared with the level before the differentiation. What do these facts signify with regard to the strength of the nervous processes? It can be assumed that here it is a question of the strength or weakness precisely of the inhibitory process. In the first case a strong inhibitory process concentrates and causes a positive induction; in the second case, being weak, it irradiates and continuously reduces the effect of its positive stimulus. A comparison with other more precise indicators of the strength of the nervous processes may help to establish exactly the mechanism of this phenomenon.

As regards determining the mobility of the nervous processes, until recently we, as mentioned above, did not pay special attention to this particular property of the nervous processes: hence, we do not possess, or to be more exact, have not contemplated any special methods for determining it. Consequently, the job of elaborating them still remains, or the corresponding experimental forms must be selected from among those already at our disposal.

Perhaps a special and most precise method could be elaborated by means of trace conditioned reflexes. By changing, on the one hand, the duration of the indifferent stimulus, which must be turned into a special trace conditioned stimulus, and, on the other hand, the interval between the end of the indifferent agent and the beginning of the unconditioned stimulus that reinforces it, we shall be able directly to measure the degree of inertness or lability of the given nervous system. It can be anticipated, for instance, that, depending on the time needed for the disappearance of the trace of the stimulus which has ceased to act, the above indicated interval will be of essential importance for a quicker or slower elaboration of a trace conditioned reflex, or even for the possibility of its elaboration in general. The duration of the indifferent stimulus will likewise make itself felt. It is conceivable that in a particularly inert nervous system there will be specially and rapidly revealed for this stimulus the minimum duration under which it is still possible to elaborate a trace reflex.

Next come the methods already tried on two of our dogs which exhibited a striking contrast with regard to the mobility of their nervous processes and which have been cited above as examples. We shall now dwell on them in more detail, partly for the purpose of their further methodical examination and possible perfection, and partly, with the object of elucidating the mechanism of their action.

It might seem that the last method, applied to the inert dog and consisting in a regular rhythmic reinforcement or non-reinforcement of one and the same stimulus, which determined the elaboration of the respectively interchanging excitatory and inhibitory processes, is specially designed to reveal the mobility of these processes. However, this must be proved in a more precise way. By varying systematically in one and the same dog, as well as in dogs belonging to different types of nervous system, the duration of the interval between the reinforced and non-reinforced stimuli and by comparing the results, one can become fully convinced of the essential role played in this respect precisely by the mobility of the nervous processes. This has been just tested on the dog in question. After the summer recess last year the dog finally coped with the required rhythm at usual intervals of five minutes between the stimuli. When the intervals were reduced to three minutes, the rhythm became markedly disturbed. Consequently, the successful elaboration of a rhythm in different animals depends on the intervals, that is, on the degree of mobility of the nervous processes. The longer the required interval, the lower the mobility, and vice versa.

In order to elucidate the mechanism, I must speak in more detail about the complicated experiment (unsuccessfully performed on the same dog) consisting in an unusual elaboration of a conditioned stimulus from an external agent; this stimulus repeated several times in the course of the experiment among other elaborated conditioned stimuli was reinforced only when applied the fourth time. Successful solution of the problem could be attained subject to complete exclusion of the action of all other reflexes on the repeatedly applied agent. Only on this condition was it possible to establish a differentiation between the first repetitions of the agent and its last application. This probably occurs in the same way as the elaboration of a differentiation between particular moments of a protractedly acting stimulus in the case of a considerably delayed conditioned reflex, when at the initial phases of the action of one and the same prolonged stimulus there develops an inhibitory reflex, and at the later phases—a positive reflex. Otherwise, i.e., under the action of other stimuli, the excitatory process evoked by the repeatedly applied agent would not show regular fluctuations depending exclusively on the repetition of the agent, but would fluctuate accidentally and irregularly, depending in each case on the diverse influences of previously applied changing stimuli; hence, no differentiation between particular applications of the repeated agent could be elaborated. Consequently, only a high mobility of the nervous processes, i.e., a rapid development and discontinuance of the processes caused by all the other stimuli applied in the experiment, including, of course, the process of eating, could ensure the successful solution of the problem. It should be added that this difficult problem was, nevertheless, solved by another dog, although after a longer period of time and with much greater and more painful strain (experiments of Vyrzhikovsky). The effect produced by the first three applications of one and the same new external agent, varying its place in the system of other positive and negative conditioned stimuli, was inhibited; only the last, fourth, application became a constant, durable conditioned stimulus. Since in this dog the conditioned salivary reaction always preceded the addition of the unconditioned stimulus, our inert dog naturally could not make use of any extraneous signals, and consequently, the differentiation between particular applications of one and the same agent could take place only due to the distinction made by the peripheral receptor and the corresponding nerve cell between the last and the first three applications.

Hardly anything can be added to what has already been said about the methods and experimental forms testifying to the lability of the nervous processes in our first dog. The transformation of contrary conditioned stimuli into stimuli of opposite action is obviously determined, above all, by the mobility of the nervous processes which rapidly adapt themselves to the requirements of the new external conditions. This is generally proved by the greater or lesser difficulty with which this procedure is endured even by many strong equilibrated animals, to say nothing of weak and almost all castrated animals, which, as a rule, fall into a chronic morbid state. Similarly the other experimental form applied to this dog, namely, the rapid elaboration of a considerably delayed conditioned reflex among other short-delayed conditioned reflexes applied much earlier, of course, directly testifies to the high mobility of its nervous processes. The new excitatory process, despite the firmly established stereotype in the action of other stimuli, rapidly adapted itself to the requirements of the new condition, at first being replaced by a durable inhibitory process and then just as quickly reappearing after slight modification in the course of its development, a modification which more closely coincided with the application of the unconditioned stimulus.

Experiments with a direct transition from an inhibitory to an excitatory process and vice versa should likewise be included in the category of experimental forms ascertaining the mobility of the nervous processes. We know that in certain dogs this transition is accomplished easily and with exactitude. Sometimes, in particularly perfect types, the direct precedence of the inhibitory process, owing to its positive induction, determines even an increased effect of the positive stimulus; but in weak types this is usually accompanied by a breakdown, i.e., by a more or less serious nervous disorder.

The so-called reshaping of the stereotype, that is, a certain change in the sequence of a repeatedly applied system of the same conditioned reflexes (for example, a fully inverted sequence) must also be related to this category of experimental forms. In some dogs this change does not exert even the slightest influence on the effects of the different stimuli; in others it is sometimes accompanied by complete disappearance of the conditioned salivary reaction for days (in the case of food conditioned reflexes).

In old age it often happens that the systems of conditioned reflexes, previously reproduced in a regular and stereotype way, i.e., with precise effects of the stimuli, become irregular and chaotic; the precision and constancy of the effect can be re-established only by a simplification of the system—either by the exclusion of negative reflexes, or by a simultaneous reduction of the number of positive reflexes. It would be most natural to explain the mechanism of these facts by a decline, above all, in the mobility of the nervous processes, brought about by old age, as a result of which the inertness and duration of the processes, at previously established intervals, lead to a confusion and collision of the effects produced by the different stimuli.

Certain morbid disturbances observed in our dogs when they have to solve difficult nervous tasks, expressed in pathological states of definite cortical points, should be also ascribed to pathological changes in the mobility of the nervous processes; such are the inertness and explosiveness of the excitatory process. On the one hand, it was frequently observed that the excitatory process of an isolated point of the cortex became abnormally tenacious: the effect of the conditioned stimulus connected with it was not susceptible to inhibition by preceding inhibitory reflexes to such a degree as the effects of other stimuli; its extinction proceeded much more leisurely, and this stimulus did not lose its positive action, in spite of the fact that it was not reinforced systematically for weeks and months (Filaretov, Petrova). On the other hand, the previous stimulus, which had acted normally and whose moderate effect appeared after a certain delay, increasing after the addition of natural food stimuli and ending in the normal act of eating upon presentation of food, now, under a pathological state of the corresponding point of the cortex, began to produce a tremendous (secretory and motor) effect, arising and ending abruptly. When food was offered, the dog violently and obstinately rejected it (experiments of Petrova). It is clear that an extreme lability of the excitatory process was in evidence and that the latter, especially due to its summation with natural food stimuli, rapidly reached the limit of working capacity of the cortical cell and evoked a very strong transmarginal inhibition.

Thus, I repeat, the possible variations of the basic properties of the nervous system, as well as the possible combinations of these variations, determine the types of nervous system; as calculated, their number amounts at least to twenty-four. But life shows that the actual number is considerably smaller: we distinguish four types which are particularly distinct and strongly pronounced, and, what is most important, differ in their adaptability to the external environment and their resistibility to morbific agents.

We must admit a type of *weak* animals, characterised by a manifest weakness both of the excitatory and inhibitory processes; they never fully adapt themselves to the conditions of life, are easily broken, often and quickly become ill and neurotic as a result of difficult life situations, or, what is the same thing, of the difficult nervous tasks which we place before them. But of still greater importance is the fact that this type, as a rule, cannot be improved to any considerable degree by training and discipline; it becomes fit only under particularly favourable, deliberately created, conditions, or, as we usually say, in hot-house conditions.

The type is in contrast to the types of *strong* animals which in their turn markedly differ.

Among the latter, in the first place, is the *strong*, but *unbalanced* type with a strong excitatory process, but with a weaker, and sometimes even a considerably weaker, inhibitory process, in view of which this type is also easily subject to pathological disturbances when inhibition is required. This, predominantly, is a fighting type, but not adapted to everyday life with all its fortuities and exigencies. Nevertheless, being strong, it is capable of disciplining itself to a considerable degree, improving thereby the originally insufficient inhibition. We term it the *excitable type*, but to avoid misunderstanding and confusion it would be better to use the adjective *i m p e t u o u s*, which directly stresses its defect and at the same time obliges us to regard it as a strong type.

From this strong type one must single out the *strong* and *equilibrated* animals.

But these animals, in their turn, differ greatly, first of all in external behaviour, and this, as we already know, is precisely due to the mobility of the nervous processes. In order to designate these *strong* and *equilibrated* types we can correctly accord them the attributes *c a l m* and *l i v e l y*, in conformity with their mobility.

Such are the principal types which exactly correspond to the ancient classification of the so-called human temperaments—melancholic, choleric, phlegmatic and sanguine.

As for the less significant variations, they are most frequently met with, as already mentioned, in the weak type, but they have not yet been fully investigated and systematised by us.

In conclusion I wish to say a few words about the frequency of these types among the multitude of dogs of various breeds that have passed through our laboratories during our study of the conditioned reflexes. The *w e a k* type in all its variations and the *l i v e l y*, sanguine type are the most frequent; then comes the *impetuous*, choleric type; rarest is the *c a l m*, phlegmatic type.

Basing ourselves on the elementary physiological principles underlying the classification of the types of nervous system in animals, we must admit the same types in the mass of human beings—a classification already made by Greek classical thought. Thus, Kretschmer's classification of nervous types, which has obtained almost universal recognition, especially among psychiatrists, must be regarded as mistaken or inadequate. Kretschmer found his types in the clinic, among the ill. But are there not absolutely healthy individuals? And why must all human beings indispensably carry nervous and mental disorders in embryo?

Kretschmer's types represent only a part of all human types. His cyclothymics are closest to our excitable, impetuous type, or to Hippocrates' cholerics, and his schizothymics—to our weak type, or to Hippocrates' melancholics.

Since the first type lacks a proper abating and restorative process—the process of inhibition—its excitatory process often considerably exceeds the working capacity of the cortical cells. This causes a derangement of the proper interchange of normal work and rest, which manifests itself in extreme morbid phases of the excitatory and inhibitory states, both with regard to intensity and duration. Hence, the eventual development of a manic-depressive psychosis under particularly difficult circumstances of life, or under certain unfavourable conditions of the organism.

In the second type both processes are weak, and because of this it cannot endure individual and social life with its severe crises, which mostly fall on a still young, not sufficiently adjusted and hardened organism. This may lead, and often does lead, to a complete destruction of the higher part of the central nervous system, unless some lucky chance in life, or, more often, the protective function of the inhibitory process, does not save it from disastrous overstrain during this difficult period. It can be rightfully assumed that for those representatives of the weak type who end up with schizophrenia there are certain specific conditions, such as a particularly irregular course of development, or permanent auto-intoxication, causing extreme fragility of the nervous apparatus. Aloofness or reticence which, according to Kretschmer, is the main feature of schizothymics from childhood, does not present anything specific; in the case of a weak nervous system it is merely a general indication of the extreme complexity of the social environment; hence the natural withdrawal from it. Is it not a widely recognised and current fact that the mere transfer of a nervous person to a clinic or sanatorium, that is, the simple act of removing the patient from his everyday surroundings, affords relief and is even of curative importance?

It should be added that reticence or aloofness from society is by no means an exceptional feature of schizothymics, i.e., of weak individuals. Even strong persons may be reserved, but for quite different reasons. This type of person leads a strenuous but at the same time one-sided subjective life; he early becomes possessed by a certain inclination, concentrates on a single aim and is dominated and carried away by a single idea. Other people are not only undesirable; they even disturb him and distract him from the principal object of life.

Naturally, there are many great men also among cyclothymics (the strong type). But it is understandable, that, being unequilibrated, they possess a particularly fragile nervous system. Hence, the widespread and vividly discussed problem: genius or insanity?

And then comes, of course, the multitude of human beings more or less strong and even exceedingly so, and at the same time equilibrated, the phlegmatics and the sanguines, the people who make the history of mankind either by their systematic mundane but indispensable labour in all branches of life, or by the exploits of their mind, lofty emotions and iron will. Of course, as far as great men are concerned, no matter how strong they may be, they are also subject to breakdowns, since the scale of their activity is extraordinary, and there is a limit to any strength.

EXPERIMENTAL PATHOLOGY OF THE HIGHER NERVOUS ACTIVITY[71]

First I should like to say a few introductory words concerning the complicated fate of our work in the sphere of physiology and pathology of the higher nervous activity, assuming that the adjectives "higher nervous" conform to the adjective "psychical".

Thirty-five years ago I was engaged in the investigation of digestion—previously a special subject of mine—and among other things I investigated the so-called "psychical secretion of saliva". Intending to subject it to further analysis, I soon became convinced that if we adopted the psychological standpoint, that is, if we started guessing what the dog feels, thinks, etc., nothing would come of it and no exact knowledge could be obtained. It was then that I first decided to treat this psychical phenomenon, this "psychical salivation" as objectively, that is, solely from without, as everything else is studied in physiology. Soon Dr. Tolochinov became my associate and we began this work together. Helped by numerous collaborators we have been carrying on this work incessantly for the last thirty-five years.

At the outset the work was marked by a slight but interesting occurrence in our laboratory life. When I decided to continue the work along those lines, one of my collaborators, a very clever and alert young man who had worked with me on another, ordinary physiological subject, expressed his astonishment and even indignation. "How is that?" he said. "For goodness' sake! Is it conceivable to study psychical activity on dogs, and in the laboratory?" And this, as it appeared subsequently, was very significant. Twelve years later, when I travelled to London for the jubilee celebrations of the Royal Society, I met the leading British neurophysiologist Sherrington. "You know," he said to me, "your conditioned reflexes would hardly be popular in England, since they have a materialistic flavour."

Well, and how do matters stand at present? I must tell you that these first impressions of our new work are still typical of the attitude to it of a considerable part of the educated public; and because of this work I am regarded by many as a very odious person.

Now, what about science? Here, too, the situation is far from being definite. True, in England, the country with which Sherrington tried to frighten me, there is an altogether different situation. There, the theory of the conditioned reflexes is now taught in all schools. It has been widely recognised also in the United States. But this is a long way from being the case in all countries. In Germany, for instance, the approach towards this theory is far from being such. Not very long ago a German professor of physiology visited Kharkov: in the course of a conversation with Professor Volborth—one of my former assistants—about conditioned reflexes, he plainly stated that this was "keine Physiologie".

It should be added that in general physiologists still cannot exactly determine the proper place of conditioned reflexes in the textbooks on physiology. It seems to me that these reflexes must be rightfully advanced to the fore when expounding the physiology of the cerebral hemispheres, since they represent the normal, objectively established work of these hemispheres. Analytical data accumulated up to the present time by means of stimulations, extirpation and other methods of investigating the cerebral cortex, must follow, naturally, the description of the normal activity.

I do not know what impression our modern physiology of conditioned reflexes expounded by Prof. Podkopayev has made on you, but in submitting the pathology of these reflexes, I make so bold as to think that you will see for yourselves how expedient and fruitful our method of treating the subject is. That is why I deemed it necessary to begin with this short introduction.

Now for the subject itself. I am very glad that Prof. Podkopayev delivered his lectures on the physiology of conditioned reflexes, prior to me, before this very audience; this relieves me of the need to make any preliminary explanations. I take it for granted that all of you are in possession of the basic physiological data, and so I shall proceed directly to an exposition of the purely pathological facts.

The nervous activity, as all physicians are aware, consists of two mechanisms, or two processes—excitatory and inhibitory. With regard to these two processes we distinguish three fundamental elements, namely, the strength of both the excitatory and inhibitory nervous processes, the mobility of these processes—their inertness or lability—and finally, the equilibrium between these processes.

Certainly, the entire normal higher nervous activity, or in the usual terminology, the psychical activity, not only of animals, but also of man, is based on the normal course of these processes with their inherent properties. At least our experiments with dogs, our usual objects of investigation, have convinced us that all their intricate and highly complex relations with the surrounding world fully come within the bounds of our research into the above-mentioned processes and their properties; they are comprehended by us to the extent permitted by the possibilities of our experiments.

We can divert all these processes with their basic properties from their normal path and cause them to become pathological. For this purpose we have quite definite methods at our disposal. There are three of these methods —overstrain of the excitatory process, overstrain of the inhibitory process and overstrain of the mobility of the nervous processes. As to the latter methods, it should be pointed out that the expression "overstrain of the mobility of the nervous processes" is actually used by me for the first time; usually we referred to it as collision of the excitatory and inhibitory processes.

How to weaken the excitatory process, to make it pathological? For this purpose it is necessary to act upon the cell, within which the excitatory process is produced, by an external agent of a very great, extraordinary strength; by doing so we overstrain the work of the cell, its excitatory process, as a result of which the latter becomes pathological.

In a similar way, that is, by overstrain, the inhibitory process can also be made pathological.

You already know how we obtain inhibition by means of negative conditioned stimuli. Let us suppose that a given conditioned inhibitory stimulus has constantly evoked in its cell inhibition of half a minute duration and that the cell has endured it very well. I then expressly prolong the action of the same stimulus for five or ten minutes. A strong cell is able to sustain it, but in a weak cell the inhibition breaks down; the work of the cell becomes pathological and changes in different ways.

Finally, the third method. It is possible to make both the excitatory and inhibitory processes pathological by means of abruptly transforming, without any intervals, the inhibitory state of the cell into a state of excitation, or vice versa. We usually refer to this as a collision between the excitatory and inhibitory processes. It is obvious that a certain amount of time is required for a corresponding change in the activity of the cerebral cells, just as it is required for any other activity. Under such collisions only those cells may remain unaffected and intact where the basic nervous processes are strong and especially where these processes are highly labile.

Now, what results from the action of these morbific methods? How does deviation from the normal occur? How is the pathological state of the cells originated? A general weakening of the cell takes place. As to the excitatory process, the cell becomes incapable of performing the work which it performed previously, i.e., the limit of its working capacity decreases, and this manifests itself in the following pathological phenomena.

You are aware that if we have before us an absolutely normal cell and that if we apply external agents of different physical strength as conditioned stimuli, the conditioned effects of these stimuli more or less correspond to their physical strength.

Now, if we break this cell down, i.e., if we overstrain it and thus make it pathological, its relation to the stimuli becomes different. In some cases conditioned positive stimuli of different physical strength produce an equal effect, and then we say that this is the equalisation phase of the cell's activity. In other cases, when the weakening of the cell, i.e., the decrease in the limit of its working capacity, is progressing, a state sets in in which strong stimuli produce a lesser effect than weak ones; this is the paradoxical phase. Finally, a further disturbance of the cell's activity manifests itself in the fact that the cell no longer responds to the positive stimulus, whereas the inhibitory stimulus produces a positive effect; we have termed this phase the ultraparadoxical phase.

Besides the decline in the limit of working capacity, i.e., the weakening of the excitatory process in the cell, there can also be observed other changes of the excitatory process. One of the most striking of these—particularly interesting and particularly applicable in neurology and psychiatry—is the inert state of the excitatory process, i.e., a state in which the excitatory process becomes more tenacious, persistent, and gives way more slowly to normally arising inhibitory influences.

I shall dwell for a while on inertness. The excitatory process normally, even in healthy people, varies not only in strength, but also in another respect—in mobility. With some people the excitatory process is less mobile, i.e., it is more susceptible to stimulation, reacts more quickly under the influence of stimulation; at the same time, when the stimulation is over, its effect disappears sooner than with other types of normal people.

On this basis we, like Hippocrates, divide the equilibrated, strong animals into two categories—the phlegmatic and the sanguine. The phlegmatics, it follows, will be characterised by a relatively slow development of the excitatory process, the sanguines—by a quick one.

But this is within the bounds of normalcy. If, however, I act on the cell by means of morbific methods, I can make the inertness of its excitatory process excessive and pathological so that its state of excitation becomes exceedingly persistent.

Concerning the pathological changes of the excitatory process the following addition should be made. Two morbid changes in its mobility are observed. One of these I have just mentioned—pathological stagnation. Given other morbific conditions we get a diametrically opposite state of the nerve cell, namely, pathological lability. In neurology this is known as excitatory weakness, i.e., a state in which the cell becomes very alert, very rapidly reacts to stimulation, and at the same time quickly becomes bankrupt and weakens. We call this the state of explosiveness.

In the same way it is possible to break down (in our usual laboratory terminology) the inhibitory process as well, to make it pathological. By means of a sudden, and not gradual, considerable extension of the duration of the inhibitory state in a cell through the action of a corresponding external stimulus, we can greatly weaken the inhibitory function of the cell and almost fully destroy it.

It should be pointed out that in this respect the inhibitory process has been investigated to a lesser degree than the excitatory one.

The inhibitory process, too, usually manifests itself in different ways with regard to its mobility. Sometimes it develops rapidly and just as rapidly vanishes; sometimes, on the contrary, it assumes a more protracted character.

Thus, the inhibitory process is either normally inert or normally labile. However, it can also be brought to a pathological state with regard to inertness. In our laboratory there is a dog which has been exhibiting pathological inertness for the past three years. In this animal under the influence of frequent collisions, the positive stimulus began to evoke, instead of the normal excitatory process, an inhibitory one, and of such a persistent nature that although we constantly reinforced it under favourable conditions in the course of the three years, we just could not restore its initial positive effect. Only recently did we find a means of changing this state of affairs, but I shall speak about that at the end.

Thus, you have before you, in general outline, the changes which occur under the action of morbific agents—the change in the excitatory process, the change in the inhibitory process and, hence, as a result, a derangement of the proper correlations between the excitatory and inhibitory processes. But the normal activity of the nervous system is, of course, determined by an equilibrium between these basic processes with their normal properties.

I must tell you that often it is quite easy to obtain a pathological state of the higher nervous activity with the help of the methods I have just mentioned. But, depending on the types of nervous system, one can observe a great difference in the facility with which this pathological state is attained.

In equilibrated and strong animals, i.e., those in which both the excitatory and inhibitory processes are of equal strength and whose lability is normal, it is, of course, likewise possible to produce a nervous disorder; however, it would take considerable time and labour, since it necessitates trying different methods. In excitable and weak animals this is very easily attained. As you already know, we classify as "excitable" that type of animal in which the excitatory process is very strong; the inhibitory process is probably also considerable, but the two processes do not conform. The excitatory process strongly predominates, and therefore in this type the negative stimuli hardly ever reach zero. This type can be broken down rather easily, i.e., made pathological. As soon as it is offered a series of tasks calling for a considerable degree of inhibition, it becomes quite weak—the animal can no longer discern anything, inhibit anything, i.e., it becomes neurotic.

As regards animals of the weak type, they can be easily made abnormal by all our methods.

The neurotic state manifests itself in the fact that the animal does not properly respond to the conditions in which it exists. This relates both to its laboratory characteristics and general behaviour. With regard to the latter everyone will admit that whereas previously the dog was normal, it is now ill.

In the laboratory we usually apply a system of conditioned reflexes—positive and negative—which are elaborated on the basis of various unconditioned stimuli: positive reflexes to stimuli of different physical strength and negative reflexes of different kinds. This entire system is normally governed by strict rules: the positive effect depends on the strength of stimulation; the inhibitory stimulus produces a greatly diminished or a zero effect, etc. Under the influence of our morbific methods all or many of the normal reactions become weakened and distorted.

The disturbed nervous equilibrium is clearly observed not only by us in the system of conditioned reflexes; our attendants also notice it. The dog obeyed them previously, behaved orderly, it knew where to go when led to an experiment. Now everything has abruptly changed. And the attendants simply say that the dog has become stupid and even has gone mad.

The pictures of neuroses in diseased animals vary considerably owing either to the different intensity of the disorder, or to the appearance in the foreground of this or that pathological symptom. Recently we have observed a particularly large number of such neuroses and neurotic symptoms on an organically pathological basis, namely, on castrated animals. It goes without saying that castration itself disturbs the normal relations within the nervous system. I shall, therefore, briefly touch on the postoperative state of our dogs, as far as their nervous system is concerned.

One of the most striking of the morbid, neuropathological symptoms appearing almost immediately after castration is an enormous decline of the inhibitory process, of the inhibitory function, so that the dog, which prior to the operation acted in an exemplary manner, in full accordance with the conditions influencing its nervous system, now becomes quite chaotic. Normally one sees day after day an absolutely uniform and perfectly exact system of conditioned reflexes, but after castration no day is similar to another; there is a series of entirely different days and there is no order whatsoever.

One more very important detail manifested itself shortly after castration and surprised even us. In the case of strong types, the action of the animals after castration, as I have just said, is extremely distorted and instead of being strictly regular, becomes chaotic. In the case of weak types the reverse is the case. For some time after the operation the dogs behave better and more orderly than before. True, this different condition exists only temporarily—for one, one and a half or two months. Then the nervous activity in these dogs, too, becomes weakened just as that in strong dogs. I shall revert to this question later and show on what this difference is based and how we interpret it.

Then, after months of entirely chaotic activity a circularity sets in which did not exist before, i.e., the dogs do not work and manifest their system of conditioned reflexes in a disorderly manner constantly, i.e., from day to day, but their activity now periodically changes. It is chaotic for a while and then for a certain period it greatly improves in a spontaneous way and becomes more orderly. And as time goes on, the more distinct this periodicity becomes; the periods of better work are more frequent and of larger duration, until after some years everything becomes normal. This, obviously, denotes the existence of certain adaptability in the organism.

Of course, since we know the system of endocrine glands, which to a certain degree assist and replace one another, it is conceivable that in time the defect sustained by the organism immediately after castration becomes more or less levelled out. But the return to the apparent normal after castration takes place in different dogs after different periods; with some it occurs after one month, with others it takes years, and there are dogs in which this state has so far not set in at all. This is obviously connected with the initial strength of the nervous system.

It is clear that in these castrated dogs, after their full or partial recovery, it is possible to produce various neuroses much more easily than in absolutely normal dogs, since in the former the equilibrium has already been disturbed, and naturally they are, so to speak, more fragile than normal dogs. Thus, we can produce in them numerous neurotic disturbances by means of the above-mentioned morbific methods.

To a considerable degree the pathological nervous states produced by us conform to the so-called psychogenic diseases in human beings. The same overstrain and the same collisions of the excitatory and inhibitory processes are also encountered in our own lives. For instance, somebody has deeply insulted me and I for some reason or other have not been able to respond to it by corresponding words, or, moreover, by a certain action, with the result that I had to overcome the struggle or conflict between the excitatory and inhibitory processes within myself. And this was repeated more than once. Or let us take another case from the literature on neuroses. A daughter is at the sick-bed of her father whom she loves deeply and who is living his last days; however, she must pretend that everything is all right and that everybody expects his recovery, whereas in reality she is weighed down by unbearable anguish and sorrow. This often leads to breakdowns, to neuroses.

Indeed, can we find any essential physiological difference between such breakdowns and those which we obtain in our experimental animals by colliding the excitatory and inhibitory processes?

But in addition to these neuroses, there must be, owing to the extreme complexity of our brain in comparison with that of the higher animals, special human neuroses, to which I ascribe psychasthenia and hysteria. These states cannot be produced in dogs, since in cases of this kind the division of the human brain into a higher, purely human part, connected with speech, and a lower part, which, just as in animals, receives the external impressions and directly analyses and synthesises them in a certain way, makes itself felt. But neurasthenic states of different kinds can be fully reproduced in animals.

In view of the fact that our data seemed to me sufficient for a physiological interpretation of the mechanisms of nervous diseases, I decided, two or three years ago, to visit the neurological and the psychiatric clinics (of course, devoting only a little time to the matter). As far as the neurological clinic is concerned, I can say that practically all the neurotic symptoms and pictures observed there can be understood and connected with our pathophysiological laboratory facts. And this is not only my personal opinion, the opinion of a physiologist, it is also the opinion of neuropathologists who acquainted me with the clinic and who admit that our physiological interpretation of neuroses is not fantastic, that we are really laying a solid foundation for constant contact between our laboratory facts and human neuropathological phenomena.

Before passing to another category of our facts I shall explain a phenomenon which I have mentioned but have not analysed in detail.

Why is it that animals with strong nervous systems immediately after castration become chaotic, and only later, after a certain time, does their behaviour more or less level out, while animals with weak nervous systems, on the contrary, immediately after castration behave better, in a more regular manner than before castration, and only later become disabled?

We think that this phenomenon should be explained in the following way. Since an animal possesses sex glands, it experiences sexual excitation; consequently, additional impulses come to the brain and tonify it; but the brain is weak. Hence the deficiency in the general nervous activity. With the removal of the sex glands the additional stimuli disappear, the nervous system is eased, and its activity in all other respects assumes a more expedient character. There is nothing fantastic in this explanation. We clearly observe the same in another, more tangible case. The degree of appetite in the experimental dog is of great importance in our system of conditioned reflexes. If you have a strong dog and increase its food excitability by means of a certain method (while performing experiments with food reflexes), then all its conditioned effects are increased. On the contrary, with a weak dog a heightened food excitability usually leads to a decline of the conditioned reflexes, i.e., the additional excitation cannot be endured by the dog, and is accompanied by inhibition, which we, therefore, call protective.

Now I shall proceed to another category of facts. The development of definite pathological states in the nervous system with the aid of our definite methods is, of course, based on the fact that our concept of the mechanism of this system is to a certain degree correct. The power of our knowledge over the nervous system will, of course, appear to much greater advantage if we learn not only to injure the nervous system but also to restore it at will. It will then have been really proved that we have mastered the processes and that we can control them. Actually, this is the case. In many instances we not only bring on disease, but eliminate it with great exactitude, one might say, to order. Of course, in this case it was necessary, above all, instead of reasoning and searching for various remedies at random, to be guided by the indications of medicine. Thus, bromide plays a very important role with us. But in order to apply this remedy accurately thorough knowledge of the mechanism of its action was necessary.

With regard to bromide we have definitely established, without the least doubt, that its action is quite different from that hitherto assumed and possibly still assumed by pharmacologists. The physiological effect of bromide consists not in decreasing excitability or in weakening the excitatory process, but in intensifying the inhibitory process. Bromide bears a special relation to the inhibitory process, and this can be proved by numerous experiments. Here, for example, is a very simple experiment which we always apply when need arises.

You have an excitable type of dog—the type in which the excitatory process is extremely strong and the inhibitory process relatively weak. Consequently, the dog cannot bring its inhibitory reflexes to a complete zero—its inhibition is insufficient. You administer bromide to the dog and immediately obtain complete inhibition. You often observe in this case also a greater positive effect than previously, before the administration of bromide. But there is another, no less important side to the effect of bromide.

Although bromide has been rightly used as a remedy for nervous diseases for years (I do not know exactly for how many years but not less than sixty or seventy), it is an absolute truth that to this day medicine has not always used this powerful instrument of nervous therapy in a proper way, often committing a very serious error.

You administer bromide in a case of a neurotic state. Let us suppose that the bromide produces no effect. Then you increase the dose thinking that the previous dose was too small. But this is true only in one series of cases. In other cases, and probably in the overwhelming majority of them, the dose must be decreased and not augmented. Often you must even decrease the dose to a very considerable degree. The gradation of the useful doses of bromide is highly extensive; in our dogs its limits are approximated to a thousandfold. This is absolutely true and we all guarantee it. Consequently, a very important correction must be made in medicine in this respect. If you administer an excessively large dose, you may obtain an injurious instead of a beneficial effect; you may cause the patient serious injury.

There can be no question, of course, that this is true only of dogs, and that with nervous people matters are different. The neuropathologists in our clinic have observed that when they took these facts into consideration it turned out that in many cases successful treatment necessitated not an increase in the doses of bromide but reduction to decigrammes and centigrammes. The general laboratory rule is: the weaker the type of nervous system and the given nervous state, the smaller must be the dose of bromide.

As is also well known in medicine, rest, too, provides a certain curative effect in laboratory neuroses. If a dog has been made neurotic by us, it is often helpful not to work with this dog every day, since a daily system of our conditioned reflexes is undoubtedly a difficult task, which in this state is beyond the dog's strength. As soon as you introduce a regular two-or three-day recess between the experiments, the nervous system begins to recover.

In some cases it has been observed that rest, as it were, substitutes bromide. Suppose you have a dog whose work after castration is chaotic. You can help it in two ways: either you make it work (that is, you experiment with it) not every day, but once in two or three days, with the result that its work considerably improves; or you administer a suitable dose of bromide which produces the same effect.

It should be pointed out that we are now applying another extremely important method of treatment, but as yet we are not entitled to say definitely that it is an agent of radical treatment. Still, it is impossible not to pay attention to it and not to look upon it with great hope.

With the help of our morbific methods, which make the whole cerebral cortex pathological, it is also possible to cause a completely isolated region of the cortex to become ill; this is an extremely important and highly impressive fact. Suppose you have a dog with a series of different acoustic conditioned stimuli: beats of the metronome, a noise, a tone, a crackling or a gurgling sound, etc. From all these stimuli it is not difficult to obtain only one which would prove noxious and evoke a sharp deviation from the normal. So long as you apply the other acoustic stimuli, the animal's behaviour is orderly and its work is quite regular. But the moment you touch the point of application of the morbific stimulus, not only is the reaction to it distorted in one degree or another, but thereafter the entire system of conditioned reflexes becomes deranged, and its harmful effect spreads over the whole cerebral cortex. This fact in itself leaves no room for doubts, since it has been frequently produced and is being produced now by many experimenters.

But here I would like to draw your attention to the following. When I enumerated all our sounds, it was obvious that they were of a more or less complex nature. How, then, are we to picture the disorder of the cerebral cortex in relation to separate sounds? It can hardly be assumed that to each sound applied by us there corresponds a particular group of nerve cells receiving the elementary acoustic stimuli of which the sound is formed. It is more probable that in the case of each of our acoustic stimuli it is a question of a dynamic structural complex, whose elements, the corresponding cells, enter also into other dynamic complexes when other complex sounds are applied. And it is the results of the difficulties created by our morbific methods in the process connecting and systematising the dynamic complexes that are responsible for the destruction and disturbances in those complexes.

Isolated pathological points can be obtained in all parts of the cerebral hemispheres. Here is an example. You elaborate conditioned positive stimuli from a mechanical stimulation of different spots of the skin. You can obtain such a state when in two points of the skin the excitatory process does not call forth any pathological effect while the third is functionally pathological.

We now have a dog of the excitable type, i.e., one in which the excitatory process is extremely strong but in which the corresponding inhibition is insufficient. This dog has been castrated. Being of a strong type it recovered rather quickly. Since it was excitable much time and effort was required prior to castration to elaborate in it a differentiation to the metronome. For a period after castration our laboratory sustained some trouble: there was a shortage of food for the animals and they became emaciated. Due to the general nervous exhaustion the reflex of our dog to the metronome, which had been complicated by a difficult differentiation, became morbid, while all other conditioned reflexes remained unaffected. As soon as metronomes were applied, normal work with conditioned reflexes became impossible. We tried to exclude the inhibitory metroncme as the more difficult one, and to make use only of the positive metronome, but that did not change the picture. Bromide proved ineffective, which, for some unknown reason, is generally the case in disorders of isolated points of the cerebral hemispheres.

Then the question arose whether the same thing would occur in another part, in another analyser of the cerebral hemispheres where the excitatory and the inhibitory processes would collide. In order to obtain an answer to this question we selected the cutaneous region, where we could apply an easier differentiation, i.e., make one spot of the skin positive and another inhibitory. The stimulation of one spot was reinforced by feeding, while that of the other spot was not. The effect was the same. So long as the positive conditioned stimulus alone was being elaborated, the dog behaved quite normally, and the entire system of reflexes was in order. But as soon as the inhibitory stimulus began to manifest itself, all the reflexes diminished and became distorted; the dog became extremely violent, so that the experimenter could not attach the apparatus to the skin or take it off without the risk of being bitten.

Now I wish to direct your attention to the following interesting phenomenon. When we had such isolated points in the cerebral cortex of other dogs, their harmfulness and morbidness were expressed only in the fact that their stimulation resulted in the derangement or destruction of our entire system; but our observations showed that this was never accompanied by a manifestation of pain in the animals. However, in this case there was a distinct impression that the touch to the skin became painful. How is this phenomenon to be explained?

As a matter of fact the only difficulty during the collision of the excitatory and inhibitory processes was in the brain, and this difficulty made itself felt in the system of conditioned reflexes. What, then, caused the pain in the skin? Apparently this may, and should, be explained in the following way. In a certain point of the cerebral cortex of the dog there arises a considerable difficulty, which must cause pain, just as you feel a kind of heaviness, a very disagreeable sensation in your head when you tackle an extraordinary difficult problem. We must assume a similar state in our dog. But in the course of these experiments the dog apparently formed a conditioned connection between the attaching of the apparatus to the skin and the difficult state of the cutaneous analyser in the brain; conditionally the dog transfers the struggle against this difficult state in the brain to the moment of skin stimulation, exhibiting resistance to any contact with the skin. However, this is not a hyperaesthesia of the skin. Consequently, this is an extremely interesting case of objectification of an internal cerebral process, a manifestation of the strength of its connection with the stimulation of the skin. As for the brain, we must assume merely a special kind of heavy sensation in it, a peculiar kind of pain. It is not without reason that psychiatrists have described melancholia as a mental pain, or a cortical pain, the sensation of which differs from the pain caused by wounds or disorders of different parts of the organism.

Thus, for a long time we could not do anything with this dog. At last, however, a favourable way out was found thanks to the good fortune of one of my oldest and most valuable associates, Dr. Petrova. Formerly Petrova worked as a therapist, but later she was enticed into the study of conditioned reflexes and has devoted herself entirely to it for many years. I had an interesting experience in this connection. I must tell you that although I began my professorship as a pharmacologist, I have always had a strong prejudice against introducing several substances at a time into the organism. It always struck me as strange whenever I saw a prescription containing three and more drugs. What a brew! And I had always been against such combinations of pharmaceutical remedies in the physiological analysis of phenomena; in this I proceeded from the principle that the simpler the conditions of the phenomena are, the better the chances for elucidating them. I admitted bromide to our laboratory as a single drug basing myself on medical practice; caffeine was also introduced as a separate stimulant related to the excitatory process. But I was always against using them in combination. However, the therapist, being used to combinations, insisted on a trial, and proved to be right. The effect was extraordinary and miraculous. When a mixture of bromide and caffeine was given to the dog mentioned above, the persistent neurosis immediately disappeared without leaving the slightest trace. We acted carefully. Having administered the mixture of bromide and caffeine for two days, we at first tried only the positive mechanical stimulation of the skin. The effect proved to be normal; the animal was absolutely quiet and no derangement of the system of conditioned reflexes was observed. A little later, being encouraged by the results of the trial of the positive stimulus, we applied the negative one. In this case too the effect proved to be the same—there was not the slightest trace of the former morbid reaction.

Post factum it was not difficult for me to build a respective theory. Now I presented the matter to myself in the following way. Certainly it must be assumed that in the overwhelming majority of cases a disorder of the nervous system is a disturbance of the proper correlations between the excitatory and inhibitory processes, as it appeared in the course of application of our morbific methods. Now since we have, so to speak, two levers in the form of pharmaceutical remedies, two communicators towards the two chief apparatus, i.e., towards the two processes of nervous activity, then by putting into action and correspondingly changing the strength now of one, now of the other lever, we have a chance of restoring the disturbed processes to their former place, to their proper correlations.

We have another similar case. I have already mentioned the case of the dog in which the pathological inertness of the inhibitory process lasted for three years, i.e., its positive process became pathological and the positive stimulus turned into an inhibitory one. Although we have been constantly reinforcing this stimulus for three years now, i.e., we have been creating the conditions under which it ought to be positive, we have always had it inhibitory. No matter what we tried—bromide, rest, etc.—nothing helped. Under the influence of the mixture of bromide and caffeine this stimulus which for such a long time produced a morbid reaction, has now assumed a normal positive effect.

In the same dog, parallel with the pathological inertness of the inhibitory process, there was pathological lability of the excitatory process on another stimulus, i.e., it developed its action not gradually but impetuously, in an explosive manner; but a negative phase set in quickly in the course of the excitation. At the first moment of the application of this conditioned stimulus the dog makes a violent effort to reach the food receptacle and exhibits a profuse salivary secretion, but soon, already in the course of excitation, the salivation stops; when you begin to reinforce the stimulus and offer food, it does not take it and turns away. This pathological phenomenon, too, disappears under the action of our mixture, the morbific stimulus becoming quite normal in its action.

Interesting too is the following fact. We administered the mixture to this dog for ten days and then decided to find out whether the cure was radical. But this was not the case. When we ceased to administer the mixture the old relations returned. Of course, much more time is probably required to eliminate the disturbances entirely. But one can also assume that we really establish correct relations between both processes changing them temporarily, but do not treat the processes themselves, or at least both of them simultaneously. It is clear that should it be the first case, it is a great triumph for therapy. In any event, in the present-day palliative, and possibly future radical treatment by means of a mixture of bromide and caffeine, it is necessary to take into account the extreme precision of the dosage of both drugs, reducing them, especially in the case of caffeine, even to milligrammes.

In conclusion, I shall briefly touch on the question of the application of our laboratory results to the neuropathological and psychiatric clinics. As for the first, there is no doubt that our human neuroses can be explained quite satisfactorily in the light of the laboratory analysis. But it seems to me that in psychiatry, too, certain things have been clarified by our laboratory research.

At present I am writing a series of booklets entitled *Latest Papers on the Physiology and Pathology of the Higher Nervous Activity*. Two brief articles published in the last issue have been translated into foreign languages. One of them has already been published in French, the other has been sent to an English psychiatric journal, and it goes without saying that I eagerly await the reaction of our own and foreign experts.

Now you are aware that in the laboratory we are able to make pathological, and besides, in a functional way, an isolated point of the cerebral cortex, leaving all other points absolutely intact. I wish to make use of this phenomenon of isolated disorders for interpreting a very interesting and very enigmatic psychiatric form, namely paranoia. As is known, paranoia is characterised by the fact that a mentally normal person, who, like all healthy people, reckons with logic and reality, and sometimes may even be gifted, as soon as it comes to one definite subject, distinctly turns into a lunatic, acknowledging neither logic, nor reality. It seems to me that this form can be understood on the basis of our laboratory findings relating to isolated disorders of separate points in the cerebral cortex.

One can hardly dispute that the stereotypies of skeletal movement can and should be understood as the expression of the pathological inertness of the excitatory process in the cortical cells which are connected with movement, and that perseverations should be similarly looked upon only in the cells of speech movement. But at first sight it is more difficult to explain obsessive ideas and **paranoia** in the same way. However, it seems to me that the understanding of isolated pathological points of the cerebral cortex not only in a purely crude anatomical sense, but also in a structurally-dynamic one (as mentioned above) has eliminated this difficulty to a sufficient degree.

Here is another case of a neurosis which is very close to a psychosis.

In persecution mania the patient sometimes firmly regards as reality that which he fears and wants to avoid. For example, he wants to have a secret and it seems to him that all his secrets are constantly being disclosed in some way. He wants to be alone, and although he is alone in his room and everything lies open before his eyes, he still imagines that somebody else is with him. He wants to be respected, and it seems to him that at every moment he is being insulted in some way or other by signs, words, or facial expressions. Pierre Janet has described this as feelings of possession, as if somebody is taking hold of the patient.

In my view, this case is based physiologically on the ultraparadoxical phase, which I have already mentioned and which, as you know, consists of the following.

Suppose we have two metronomes of different frequency which act as conditioned stimuli, one of them with 200 beats per minute being the positive stimulus and the other with 50 beats—the negative one. Now, if the nerve cell becomes pathological or simply falls into a hypnotic state, the effect is reverse: the positive stimulus turns into an inhibitory one, and the inhibitory becomes positive. This is an absolutely exact and constantly recurring laboratory phenomenon. Therefore, I interpret the state of the above patient in the following way: when he wanted to be respected or to remain alone, this was a strong positive stimulus, which evoked in him an opposite idea involuntarily and irresistibly in accordance with the rule of ultraparadoxicality.

Thus you see that in the field of pathology our method of work, the method of an objective attitude towards the higher phenomena of the nervous activity, is fully justifiable for animals, and the more we apply it the more it is justified. At present we are making, as it seems to me, warrantable attempts to apply the same method to human higher nervous activity which is usually called psychical activity.

That is all I wanted to tell you.

THE CONDITIONED REFLEX[72]

When the developing animal world reached the stage of man, an extremely important addition was made to the mechanisms of the nervous activity. In the animal, reality is signalised almost exclusively by stimulations and by the traces they leave in the cerebral hemispheres, which come directly to the special cells of the visual, auditory or other receptors of the organism. This is what we, too, possess as impressions, sensations and notions of the world around us, both the natural and the social—with the exception of the words heard or seen. This is the first system of signals of reality common to man and animals. But speech constitutes a second signalling system of reality which is peculiarly ours, being the signal of the first signals. On the one hand, numerous speech stimulations have removed us from reality, and we must always remember this in order not to distort our attitude to reality. On the other hand, it is precisely speech which has made us human, a subject on which I need not dwell in detail here. However, it cannot be doubted that the fundamental laws governing the activity of the first signalling system must also govern that of the second, because it, too, is activity of the same nervous tissue.

The most convincing proof that the study of the conditioned reflexes has brought the investigation of the higher part of the brain on to the right trail and that the functions of this part of the brain and the phenomena of our subjective world have finally become united and identical, is provided by the further experiments with conditioned reflexes on animals reproducing pathological states of the human nervous system—neuroses and certain psychotic symptoms; in many cases it is also possible to attain a rational deliberate return to the normal—recovery—i.e., a truly scientific mastery of the subject. Normal nervous activity is a balance of all the above-described processes participating in this activity. Derangement of the balance is a pathological state, a disease; and often there is a certain disequilibrium even in the so-called normal, or to be more precise, in the relative normal. Hence the probability of nervous illness is manifestly connected with the type of nervous system. Under the influence of difficult experimental conditions those of our dogs are quickly and easily susceptible to nervous disorders which belong to the extreme—excitable and weak—types. Of course, even in the strong equilibrated types the equilibrium can be deranged by applying very strong, extraordinary measures. The difficult conditions, which chronically violate the nervous equilibrium, include: overstrain of the excitatory process, overstrain of the inhibitory process and a direct collision of both opposite processes, in other words, overstrain of the mobility of these processes. We have a dog with a system of conditioned reflexes to stimuli of different physical intensity, positive and negative reflexes which are called forth stereotypically in one and the same order and at the same intervals. We sometimes apply exceptionally strong conditioned stimuli, sometimes we greatly prolong the duration of the inhibitory stimuli; we now elaborate a very delicate differentiation, now increase the quantity of inhibitory stimuli in the system of reflexes; finally, we either make the opposing processes follow each other immediately, or even simultaneously apply opposite conditioned stimuli, or at once change the dynamic stereotype, i.e., convert the established system of conditioned stimuli into an opposite series of stimuli. And we see that in all these cases the above-mentioned extreme types fall with particular ease into chronic pathological states differently manifesting themselves in these types. In the excitable type the neurosis is expressed in the following way. The inhibitory process, which even in a normal state constantly lags behind the excitatory process in relation to strength, now becomes very weak, almost disappearing: the elaborated, although not absolute, differentiations become fully disinhibited; the extinction assumes an extremely protracted character, the delayed reflex is converted into a short-delayed one, etc. In general, the animal becomes highly unrestrained and nervous during the experiments in the stand: it either behaves violently, or—which is much less frequent —falls into a state of sleep; this had not been observed before. In the weak type the neurosis is almost exclusively of a depressive character. The conditioned reflex activity becomes highly confused, and more often completely vanishes; in the course of the experiment the animal is in an almost continuous hypnotic state, manifesting its various phases (there are no conditioned reflexes at all, the animal even refuses food).

Experimental neuroses in most cases assume a lingering character lasting for months and even years. Some therapeutic remedies have been successfully tested in protracted neuroses. Already long ago bromide was applied in the study of the conditioned reflexes when certain experimental animals could not cope with the tasks of inhibition. And it was of essential help to these animals. A prolonged and diverse series of experiments with conditioned reflexes on animals proved beyond all doubt that bromide bears no special relation to the excitatory process and does not decrease the latter, as was generally believed, but influences the inhibitory process, intensifying and tonifying it. It is a powerful remedy, regulating and rehabilitating the disturbed nervous activity, on the indispensable and essential condition, however, that it is exactly dosed according to the types and states of the nervous system. In the case of a strong type and when the state of the dog's nervous system is still strong enough, large doses of bromide are to be administered—from two to five grammes a day; for the weak type the dose must be reduced to centigrammes and milligrammes. Such bromisation for a period of one or two weeks sometimes proves sufficient to cure a chronic experimental neurosis. Recent experiments have shown even a greater therapeutic effect, especially in very severe cases, of a combination of bromide and caffeine, but again subject to very precise dosage of both substances. Sometimes recovery was also attained in animals, though not so quickly and fully, exclusively by means of a regular prolonged or short rest from laboratory work in general, or by the abolition of the difficult tasks in the system of conditioned reflexes.

The described neuroses in animals can best be compared with neurasthenia in human beings, especially since some neuropathologists insist on two forms of neurasthenia—excitatory and depressive. Besides, certain traumatic neuroses may correspond to them, as well as other reactive pathological states. It may be assumed that recognition of two signalling systems of reality in man will lead specially to an understanding of the mechanisms of two human neuroses—hysteria and psychasthenia. If, on the basis of the predominance of one system over the other, people can be divided into a predominantly thinking type and a predominantly artistic type, then it is clear that in pathological cases of a general disequilibrium of the nervous system, the former will become psychasthenics and the latter hysteriacs.

Along with elucidation of the mechanisms of neuroses, the physiological study of the higher nervous activity provides a clue to an understanding of certain aspects and phenomena in the pictures of psychoses. We shall dwell first of all on some forms of delusion, namely, on the variation of the persecution delusion, on what Pierre Janet calls "senses of possession", as well as on Kretschmer's "inversion". The patient is persecuted precisely by that which he particularly wants to avoid; he desires to have his own secret thoughts, but he is certain that they are constantly being disclosed and made known by others; he wishes to be alone, but he is tormented by the persistent sensation that someone else is in the room, although there is nobody there except himself, etc.; according to Janet, these are senses of possession. Kretschmer refers to two girls who, having entered the period of puberty, and being sexually attracted by certain males, for some reason suppressed this attraction. As a result, they were first seized with an obsessive idea; to their great grief, it seemed to them that their countenance betrayed their sexual excitation and that everybody noticed this; at the same time they greatly valued their chastity, their virginity. Afterwards one of the girls suddenly began to imagine and even to sense that the sexual tempter—the serpent which had seduced Eve in the Garden of Eden—was inside her and was even reaching towards her mouth. The other girl imagined that she was pregnant. It is this latter phenomenon that Kretschmer terms inversion. In respect of its mechanism it is obviously identical with the sense of possession. This pathological subjective experience can, without undue strain, be interpreted as a physiological phenomenon of the ultraparadoxical phase. The idea of sexual inviolability, being a very strong positive stimulus, on the background of the state of inhibition or depression in which both girls found themselves, turned into an equally strong opposite negative idea, reaching the level of sensation; in one girl it was the idea of a sexual tempter existing inside her body, in the other—the idea of pregnancy as a result of sexual intercourse. Exactly the same thing is experienced by the patient with the sense of possession. The strong positive idea "I am alone" turned, under the same conditions, into a similar negative idea—"there is always someone near me"!

In the course of experiments with conditioned reflexes

in various difficult and pathological states of the nervous system it is often observed that temporary inhibition leads to a temporary improvement in these states; in one dog there was twice observed a patent catatonic state, which resulted in a marked decline of a chronic and persistent nervous disorder, almost in a return to the normal for several days in succession. In general, it should be pointed out that in experimental disorders of the nervous system almost always separate phenomena of hypnosis are observed, which gives the right to assume that this is a normal physiological remedy against morbific agents. Hence, the catatonic form or phase of schizophrenia entirely consisting of hypnotic symptoms, can be regarded as physiological protective inhibition, limiting or fully excluding the work of the disordered brain which, owing to the action of a certain, still unknown, noxious agent, has been threatened by serious disturbances or complete destruction. Medicine knows very well that the first therapeutic measure, which must be applied in the treatment of almost every illness, is to ensure a state of rest for the diseased organ. That such a concept of the mechanism of catatonia in schizophrenia conforms to reality, is convincingly proved by the fact that only this form of schizophrenia shows a considerable rate of recovery, despite the protracted character of the catatonic state, which sometimes persists for years (twenty years). From this point of view any attempt to act on catatonics by means of stimulating methods and remedies is definitely injurious. On the contrary, a very considerable increase in the rate of recovery can be expected when physiological rest (inhibition) is supplemented with deliberate external rest for such patients, when they are kept away from the action of constant and strong stimuli emanating from the surroundings, kept away from other, restless patients.

In the course of the study of conditioned reflexes, along with general disorders of the cortex, there were frequently observed extremely interesting cases of disorders experimentally and functionally produced in very small points of the cortex. Let us take a dog with a system of various reflexes and among them conditioned reflexes to different sounds—a tone, a noise, the beat of a metronome, the sound of a bell, etc.; it is possible to induce a disorder only at one of the points of application of these conditioned stimuli, while all other points remain normal. The pathological state of an isolated cortical point is produced by the methods described above as morbific. The disorder manifests itself in different forms and degrees. The mildest change effected at this point is expressed in its chronic hypnotic state: instead of the normal relation between the strength of the effect induced by the stimulation and the physical intensity of the stimulus, the equalisation and paradoxical phases develop at this point. Proceeding from the above, this, too, can be interpreted as a physiological preventive measure under a difficult state of a cortical point. When the pathological state develops further, the stimulus in some cases has no positive effect at all, provoking only inhibition. In other cases the opposite occurs. The positive reflex becomes unusually stable: its extinction proceeds more slowly than that of the normal reflexes; it is less susceptible to successive inhibition by other, inhibitory conditioned stimuli; it often stands out in bold relief for its strength among all other conditioned reflexes, which was not observed prior to the disorder. This signifies that the excitatory process at the given point has become chronically and pathologically inert. The stimulation of the pathological point sometimes remains indifferent to the points of other stimuli, and sometimes it is impossible to touch this point with its stimulus without deranging in one way or another the entire system of reflexes. There are grounds for assuming that in the case of disorder of isolated points, when now the inhibitory, now the excitatory processes predominate at the diseased point, the mechanism of the pathological state consists precisely in the derangement of equilibrium between the opposed processes:

there takes place a considerable and predominant decrease now of one process, now of the other. In the case of pathological inertness of the excitatory process bromide (which reinforces the inhibitory process) often fully eliminates the inertness.

The following conclusion can hardly be considered fantastic. If stereotypy, iteration and perseveration, as is perfectly obvious, have their natural origin in the pathological inertness of the excitatory process of the different motor cells, then obsessional neurosis and paranoia must also have the same mechanism. This is simply a matter of other cells or of groups of cells connected with our sensations and notions. Thus, only one series of sensations and notions connected with the diseased cells becomes abnormally stable and resistant to the inhibitory influence of other numerous sensations and notions, which to a greater degree conform with reality because of the normal state of their cells. Another phenomenon, frequently observed in the study of pathological conditioned reflexes and having a direct bearing on human neuroses and psychoses, is circularity in the nervous activity. The disturbed nervous activity manifested more or less regular fluctuations. There was observed at first a period of extremely weakened activity (the conditioned reflexes were of a chaotic character, often fully disappeared or declined to the minimum); then, after several weeks or months, as if spontaneously, without any visible reason, there took place a greater or lesser, and even complete, return to the normal, which was again superseded by a period of pathological activity. Sometimes periods of weakened activity and abnormally increased activity alternated in this circularity. It is impossible not to see in these fluctuations an analogy with cyclothymia and the manic-depressive psychosis. The simplest way would be to ascribe this pathological periodicity to the derangement of normal relations between the excitatory and inhibitory processes, as far as their interaction is concerned. Since the opposite processes did not limit each other in due time and in the proper measure, but acted independently of each other and excessively, the result of their activity reached its maximum—and only then was one process superseded by the other. Thus, there developed a different, namely, exaggerated, periodicity, lasting a week or a month, instead of the short and very easy periodicity of one day. Finally, it is impossible not to mention a phenomenon which so far has manifested itself with exceptional force only in one dog. This is the extreme explosiveness of the excitatory process. Certain individual stimuli or all the conditioned stimuli produced an extremely violent and excessive effect (both motor and secretory), which, however, abruptly disappeared already during the action of the stimulus—when the food reflex was reinforced, the dog did not take the food. Obviously, this was because of the high pathological lability of the excitatory process, which corresponds to the excitatory weakness of the human clinic. In certain conditions a weak form of this phenomenon is often observed in dogs.

All the pathological nervous symptoms described above are manifested in corresponding conditions both in normal dogs, i.e., not subjected to surgical operation, and (especially some of these symptoms, for example, circularity) in castrated animals, being, consequently, of an organic pathological nature. Numerous experiments have shown that the most fundamental property of the nervous activity in castrated animals is a considerable and predominant decline of the inhibitory process, which in the strong type, however, is greatly levelled out with the passage of time.

To sum up, we must emphasise once more that when we compare the ultraparadoxical phase with the sense of possession and with inversion, and the pathological inertness of the excitatory process with obsessional neurosis and paranoia, we see how closely the physiological phenomena and the experiences of the subjective world are interconnected and how they merge.

TYPES OF HIGHER NERVOUS ACTIVITY, THEIR RELATIONSHIP TO NEUROSES AND PSYCHOSES AND THE PHYSIOLOGICAL MECHANISM OF NEUROTIC AND PSYCHOTIC SYMPTOMS[73]

Of the vast material relating to the study of the higher nervous activity in dogs by the method of conditioned reflexes I shall now dwell only upon three points because of their particularly close connection with morbid disturbances of this activity. They are: the strength of the two basic nervous processes—excitation and inhibition—then the correlation of their intensities, or their equilibrium, and finally their mobility. These properties constitute, on the one hand, the basis of the types of higher nervous activity, types which play an important part in the genesis of nervous and so-called mental diseases, and on the other hand, typical changes taking place under pathological states of this activity.

Two thousand years ago the great genius of ancient Greece—the artistic genius, of course, not scientific—was able to discern in the immense diversity of variations of human behaviour its fundamental features in the form of four temperaments. And only now is the study of the higher nervous activity by the method of conditioned reflexes in a position to base this systematisation on a physiological foundation.

According to the strength of the excitatory process (i.e., according to the working capacity of the cerebral cells) our dogs were divided into two groups—strong and weak. The strong group, in its turn, was divided into equilibrated and unequilibrated, depending on the correlations between the intensities of the excitatory and inhibitory processes. And finally the strong and equilibrated dogs were divided, according to the mobility of the processes, into quiet and lively ones. Thus, there are four basic types: the strong and impetuous type, the strong, equilibrated and quiet type, the strong, equilibrated and lively type, and the weak type. And they correspond to the four Greek temperaments—choleric, phlegmatic, sanguine and melancholic. Although there are different gradations of these types, life clearly shows that it is just these combinations that are more frequently met with and bear a more pronounced character. It seems to me that this coincidence of types in animals and human beings is convincing proof that such a systematisation conforms to reality.

However, to obtain a full and clear idea of the variations of human behaviour, normal and pathological, it is necessary to add to these types, which are common in man and animals, certain particular, purely human types.

Before the appearance of the family of homo sapiens the contact of the animals with the surrounding world was effected solely by means of direct impressions produced by its various agents which acted on the different receptor mechanisms of the animals and were conducted to the corresponding cells of the central nervous system. They were the sole signals of external objects. In the future human beings there emerged, developed and perfected, signals of the second order, signals of these initial signals, in the shape of speech—spoken, auditory and visible. Ultimately these new signals began to denote everything taken in by human beings directly from the outer, as well as from the inner world; they were used not only in mutual intercourse, but also in self-communion. This predominance of the new signals was conditioned, of course, by the tremendous significance of speech, although words were and remain but second signals of reality. We know, however, that there are large numbers of people who, operating exclusively with words and failing to base themselves on reality, are ready to draw from these words every possible conclusion and all knowledge, and on this basis to direct their own life as well as the life of others. However, without entering deeper into this important and very broad subject, it is necessary to state that thanks to the two signalling systems, and by virtue of the long-established different modes of life, human beings in the mass have been divided into artistic, thinking and intermediate types. The last-named combines the work of both systems in the requisite degree. This division makes itself felt both in individual human beings and in nations.

Let us pass now to pathology.

In our experiments on animals we constantly obtained convincing proof that chronic pathological derangement of the higher nervous activity under the influence of morbific agents arises with particular ease in the impetuous and the weak types, where it assumes the form of neurosis. Impetuous dogs become almost completely deprived of inhibition; in weak dogs the conditioned reflex activity either fully disappears, or is of a highly chaotic character. Kretschmer, who recognises only two general types corresponding to our impetuous and weak types, correctly, as far as I can judge, associates the first with the manic-depressive psychosis, and the second with schizophrenia.

Having some very limited clinical experience (during the last three or four years I have regularly visited the nervous and psychiatric clinics) I take the liberty of advancing the following supposition concerning human neuroses. Neurasthenia is a pathological form inherent in the feeble-general and intermediate human types. A hysterical person is the product of the feeble-general type combined with the artistic type, and the psychasthenic (to use the terminology of Pierre Janet) is the product of the feeble-general type combined with the thinking type. In hysterical persons, general weakness, naturally, has a special effect on the second signalling system, which in the artistic type in any case yields pride of place to the first system, while in normally developed persons the second signalling system is the highest regulator of human behaviour. Hence the chaotic character of the activity of the first signalling system and of the emotional fund in the form of pathological fantasies and unrestrained emotivity with profound destruction of the general nervous equilibrium (sometimes paralyses, or contractures, or convulsive fits or lethargy) and in particular, synthesis of personality. In psychasthenics the general weakness, naturally, again affects the basic foundation of the correlations between the organism and environment, namely, the first signalling system and the emotional fund. Hence the absence of a sense of reality, continual feeling of inferiority of life, complete inadequacy in life together with constant fruitless and perverted cogitation in the form of obsessions and phobias. This, in general outline, is how I conceive the genesis of neuroses and psychoses in connection with the general and particular types of human higher nervous activity.

Experimental study of pathological changes in the basic processes of the nervous activity of animals makes possible a physiological understanding of the mechanism of the mass of neurotic and psychotic symptoms, both taken separately or as components of certain pathological forms.

Weakening of the excitatory process leads to the predominance of inhibition, both general and diversely partial, in the form of sleep or of a hypnotic state with its numerous phases, of which most characteristic are the paradoxical and ultraparadoxical phases. This mechanism, I believe, is responsible for a particularly large number of pathological phenomena, such as narcolepsy, cataplexy, catalepsy, feelings of possession—*les sentiments d'emprise* (according to Pierre Janet), or inversion (according to

Kretschmer), catatonia, etc. The weakening of the excitatory process is caused either by its overstrain, or by its collision with the process of inhibition.

Under certain laboratory conditions which are not yet quite clear there takes place a change in the *mobility* of the excitatory process in the form of *pathological lability*. This phenomenon, long known in the clinic under the name of excitatory weakness, consists in an extremely high reactivity or sensitivity of the process followed by its rapid consecutive exhaustion. Our conditioned positive stimulus produces an instantaneous and extraordinary effect, which, however, falls to zero and becomes inhibited already during the normal period of stimulation. We sometimes call this phenomenon explosiveness.

But in our experimental practice we also meet with quite the opposite pathological change in the *mobility* of the excitatory process—with *pathological inertness*. The excitatory process persists despite a prolonged application of conditions, under which normally the excitatory process is superseded by inhibition. The positive stimulus is not susceptible or slightly susceptible to successive inhibition evoked by preceding inhibitory stimuli. This pathological state is in some cases caused by a moderate, but continuously growing intensity of the excitatory process, and in other cases by collisions with the inhibitory process. It is quite natural to attribute the phenomena of stereotypy, obsessive ideas, paranoia, etc., to this pathological inertness of the excitatory process.

The inhibitory process can also be *weakened* either by its overstrain, or by collisions with the excitatory process. This weakening leads to an abnormal predominance of the excitatory process in the form of a derangement of differentiations, retardation and other normal phenomena in which inhibition intervenes; it also manifests itself in the animal's general behaviour in the form of fussiness, impatience and violence, and finally in the form of pathological phenomena, for example, neurasthenic irritability.

In man it takes the form of submanic and manic states, etc.

This year phenomena of pathological lability of the inhibitory process have been observed in our animals by my old colleague, Prof. Petrova, who has enriched experimental pathology and therapy of the higher nervous activity with quite a considerable number of important facts. A dog which previously took its food, placed at the edge of a staircase, with ease, without any hesitation, ceases to do so, hurriedly avoids the food and moves away from the edge. The matter is quite clear. When a normal animal, approaching the edge of a staircase, stops and does not move farther, this means that it is able confidently to hold itself back, as much as is necessary to prevent it from falling down. In our case this retention is exaggerated; the reaction to depth is excessive and keeps the dog, to the detriment of its interests, much farther from the edge of the staircase than is actually necessary. Subjectively this is an obvious state of dread or fear, a phobia of depth. The phobia could be induced, and could be eliminated, i.e., it was under the experimenter's control. The condition responsible for its emergence is what we may call the torture of the inhibitory process. I will demonstrate this fact in a few days' time at the international physiological congress in Leningrad. I think that in many cases persecution mania can also be accounted for by the pathological lability of inhibition.

We have already examined the pathological *inertness* of the inhibitory process.

A difficult task still remains to be accomplished—it is necessary to determine with precision and in all cases when and in what particular conditions one or another pathological change arises in the basic nervous processes.

THE PROBLEM OF SLEEP[74]

Dear Comrades,

Although something extraordinary, one might say, even distressing, befell me yesterday, with the result that I am now, so to speak, not quite myself, I thought it necessary, nevertheless, to be present at the conference. Why? Because I believe that in a discussion of a scientific matter such as sleep, which is essential both from the practical and clinical points of view, my judgement will be not without interest, especially since I, jointly with my colleagues, have been studying the phenomena of sleep for thirty-five years in the course of our research into the higher nervous activity of dogs.

We came up against the phenomena of sleep at an early stage in our research; we were obliged to consider it, to subject it to special investigation, which now gives me the right to speak on this subject. That is why, despite my somewhat disturbed state, I decided to come here and to say a few words.

I

I should like first of all to make a general remark. The more perfect the nervous system of the animal organism, the more centralised it is, the more its higher part controls and regulates the entire activity of the organism, even though this is not clearly manifest. It might seem to us that in higher animals many functions are effected independently of the influence of the cerebral hemispheres, but this is not so in reality. The higher part controls all the phenomena which develop in the organism. This was established long ago in the phenomena of hypnotic suggestion and auto-suggestion. It is well known that during hypnotic sleep it is possible to influence many vegetative processes by means of suggestion. On the other hand, we know of cases of auto-suggestion, such as symptoms of phantom pregnancy, accompanied by an active state of the lacteal glands and the accumulation of fat in the abdominal walls, simulating pregnancy. All this originates from the head, from thoughts and words, from the cerebral hemispheres in order to influence such a peaceful and genuinely vegetative process as the growth of the adipose tissue.

If the cerebral hemispheres, as everybody knows, are concerned with the slightest details of our movements, bringing some into action and suppressing others, just as it takes place, for example, when one plays the piano, one can easily imagine the minuteness of the degree of inhibition: one movement of a certain intensity is effected, while another, neighbouring movement, even the smallest one, is suppressed and retained. Or take, for example, our speech movements. What a multitude of words we have for expressing our thoughts! Nevertheless, we are precise in conveying the sense; we never use unnecessary words, employing only those which are most suitable in the given case, etc. Consequently, if the cerebral hemispheres constantly interfere even with these minute everyday activities and regulate them, it would be strange to suppose that the division of our activity into wakeful and sleeping states does not depend on the cerebral hemispheres. It is clear that here, too, supreme power belongs to the cerebral hemispheres and all of us are well aware of this.

Now, at a certain time of the day we become drowsy, and, since we are tired, sleep sets in. But we can do without sleep a whole night, and even for two or three nights in succession. And it is our head, our cerebral hemispheres which, of course, control this phenomenon.

I shall now turn to the details.

It is clear, and everybody is aware of this now, since it has become a widespread and established physiological truth—that our entire nervous activity consists of two processes—excitatory and inhibitory—and that our whole life is a continuous interaction of these two processes.

When we began our objective study of the higher nervous activity by the method of conditioned reflexes, and began to elucidate the laws of the particular functions and tasks accomplished by the cerebral hemispheres, we, of course, immediately encountered the two processes. Every physiologist knows that these processes are inseparable, that they are always present not only in the nerve cell, but in each nerve fibre.

I must make a certain reservation. If I begin to speak about conditioned reflexes this would take a lot of time, and I do not know when I would end. Since we have been working on conditioned reflexes for thirty-five years and have published the results of our work in special papers and books, allow me to assume that knowledge of conditioned reflexes is widespread and consequently, there is no need to treat this subject in an elementary way, i.e., to begin all over again.

When we applied our conditioned stimuli and then carried out a detailed investigation of the activity evoked by them at every given moment, we constantly observed a spontaneous development of inhibition side by side with excitation. In other cases we produced the inhibition ourselves when we wanted to separate different phenomena.

Since you are acquainted to a degree with the conditioned reflexes, you undoubtedly know that we have, on the one hand, external stimuli which produce an excitatory process in the central nervous system, and, on the other hand, stimuli which produce an inhibitory process in the cerebral hemispheres. Right at the beginning of our research we observed that as soon as we applied the inhibitory stimulus, a somnolent state of the animal, in the form of drowsiness or sleep, immediately intervened. This was of a constant character. We had to conclude, therefore, that these phenomena are closely interconnected and that certain efforts and resources are necessary to get rid of this drowsiness or sleep in the course of experimentation. Thus, when an inhibitory process arises in the cerebral hemispheres, establishing in them a certain differentiation either between the stimuli or between different moments of stimulation, etc., a state of drowsiness inevitably develops.

You can see, as we have seen during the past thirty-five years, that every time a cortical inhibition sets in which analytically assigns its proper place to everything, giving free rein to one process and suppressing the other, a state of drowsiness or in its ultimate stage of development—a state of sleep—simultaneously and invariably appears. The view that drowsiness and sleep are phenomena related to the cerebral hemispheres and that they are the result of the action of definite stimuli, is strictly obligatory for us. Surely a phenomenon observed every day is beyond any doubt.

That, of course, leads to the next question. How does this come about? What has this to do with sleep when it is simply a matter of differentiation between stimuli? They appear to be different things having nothing in common.

But the matter is quite simple. If we admit that everything can be explained by a constant interaction between the excitatory and inhibitory processes, then we shall have no difficulty in understanding the phenomena. Every time you produce an inhibition, a physiological inhibition, i.e., when you want to separate the active state from the inactive, drowsiness, as I have already said, immediately begins to manifest itself. But you can always eliminate this drowsiness, suppress it, and, on the contrary, ensure the predominance of the excitatory process. This is within your power, within your experimental possibilities, and it is what we do. The moment a state of drowsiness develops in the dog during an experiment, i.e., the moment inhibition takes the upper hand, we apply a stimulation, thereby eliminating the drowsiness, limiting the inhibition and confining it within definite bounds.

How, then, is this matter to be further interpreted? It must be admitted that both excitation and inhibition are dynamic processes, which, on the one hand, may irradiate and spread, and, on the other, may be driven into definite narrow confines and concentrated there. This is the main point, the whole secret, and it is this that we use in all our physiological activity.

The basic property of both processes consists in the fact that on the one hand, when they arise, they tend to spread, to occupy an undue area; on the other hand, they can, given the corresponding conditions, concentrate in definite regions and remain there. When the inhibition is irradiated, diffused, you have the phenomenon of drowsiness or sleep.

Everybody knows, of course, that sleep does not set in instantaneously, that it is a gradual process. Similarly one does not awake all of a sudden; certain time is required before one gradually becomes active and, so to speak, completely throws off the fetters of sleep.

I advise everybody who values scientific truth, who does not want to reconcile himself to superficial knowledge, who is tormented by the thought "is this right or not?", to make a thorough study of two articles in my book *Twenty Years of Objective Study of the Higher Nervous Activity (Behaviour) of Animals* which is the result of thirty-five years of intense reflections. One of the articles is entitled "On Inhibition and Sleep" and the other, written jointly with M. K. Petrova,—"Physiology of the Hypnotic State of the Dog".

In any case, in order to give you a more or less clear illustration of this phenomenon, I shall cite one of our experiments.

I must tell you that when you observe the genesis of drowsiness and its first manifestations, you become convinced, and unshakably so, that hypnosis and sleep are, of course, one and the same process. In essence, hypnosis does not differ from sleep; it differs only in certain peculiarities. Hypnosis, for example, is sleep which develops very slowly, i.e., it is at first confined to a very small and restricted area and then begins to spread farther and farther until it finally descends from the cerebral hemispheres to the subcortex, leaving untouched only the centres of respiration, of the heart-beat, etc., though somewhat weakening these too.

I shall now submit to you one of the numerous cases investigated by us in the course of thirty-five years. Let us take a dog which is falling into a state of drowsiness, sleep or hypnosis. What do we observe in this animal? Our experiments with conditioned food reflexes show the following: at first the dog works and eats quite normally; then its tongue comes out of the mouth in a strange manner, and gradually begins to fall down. This is the first manifestation of a certain functional paralysis, of a diminution of activity, of inhibition of the minute centre in the motor region of the cortex which controls the movement of the tongue. This centre becomes inactive, as a result of which the tongue is paralysed and falls out of the mouth.

A certain period of time passes, and you give the dog food. You see that its tongue functions very slowly and awkwardly; later, you also observe—not at once, but perhaps after the second or third offering of food—that the dog uses its jaws with difficulty, that its mastication is utterly impeded, since the mouth opens and closes very slowly. Thus you witness a weakening of the activity of the masticating musculature, its inhibition or sleep.

At the same time, however, you notice that when food is offered to the dog, which until then was standing with its head turned away or with its eyes fixed on the ceiling, it easily and quickly turns its head towards you and falls upon the food.

But as time goes on, you observe in the course of the experiment that although the dog turns towards you, it brings its head to the food with great difficulty. Consequently, the inhibition or sleep has already seized other points of the skeletal movement, namely, those which control the movement of the neck.

You then see that the dog is unable even to turn towards the food, that it does not move the neck and does not take the food. And finally, you observe the onset of a general passivity of the skeletal musculature: the dog hangs limply in the straps, it is in a state of sleep. Thus, inhibition gradually develops before your eyes in a very obvious and concrete manner; at first it affects the tongue, then it spreads to the cervical muscles, from there to the general skeletal musculature until, finally, sleep sets in.

When you observe this development you can hardly doubt that inhibition and sleep are one and the same process.

The articles to which I have just referred contain numerous similar facts. And anyone who makes a thorough study of them will be convinced that inhibition and sleep are one and the same phenomenon. The only difference is that when the most minute points of the cerebral hemispheres are inactive, it is inhibition and, at the same time, sleep of an isolated cell; but when this inhibition, duly or unduly, spreads under the influence of certain conditions, it embraces more and more new areas of cells and is manifested in a passive, inactive state of the numerous organs dependent on these regions.

It is a pity that cinematography appeared too late and could not be utilised by us and our physiological laboratories. Had it been as accessible then as it is now, all these phenomena could have been very easily comprehended. We could now demonstrate them to you in the space of fifteen minutes, and you would leave us with the deep conviction that inhibition and sleep are one and the same process. But while inhibition is a concentrated process, hypnosis and sleep represent an inhibition which spreads over more or less vast areas.

This spread of inhibition is of great importance for the comprehension of numerous nervous phenomena.

The British mind, as far as I have been able to follow it, has fully realised and caught up this idea. Thus, Wilson, one of the outstanding British neurologists, now considers all cases of narcolepsy and cataplexy precisely from this point of view. And we, who have observed all these phenomena in dogs, fully agree with him. In our opinion, Wilson is undoubtedly on the right trail.

Such, in general outline, of course, is our understanding of the phenomena relating to alternating sleep in the cerebral hemispheres, as well as to the sleep of the entire brain, following the mobile inhibition.

II

I shall pass now to other facts which to a certain degree compete with the concept just developed by me.

First of all I draw your attention to an extremely important fact recently obtained in the Soviet Union by Prof. Galkin, in A. D. Speransky's laboratory. It should be pointed out that this fact had been observed long ago in the clinic, but only once. Of course, much consideration was given to it at the time, and it was even properly understood by some researchers; but a single fact is not sufficiently convincing. This fact concerns an observation made long ago by Strümpell on a patient, in whom most of the sense organs were damaged and who could communicate with the external world only through two openings which remained intact—one eye and one ear. When he covered these openings with his hands he inevitably fell asleep.

This phenomenon is now being reproduced in the laboratory, and in the following way. We destroy three distant receptors in the dog, namely, smell, hearing and sight; this means that we section the *fili olfactorii*, sever the *n. optici* or extirpate the eyes and damage both cochleae. After this operation the dog sleeps twenty-three and a half hours a day. It wakens only when the elementary functions of the organism begin to annoy it—the necessity to eat, to evacuate the urinary bladder or the bowels, etc. But it is extremely difficult to awake the animal in the middle of the day. For this purpose it is not sufficient to stroke the dog, it is absolutely necessary to shake it; and then, before your eyes, it slowly awakens, stretches itself, yawns, and finally stands up. Such is the fact, and it is an exact fact. We repeated the experiment several times and the result was always the same.

The character of the operation performed on the dog excludes any supposition that its nervous system has been damaged. If the operation is done thoroughly, the dog comes through it more or less easily; the fact that two days after the operation it is able to eat shows best the ease with which it endures the loss of the above-mentioned receptors.

However, I must direct your attention to a minor detail. If you destroy the receptors gradually, i.e., at first one of them, the second two or three months later, and in another period of three months the third, then sleep does not set in. The dog, of course, is not as active as the animal which sees and hears normally; indeed, if it has lost the sense of smell and is unable to see, what can make it move? And it is perfectly understandable that for the most part it lies rolled up. But the moment you touch the intact receptor, for example, by stroking the dog, it immediately rises and begins to act.

When, however, you deprive the cerebral hemispheres of a large quantity of stimulations at once, the dog falls into a state of deep sleep. This indubitable fact, which must be reckoned with, naturally gives rise to the following question: How is this phenomenon to be interpreted? And in this connection there arises the problem of two kinds of sleep—the passive sleep caused by the abolition of a large quantity of stimulations usually reaching the cerebral hemispheres, and the active sleep which, in my understanding, is an inhibitory process, since the latter must be undoubtedly regarded as an active process and not as a state of inactivity.

Then the following question of principle arises: Does not the nervous system experience three different states—excitation, inhibition, and a certain indifferent state, when the first two are absent?

But proceeding from the general biological data we have grounds for doubting the existence of a neutral state. Life is a continuous interchange of destruction and restoration, in view of which a neutral state is simply inconceivable. On the whole, the problem can be reduced to the following: Is not the passive sleep, which differs from the usual sleep developing under the above-mentioned conditions, also a result of active inhibition?

I think that certain considerations can be submitted which make it clear that the case of sleep observed in dogs, operated upon in accordance with the method of Speransky and Galkin, could be also accounted for by inhibition; it is an active inhibition greatly favoured by the circumstances, since now there is no need for the inhibition to struggle against an extensive excitatory process and train itself, and as a result the stimulations falling upon the dog extremely facilitate the sleep. Why is this so? Because when the dog is mostly in a lying posture, certain points of its skin are continuously stimulated both mechanically and thermally. It is, therefore, conceivable that the passive sleep is evoked by a continuous and monotonous stimulation of the remaining receptors. And we know the fundamental rule according to which each cell, under the influence of continuous and monotonous stimulations, inevitably becomes inhibited. Consequently, it is possible to interpret this sleep as a result of inhibition proceeding from the remaining receptors subjected to a prolonged monotonous stimulation.

This is partially confirmed also by the following fact. When these dogs are transferred to new surroundings, they at first become more active, are wakened more easily, etc.; in other words, for a time they appear to be more lively.

It can be assumed, therefore, that here, too, due to a decline of the tonus, to the weakening of the excitatory process, the inhibition easily takes possession of the cerebral hemispheres and that weak, monotonous stimulations arise provoking an inhibitory process.

Then comes the following question: What happens to the dogs in which the cerebral hemispheres are extirpated? As a matter of fact, they, too, fall into a state of sleep. And this circumstance is often used as a serious objection to what I have just said, namely, to the statement that normally sleep originates in the cerebral hemispheres.

But I do not regard this objection as being physiologically grounded. It is clear that since sleep is a diffused inhibition, and the latter spreads over the nervous system up to the lower limit of the spinal cord, and since there is a central system and a nerve fibre, inhibition must indispensably take place. In cases when the cerebral hemispheres are absent, why should the inhibition not develop in the lower parts of the central nervous system, now in a concentrated, now in an irradiated form? This is all the more likely since dogs possess lower levels of distant receptors—*corpora geniculata* (one relating to the ear, and the other—to the eye), and we know that a dog deprived of the cerebral hemispheres reacts to acoustic and visual stimuli. Consequently, the conditions remain the same as when the cerebral hemispheres are intact, and sleep in this case is not excluded—it must inevitably manifest itself. So long as there exists inhibition and there is a cell which, as a result of excitation, is bound to become fatigued and fall into a state of inhibition, all the conditions for the development of inhibition are present. But in the absence of the cortex sleep begins from the subcortical formations. Hence, there is no contradiction here as far as the fundamental facts are concerned, that is, the interchange of excitation and inhibition, their concentration and irradiation. If all these phenomena take place also in the lower part of the central nervous system, then why should sleep not develop there as well? Therefore, I regard these objections as being physiologically groundless; they cannot refute our statement about the initiative of the cerebral hemispheres in the development of sleep in normal conditions.

Next come more important facts. On the one hand, a clinical fact—the encephalitic sleep or somnolence, and on the other, the physiological apparatus advanced by the Swiss physiologist Hess, which, as it were, rivals my concept about sleep originating in the cerebral hemispheres.

As for clinical sleep, the clinical concept of the centre of sleep is well known to clinicians; it is based on the fact that after an infection of the brain, the so-called encephalitis, which is accompanied by somnolence, considerable changes take place in the hypothalamus. On the basis of this fact the simple conclusion is made that the centre of sleep must be located there.

However, I make bold to say that this reasoning, which is based on the fact that there is, on the one hand, sleep, and on the other, a destruction of the hypothalamus, is oversimplified. The above conclusion is, therefore, too hasty.

Firstly, all that we know about the work of the cerebral hemispheres makes the concept of the hypothalamus as the actual centre of sleep doubtful and incomprehensible. It is difficult to assume that an infectious process arising in the brain should in no way tell upon its most reactive part—the cerebral hemispheres. It is likewise difficult to assume that the toxins should remain exclusively in the subcortex, without spreading to the cerebral hemispheres. I fully realise, of course, that bacteria favour definite chemical media, and that there must be a very delicate difference between the above-mentioned parts of the brain in respect of their chemical composition. It is quite conceivable that this is true, that the process in question concentrates mainly in the hypothalamus and produces in the nerve cells changes which can be afterwards revealed microscopically. But it may be that in the cerebral hemispheres these changes have only a functional character and manifest themselves in the weakening of the excitability of the hemispheres; at the same time they may be inaccessible to microscopic investigation. It can be supposed that there is a certain gradation of the patho-anatomical changes—from visible phenomena to purely functional, and, finally, invisible ones.

On the basis of what we observe in the hypothalamus it is difficult to assert with confidence that these infections do not exert any influence on the cerebral hemispheres. I would regard such a conclusion as being too hasty.

Secondly, I do not contest the fact that encephalitis is accompanied by sleep, and that this phenomenon is related to the hypothalamus and complies with it. However, I am inclined to interpret this fact in the same way as I have done with regard to the fact established by Speransky and Galkin. Here is what I have to say in this connection. There is no doubt that the hypothalamus is a wide route with definite centres where the stimulations coming from the internal world, i.e., from all the internal organs, are accumulated; its destruction leads to the isolation of the cerebral hemispheres from the entire internal world, from the entire activity of the organs; in other words, it provokes a state analogous to that which arises when all three receptors are destroyed, i.e., when the cerebral hemispheres are deprived of external stimulations. The stimulations proceeding from the internal organs, although we are not conscious of them, constantly maintain a heightened tonus of the cerebral hemispheres. This is proved in the first place by the fact that, as I have already mentioned, dogs with extirpated cerebral hemispheres are in a continuous state of sleep. Further proof is provided by a pigeon deprived of the cerebral hemispheres and remaining constantly immobile and somnolent. But the moment there arises the necessity to eat or to evacuate the excretory organs, the pigeon awakes. Consequently, there is no doubt that these stimulations act on the cerebral hemispheres and bring it to a state of wakefulness.

On the other hand, we know very well that in certain, particular cases, we feel the heart-beat, the movements of the intestines, etc.

Another long-established fact shows that internal stimulations contribute to the maintenance of the cortex in an alert state, to its tonus. This fact was recently confirmed in America, in laboratory conditions, on a person in whom the ability to resist sleep for a long time was investigated. The following phenomenon was observed. A person who like yourself is interested in this particular investigation and who tries hard to keep awake as long as possible, despite a strong desire for sleep, successfully resists the state of somnolence only when he walks or when he is in sitting posture. The moment he lies down, i.e., relaxes the musculature, he immediately falls asleep.

Thus you clearly see that our internal stimulations greatly contribute to the maintenace of a certain tonus in the cortex.

In my view, encephalitic sleep is caused by the separation of all internal stimulations from the cerebral hemispheres due to an affection of the hypothalamus; it is, consequently, the same drastic decline of the tonus that is observed when the external receptors are destroyed.

There remains one more important fact which supports the reasoning of the clinicians concerning the centre of sleep. I have in mind the experiments of Hess, in the course of which sleep was evoked by electric stimulation of definite parts of the brain. I am not going to contest this fact either. I fully admit it and believe that it will be reproduced by other investigators; but I consider it necessary to say a few words about its proper interpretation and the objections which can be raised to the conclusion drawn by Hess.

The first thing which attracts attention is that the above fact does not fully accord with the clinical fact, since the points in the latter case do not coincide with those stimulated by Hess.

Hess himself emphasised this circumstance and stated that his experiments would disappoint the clinicians, since anatomically the points which produced sleep did not coincide.

Whereas the lesions caused by encephalitis are located in the region of the third ventricle, in its lateral walls, etc., Hess subjected to stimulation the lowest part of the brain, almost reaching the brain stem.

How is this fact to be interpreted? It must be pointed out that a phenomenon observed in the given organism under normal conditions, as in our case, is one thing, and a phenomenon observed under pathological conditions, especially when they are artificially produced in the laboratory, as, for example, the stimulation of the brain, is another thing. They are, of course, absolutely different phenomena. While in the latter case maximum simplicity can be attained, in the normal state the phenomena become complicated. But in the given case even Hess, who obtained a definite state in dogs by stimulating certain points in the brain, stated that this could be an excitation not only of the cells of an imaginary, fantastic "centre of sleep", but of centrifugal or centripetal fibres; at the same time he drew attention to the fact that the points used by him for producing a state of sleep had been very limited.

Then I am fully entitled to ask the following question:

Is not this simply a reflex sleep originating from the same cerebral hemispheres? Indeed, we know very well that a monotonous irritation of the skin, both in our laboratory experiments on dogs and in our experiments on human beings, produces a hypnotic state, a state of sleep. There is nothing surprising in the fact that certain stimulations of the nerve paths may provoke sleep. Consequently, these experiments do not prove that sleep is a stimulation of a definite centre. Along with hypnotisation by means of passes, which, undoubtedly, is a reflex inhibition caused by monotonous stimulations, a hypnotic state can also be evoked with the help of the verbal method. The latter is addressed to the cerebral hemispheres. In our laboratory we produce a state of sleep in dogs by means of a weak electric stimulation of the skin; this sleep is so persistent that after several experiments the place where the electrodes were fixed becomes a conditioned hypnogenous stimulus: it suffices to touch this place or to cut the hair on it, and the dog immediately subsides into deep sleep. Such is the effect of peripheral stimulations.

What, then, is the value of Hess' proof, especially since he himself states that his sleep is produced with the help of a weak electric current, and besides, a special (faradic, and not direct) one? Consequently, this could be a very weak stimulation corresponding to that which we obtain in the laboratory by means of a weak electric current.

I find, therefore, that the Hess experiment, which was so highly convincing in the eyes of the author himself, and even more so in the eyes of the clinicians, can be rightfully contested and reduced to what I have already said, the existence of a special centre of sleep being out of the question. In my opinion, the crude idea that there is a special group of nerve cells which produce sleep, while another group produces the state of wakefulness, is, from the physiological point of view, contradictory. We observe the phenomenon of sleep in every cell; what reason have we, then, for asserting that there is a special group of

hypnogenous cells? If a cell exists, it inevitably produces a state of inhibition, which irradiates and renders all the neighbouring cells inactive; and when inhibition continues to spread, it produces sleep.
Such is my firm conviction.

DISCUSSION

Question: What is responsible for the absence of sleep in dogs whose distant receptors were extirpated at different times?

Answer: As you know, the inaction of one receptor always leads to an intense training of all others. It is a well-known fact, for example, that blind people have a highly sensitive touch. The same thing occurs in the given case with the reception of the external world when the olfactory receptor is removed; the activity of the latter is made up by the reinforced activity of the ear or the eye. It is, therefore, obvious that successive extirpation of the receptors makes possible such a training, while simultaneous extirpation excludes it.

It should be pointed out that there are indications which show that with the lapse of time, in the course of years, the dogs to a certain extent train themselves with the help of the remaining receptors (that is of the oral and cutaneous receptors) and in the end become more active. In any case this fact was manifested in dogs which have been used for these operations.

Question: From the point of view of inhibition how do you explain a sleep accompanied by abundant dreams?

Answer: As I have already said, sleep is an inhibition which gradually and steadily spreads to the lower levels of the brain. It is clear, therefore, that when sleep and fatigue begin to set in, the highest part of the cerebral hemispheres, which controls verbal activity (I call it the second signalling system of reality), becomes inhibited first, since we constantly operate with words.

I can add now—for the sake of brevity I omitted it in my talk—that this inhibitory process has its external and internal stimuli.

Among the internal stimuli of inhibition is the humoral element, or consequently, certain cellular metabolites, which evoke this inhibition. On the other hand, the external inhibitory stimuli, as I have already mentioned, are monotonous and weak. Naturally, it is the highest part of our brain, the verbal part of our higher cortical activity which functions in the daytime. Fatigue calls forth inhibition, and this part becomes inactive. But along with the verbal function of the cerebral hemispheres there is a function which we share with animals and which is termed by me the first signalling system, i.e., the reception of impressions produced by all the stimuli acting on us.

It is quite clear that when we are in an alert state, the part of the cortex controlling our speech, inhibits the first signalling system; that is why in the alert state we (except the artistic type of man whose constitution is of a peculiar character), when speaking, never imagine the object which we designate by words. I close my eyes and think of the person sitting in front of me, but I do not see him in my thoughts. Why? Because the excitation of the higher part inhibits the lower part. That is why when sleep begins and embraces only the higher part of the hemispheres, the adjacent lower part bearing a direct relation to impressions prevails and is manifested in dreams. When there is no pressure from above, a certain degree of freedom sets in. And even here a new fact must be added, a fact encountered in physiology, namely, positive induction. When one point becomes inhibited, the other, on the contrary, becomes excited. And if we grant this, i.e., if we assume positive induction, the phenomenon of sleep becomes particularly clear.

Question: Judging by what you have said, there is no centre of sleep. How, then, are we to explain the fact that for such an important function as sleep there is no centre, while there are centres for other, even less important functions of metabolism, for example, a sugar centre, a water centre, etc.?

Answer: The explanation is quite simple. Inhibition and sleep exist for each cell. Consequently, they do not need any special cellular groups.

Question: How should the problem of fatigue be considered from this point of view?

Answer: I have already said that fatigue is one of the automatic internal stimuli of the inhibitory process.

Question: How do you explain the occurrence of fits during sleep?

Answer: There is nothing special in this, because we are aware of the resources of our nervous system, the cerebral hemispheres. The following phenomenon is often observed: inhibition spreads over the cerebral hemispheres and sleep sets in; nevertheless, certain points, which I call points on duty or on guard, may remain active. This is observed, for example, in the sleep of the miller who wakes up when the noise of the mill ceases, or in the sleep of the mother who wakes up at the faintest sound coming from her child, but who is not disturbed by much louder sounds. So that when the conditions for the excitation of a certain part arise, sleep does not prevent the development of the process.

Question: How can all the complicated reactions of a hypnotised person be explained, if we admit that in the state of hypnosis his entire nervous system is inhibited with the exception of the one point by means of which he communicates with the hypnotist?

Answer: I have pointed out that hypnosis is a kind of sleep which gradually spreads from a basic point.

Here is a fact which was observed in our laboratory. You have a dog which long ago was deprived of three receptors and which is in a constant state of sleep. Nevertheless, you can awaken it with the help of the remaining cutaneous receptors, bring it to the laboratory, place it in the stand and perform experiments on it. Then the following, extremely interesting phenomenon is observed, a phenomenon analogous to the hypnotic state: you can elaborate only one reflex in a dog of this kind; it is impossible to form in it, as can be done in a normal animal, two, three, or four reflexes simultaneously. This is explained by the fact that the cortical tonus, i.e., the excitatory process in the entire cortex, is very weak; hence, when it concentrates on one stimulus, there is nothing left for other stimuli and they remain inactive.

In this way I explain also hypnosis and rapport. The cerebral hemispheres are not wholly embraced by inhibition, since certain points of excitation may be formed in them. Through such an excited point you evoke a response and suggest. And then the hypnotised person inevitably executes your order, for when you give it you have everything extremely restricted. Consequently, all the influence of the other parts of the cerebral hemispheres on that which is suggested by your words, on the stimulations which you produce, is fully isolated from all others. And when the hypnotised person wakes up after such suggestion, he is powerless to do anything with this isolated excitation, since it is detached from all others. Therefore, in hypnosis it is a question not of complete, but of partial sleep. That is the difference between hypnotic and natural sleep. Whereas natural sleep represents a general inhibition of the cerebral hemispheres, however, with the abovementioned exception of the so-called points on duty and points on guard, hypnosis is a partial inhibition affecting only a definite point, all others remaining in an active state.

Question: How do you explain the regular interchange of sleep and wakefulness?

Answer: It is clear that our daytime activity is the sum total of the excitations which cause a certain amount of exhaustion; when this exhaustion reaches peak, it evokes automatically, in an internal humoral way, a state of inhibition accompanied by sleep.

NOTES

[1] The article "Experimental Psychology and Psychopathology in Animals" was translated from the text published in the second edition of I. P. Pavlov's *Complete Works* (Vol. III, Book 1, Moscow and Leningrad, 1951, pp. 23-39). It is the text of the speech delivered by Pavlov at the International Medical Congress in Madrid, April, 1903. The article was first published in the *Herald of the Military Medical Academy* (1903, Vol. 7, No. 2, pp. 109-21). It is Pavlov's first report on the theory of conditioned reflexes proving the legitimacy of studying mental activity physiologically and regarding it as reflex activity. Already in this article Pavlov pointed out the possibility of employing new methods of studying higher nervous activity, but as yet mainly through mechanical destruction of different parts of the brain. This work clearly revealed Pavlov's tendency physiologically to substantiate human psychology and psychopathology by experiments on animals. However, this tendency was realised at a later period of his scientific activity. p. 13

[2] The experiments of I. F. Tolochinov, Pavlov's first collaborator, were carried out in 1901 and were summarised by him in his work "Material for the Study of the Physiology and Psychology of Salivary Glands". It was the first work on conditioned reflexes and was reported to the Congress of Naturalists and Physicians of the North in Helsinki in 1902 and published in French in the Materials of the Congress. (I. F. Tolochinov, *Contribution à l'étude de la physiologie et de la psychologie des glandes salivaires*. Törhandlinger vid Nord. Naturforscara-och Löveremot, Helsingfors, 1903.)
On Tolochinov see also Note 15. p. 20

[3] The article "On Sleep" is an excerpt from I. P. Pavlov's speech delivered at the Meeting of the Ledentsov Society for Fostering Progress in Experimental Sciences and Their Practical Application (Moscow, 1910). The article was translated from the text published in the second edition of I. P. Pavlov's *Complete Works* (Vol. III, Book 1, Moscow and Leningrad, 1951, pp. 130-32). p. 31

⁴ Here Pavlov is referring to the studies of the formation of conditioned reflexes to thermal stimuli conducted by his collaborators O. S. Solomonov and A. A. Shishlo. Pavlov's statement on sleep is essentially a summary of the data of their investigations. These investigations were set forth by the authors themselves in O. S. Solomonov's report "On Somniferous Reflexes" to the Society of Russian Physicians in Petersburg, March 25, 1910, which was published in the *Transactions of the Society of Russian Physicians* (St. Petersburg, 1911, 77th year of publication, pp. 159-71). p. 31

⁵ "On Inhibition and Sleep" is an excerpt from Pavlov's article "Basic Rules of the Function of the Cerebral Hemispheres". The excerpt was translated from the text published in the second edition of I. P. Pavlov's *Complete Works* (Vol. III, Book 1, Moscow and Leningrad, 1951, pp. 162-71). The article "Basic Rules of the Work of the Cerebral Hemispheres" is a shorthand record of the report made by Pavlov to the Meeting of the Petersburg Society of Russian Physicians, March 24, 1911 (the meeting was dedicated to I. M. Sechenov's memory). Pavlov based his report mainly on the experimental studies of his collaborators N. I. Krasnogorsky and N. A. Rozhansky who demonstrated their experiments in the course of Pavlov's report. This report was first published in the *Transactions of the Society of Russian Physicians* (St. Petersburg, 1911, pp. 175-87).

Pavlov's article "Basic Rules of the Work of the Cerebral Hemispheres" begins with a brief description of the motion of the nervous process of excitation and then deals with the main subject of the report—the experimental data on the regularities of the spread of the process of inhibition. In the present edition the first part of this article was deleted. The end of the article in which Pavlov deeply criticised the psychological, so-called subjective, method of studying the higher nervous activity of animals was also deleted.

In the deleted first part of the article Pavlov emphasises the particularly great importance of the "brilliant" discovery of central inhibition made by I. M. Sechenov.

The article develops and substantiates the proposition formulated by Pavlov in the preceding article ("On Sleep") that "sleep is a depression, an inhibition of all the activity of the higher part of the brain".

On the basis of experimental data Pavlov very convincingly proves the common nature of the phenomena of inhibition and sleep, and the possibility of transition of different forms of inhibition to sleep by way of irradiation of inhibition through the cerebral hemispheres. In this work Pavlov does not as yet touch upon the question of the character of inhibition (external and internal) which passes into sleep. p. 34

⁶ N. A. Rozhansky's experiments cited by I. P. Pavlov subsequently formed the basis of Rozhansky's dissertation. (N. A. Rozhansky, *Materials on the Physiology of Sleep.* Dissertation, St. Petersburg, 1913, 94 pages.)

Rozhansky worked on his dissertation in Pavlov's laboratories January 1910-August 1912. The dissertation contains a detailed review of the literature on problems of sleep published by that time. In his philosophical views and later also in the physiological interpretation of the phenomena of sleep Rozhansky differed with Pavlov. p.37

[7] A detailed description of Krasnogorsky's experiment performed on the dog "Gnome" and cited by Pavlov is found in N. I. Krasnogorsky's dissertation. (N. I. Krasnogorsky, *On the Process of Depression and Localisation of the Skin Motor Analyser in the Cerebral Cortex of the Dog*, St. Petersburg, 1911.) p. 38

[8] The article "Conditions for Active and Resting States of the Cerebral Hemispheres" was translated from the text published in the second edition of I. P. Pavlov's *Complete Works* (Vol. III, Book 1, Moscow and Leningrad, 1951, pp. 290-98). This article is the report (under the same title) made by Pavlov to the Petrograd Society of Biologists in 1915.

In this article Pavlov examines in detail two basic questions: 1) the conditions favouring the onset of sleep (significance of a decreased influx of external stimuli or the presence of monotonous, prolonged stimuli, the character of the stimuli and individuality of the animal) and 2) conditions impeding the onset of sleep (significance of a variety of stimuli and nervous processes, i.e., alternation of excitation and inhibition). As Pavlov directly points out in the text, I. M. Sechenov's statements in his famous *Reflexes of the Brain* were of particular importance to the question discussed in the article. It should be noted that Sechenov also dwells on the question of the onset of sleep or waking in one of his other works written much later under the title of *Participation of the Nervous System in Man's Working Movements*. In virtue of the special interest which these postulates laid down by Sechenov present we are citing the following excerpt from his works:

"*Waking*. This state is connected with the continuous effects of impulses from the external world on our sense organs and is demonstrated by accidental and, fortunately, extremely rare pathological observations on man. One such case witnessed by physicians happened in Germany. It was a case of a young man whose suffering consisted in the fact that of all the sense organs he retained functionally intact but one eye and one ear which served him as the only avenues of communication with the external world. As long as the eye could see or the ear could hear he was awake, but as soon as the physicians, by way of experiment, closed his healthy eye and stopped up the ear, the patient rapidly lapsed into sleep from which he awakened when these organs were acted upon by sensual stimuli.

"Another case occurred in Petersburg, in the Pokrovskaya community, and I was told about it by S. P. Botkin who was near and dear to all of us, Russians, during his lifetime and who still is near and dear to us by the memories he has left. A well-educated female patient retained intact only the sense of touch and the muscle sense in one of her arms. According to the hospital personnel, she was almost always asleep and communicated with people in the following manner: a pillow was placed on her abdomen and her hand which retained its sensitivity was moved along the pillow so as to write the question to which the patient's answer was wanted. To this question the patient answered in words. The patient talked similarly with S. P. Botkin. For example, the words 'Botkin has come to see you' were written with her own hand and she answered: 'I am very glad', etc.

"Can there be any doubt, after such facts, that waking with its inevitable alternation of sensations of various kinds and orders is maintained by optic, acoustic, thermal, olfactory and frequently mechanical external influences on the senses? True, we do not know what happens in the central nervous system at this time, but we cannot doubt this fact a priori: the loss of all senses must necessarily be accompanied by a total loss of consciousness, since conciousness is manifested in nothing but conscious sensations. A total loss of the senses must correspond to deep sleep without dreams." (I.M. Sechenov, *Selected Philosophical and Psychological Works*, U.S.S.R. Academy of Sciences, Moscow, 1952, p. 511.)

p. 44

[9] The case of Professor Strümpell which Pavlov mentions here and in some of his other works was the subject of a report made by Professor Strümpell to the Section of Internal Medicine at a meeting of naturalists in Munich in 1877 (this case is described in Strümpell's article "Beobachtungen über ausgebreitete Anästhesien und deren Folgen für die willkürliche Bewegung und das Bewusstsein", Deutsches Archiv für klinische Medicin, 1878, Bd. 22).

p. 44

[10] Pavlov also examines the question of the importance of the diminished influx of external stimuli to the brain for the onset of sleep in his other article "Problem of Sleep", referring to the experiments of B. S. Galkin who surgically eliminated in dogs simultaneously the visual, auditory and olfactory receptors (see I. P. Pavlov's article "The Problem of Sleep" in the present edition, p. 393).

p. 45

[11] Here Pavlov refers to M. K. Petrova's experiments summed up in her dissertation (M. K. Petrova, *On the Teaching on Irradiation of Excitation and the Inhibitory Processes*, St. Petersburg, 1914, 255 pages) and her work *Struggle Against Sleep. Work of Balancing the Stimulatory and Inhibitory Processes* (book dedicated to Pavlov's 75th birthday, Leningrad, 1924, pp. 275-85). Petrova's dissertation and her subsequent physiological investigations of sleep and related phenomena are a valuable contribution to Pavlov's teaching on sleep. The dissertation examines the different hypnotic effects of various conditioned stimuli (thermal, mechanical stimuli of the skin, acoustic, etc.), measures of struggle against sleep, transformation of strong faradic current into a somniferous agent, effect of the sentry reflex on the emergence of sleep, causes of special sleepiness of " lively", "excitable" dogs, etc.

According to M. K. Petrova, "sleep ... is characterised by a special relation of the central nervous system to external stimuli and special states of the muscles" (in the same dissertation). While sharing a number of N. A. Rozhansky's views of the physiological nature of sleep, Petrova differs with him in evaluating the significance of restraining the animal's movements for the onset of sleep, considering such restraint a secondary factor in determining the emergence of sleep. At the same time she attaches the decisive importance in the onset of sleep to the character of external stimuli, their quality, duration, strength, etc. In her opinion it is the protracted, monotonous conditioned stimuli, thermal and mechanical skin stimuli, in the first place, which have the necessary hypnotic effect. p. 51

[12] P. N. Vasilyev's experiments to which Pavlov refers are treated in Vasilyev's dissertation *Differentiation of Thermal Stimuli by the Dog (St. Petersburg, 1922)*.

In his experiments Vasilyev alternated different conditioned thermal stimuli to struggle against sleep; he also used M. N. Yerofeyeva's method and elaborated a conditioned food reflex to strong faradic current. p. 52

[13] I. P. Pavlov's article (written jointly with L. N. Voskresensky) "Some Facts About the Physiology of Sleep" was translated from the text of the work published under the same title in the second edition of I. P. Pavlov's *Complete Works* (Vol. III, Book 1, Moscow and Leningrad, 1951, pp. 299-305). This article is a report prepared for the press and made by Pavlov under the same title to the Petrograd Biological Society in 1915. It was first published in French in the journal *Comptes rendus de la Société de Biologie* (79,1079-1084, 1916). Besides, Pavlov's report "Some Facts about the Physiology of Sleep" was published in the *Herald of the Petrograd Biological Laboratory* (1917).

In this work Pavlov makes a close study of the "course of sleep", the "motion of sleep inhibition through the brain". The transitional states between sleep and waking, the phenomena of hypnosis became the object of his experimental research; by hypnosis Pavlov implies partial, limited sleep in its different manifestations. The work contains the experiments of L. N. Voskresensky who produced hypnotic states by conditioned reflexes. At the same time Pavlov also believes that hypnotic inhibition exists as an independent form of inhibition. This point of view was distinctly expressed by Pavlov in his article "Special Lability of Internal Inhibition: Hypnotic, External and Internal" (I . P. Pavlov, *Complete Works*, 2nd ed., Vol. III, Book 1, Moscow and Leningrad, 1951, p. 275). p. 53

[14] Pavlov refers to his report made to the Petrograd Society of Biologists in 1914 and published as an article entitled "Special Lability of Internal Inhibition in Dogs" (I. P. Pavlov, *Complete Works*, 2nd ed., Vol. III, Book 1, Moscow and Leningrad, 1951, p. 275).
p. 59

[15] The article "Psychiatry as an Auxiliary to the Physiology of the Cerebral Hemispheres" was translated from the text published in the second edition of I. P. Pavlov's *Complete Works* (Vol. III, Book 1, Moscow and Leningrad, 1951, pp. 346-54).

The article is a report made by Pavlov to a meeting of the Society of Psychiatrists in Petrograd in 1919. It was first published in the same year (*Russian Physiological Journal*, 1919, Vol. II, Book 4-5, p. 257).

During June-August 1918 Pavlov lived in his country home on Poklonnaya Hill in Udelnaya near Leningrad. During that period he visited the Skvortsov-Stepanov 3rd Psychiatric Hospital where, with the aid of a number of psychiatrists, mainly A. V. Timofeyev, Chief Physician of the hospital, and physician V. P. Golovina, he observed mental patients in an endeavour to understand the peculiarities of their condition and behaviour from the point of view of general physiology of the nervous system, particularly the teaching on conditioned reflexes. As L. A. Orbeli points out, "his first impressions and statements manifested his admiration of the selfless work of psychiatrists who gave all their energies and knowledge to the difficult and at times dangerous work of caring for mental patients". The report made by Pavlov to the Society of Psychiatrists in Petrograd in 1919 and published in the article "Psychiatry as an Auxiliary to the Physiology of the Cerebral Hemispheres" is a summary of these observations of the mental patients in the Udelnaya Psychiatric Hospital. Of considerable interest is the fact that the case history (described in the article) of the 60-year-old Kachalkin who was in a catatonic stupor for more than twenty years has come down to us and was recently analysed by V. I. Velikojanov, research worker at the Pavlov Institute of Physiology. (V. I. Velikojanov, "On the History of Pavlov's Teaching on the Protective Role of Transmarginal Inhibition. Patient Kachalkin". *The Korsakov Journal of Neuropathology and Psychiatry*, Vol. 60, Book 4, pp. 484-87, 1960.) This patient had been admitted to the psychiatric hospital in 1893 and was observed by Pavlov only at the end of July 1918. It should also be noted that at that time I. F. Tolochinov was the patient's attending physician; although a psychiatrist, he carried on scientific work in Pavlov's laboratory and, as was already mentioned (See Note 2), wrote, under Pavlov's supervision, the first work on conditioned reflexes. The patient Kachalkin died of heart failure in September 1918 soon after Pavlov had discontinued his visits to the hospital. This article is significant not only for its deep physiological interpretation of one of the widespread and important symptoms of catatonia, the so-called *flexibilitas cerea*, but also because it already shows the basic features of Pavlov's harmonious physiological hypothesis of the catatonic form of schizophrenia. p. 60

[16] Moritz Schiff (1823-1896), Swiss physiologist who extensively studied the central nervous system and the trophic influence of nerves on the tissues. p. 62

17 In Pavlov's attitude to the well-known British physiologist Charles Scott Sherrington the following is of some interest. Highly appraising Sherrington's works in his "Lectures on the Work of the Cerebral Hemispheres" Pavlov compares his works on the physiology of the brain with Sherrington's works on the physiology of the spinal cord (I. P. Pavlov, *Complete Works*, 2nd ed., Vol. 4, Moscow and Leningrad, 1951, pp. 18-19).

In 1934, in his work "Experimental Pathology of the Higher Nervous Activity" Pavlov reverted to Sherrington again (see present edition, p. 355). He related that, while in London at the Anniversary of the London Royal Society, he had chanced to "meet the best British physiologist and neurologist C. S. Sherrington" and the latter said to him: "You know, your conditioned reflexes would hardly be popular in England since they have a materialistic flavour." Pavlov immediately noted that Sherrington's prediction had not come true. Pavlov wrote: "... In England, the country with which Sherrington tried to frighten me, there is an altogether different situation. There, the theory of the conditioned reflexes is now taught in all schools." (Present edition, p. 356.)

After familiarising himself with Sherrington's new book *The Brain and Its Mechanisms* in 1934 Pavlov, despite his positive appraisal of Sherrington as a physiologist, expressed his sharp disapproval of this book on the "Wednesday," September 19, 1934.

Pavlov said: "Comparing the laws of the brain and its mechanisms, he (Sherrington—*Editor*) draws a very strange conclusion. It appears that up to now he is not at all sure whether the brain bears any relation to our mind.... This is clearly expressed by him in the following, words: 'If nerve activity has relation to mind...' I did not trust my knowledge of English and so I requested others to translate it for me."

"How can it be that at present time a physiologist should doubt the relation between nervous activity and the mind?" Pavlov asks and answers: "This is the result of a purely dualistic concept. This is the cartesian viewpoint, according to which the brain is a piano, a passive instrument, while the soul is a musician extracting from this piano any melodies it likes" (I. P. Pavlov, *Selected Works*, Foreign Languages Publishing House, Moscow 1955, p.563).

Pavlov also sharply criticised Sherrington's agnosticism. "I am all the more surprised," Pavlov went on to say, "that for some reason or other he regards knowledge of this soul as something pernicious and clearly expresses this point of view; according to him, if the best of us acquire some knowledge of the nervous system this would be a most dangerous thing threatening the extinction of man on earth.... Why knowledge of the soul may be pernicious? I would like to know how on earth it can lead to the extinction of man. Socrates counselled: 'Know thyself'. How, then, can a scientist, a neurologist, say: 'Do not dare know thyself'?" (*Ibid.*, pp. 563-64.) p. 62

[18] See the article "Some Facts About the Physiology of Sleep", in the present edition, p. 53, and Note 13.   p. 63

[19] The article "Concerning the So-Called Hypnotism in Animals", was translated from the second edition of I. P. Pavlov's *Complete Works* (Vol. III, Book 2, Moscow and Leningrad, 1951, pp. 359-60). It contains the report made by Pavlov to the meeting of the Branch of Physico-Mathematical Sciences of the Russian Academy of Sciences, November 9, 1921; in this report Pavlov formulates his physiological conceptions of hypnosis in animals. He considers hypnosis in animals one of the self-protective reflexes based on inhibition. The phenomena of catalepsy are regarded as inhibition of the motor area of the cortex. Pavlov also points out the transition of hypnosis to sleep during irradiation of inhibition to the other regions of the cortex.   p. 70

[20] The article "Relations Between Excitation and Inhibition, Delimitation Between Excitation and Inhibition, Experimental Neuroses in Dogs" was translated from the text published in the second edition of I. P. Pavlov's *Complete Works* (Vol. III, Book 2, Moscow and Leningrad, pp. 35-50, 1951). This article was first published in German in the *Skandinaviches Archiv für Physiologie* (Bd. XLVII, H. 1-2, 1925, S. 1-14), the journal founded by R. Tigerstedt.

Although studies of the types of higher nervous activity and of experimental neuroses in animals had been started in Pavlov's laboratory long before this article was written (as early as 1909-11), these studies made particular headway in the 1920's. Considerable attention to this problem was stimulated by the great 1924 Leningrad flood described in the article. The building housing the experimental animals of Pavlov's laboratory was flooded. The conditioned reflex activity elaborated in the rescued animals experimentally was deranged. The peculiarities of the resulting neuroses and their elimination, depending on the type of nervous system in the dogs, was the subject of all-round studies in Pavlov's laboratories.

The present article sums up the studies (mainly during 1921-23) of the conditions under which neuroses emerged. By these conditions Pavlov implied overstrain of the basic nervous processes of excitation and inhibition and of their mobility.   p. 72

[21] Reference is made to M. N. Yerofeyeva's work "Additional Data on Destructive Conditioned Reflexes", published in the *Herald of the Petrograd Lesgaft Research Institute*, Vol. III, 1921.   p. 75

[22] This refers to N. R. Shenger-Krestovnikova's work "On the Question of Differentiation of Optic Stimuli and of the Limits of Differentiation in the Visual Analyser of the Dog" published in the *Herald of the Petrograd Lesgaft Research Institute*, Vol. III, 1921.
   p. 76

[23] Reference is made to M. K. Petrova's work "Different Types of Internal Inhibition Under a Particularly Difficult Condition" published in the *Transactions of Academician Pavlov's Physiological Laboratories*, Vol. I, Leningrad, 1924.   p. 77

[24] Pavlov is referring to N. Razenkov's work "Change in the Process of Excitation in the Cerebral Cortex of the Dog Under Difficult Conditions of Work" published in the *Transactions of Academician Pavlov's Physiological Laboratories*, Vol. I, Leningrad, 1924.
p. 78

[25] A. D. Speransky's work "Changes in the Relationships Between Excitation and Inhibition in the Dog After the Flood" mentioned here was published in the *Russian Physiological Journal* (Vol. VII, Book 3-4, 1925). p. 80

[26] For I. P. Pavlov's views of the investigations of N. Y. Vvedensky and his school see Note 35. p. 86

[27] The article "Normal and Pathological States of the Cerebral Hemispheres" was translated from the text published in the second edition of I. P. Pavlov's *Complete Works* (Vol. III, Book 2, Moscow and Leningrad, 1951, pp. 51-62). It is Pavlov's report made in French at the Sorbonne, Paris, December 1925.

The article furnishes new data of the studies of experimental pathology of higher nervous activity conducted in Pavlov's laboratories. The characterisation of the reactivity of cortical nerve cells ("precipitate functional destructibility") and the indication of the significance of inhibition in limiting the afore-mentioned high reactivity, which stops "further functional destruction" deserves attention. p. 87

[28] The article "Inhibitory Type of Nervous System in Dogs" was translated from the text published in the second edition of I. P. Pavlov's *Complete Works* (Vol. III, Book 2, Moscow and Leningrad, 1951, pp. 63-70). The article is Pavlov's report made in French at the Paris Psychological Society in December, 1925.

In this report Pavlov sets forth, for the first time, the teaching on types of nervous system and outlines a classification of types according to the predominance of either excitation or inhibition. Pavlov distinguishes extreme types (sanguine and melancholic) and a balanced type. This classification of types was subsequently modified. p. 100

[29] Reference is made to A. D. Speransky's experiments described in his work "Effect of Strong Destructive Stimuli on the Dog with the Inhibitory Type of Nervous System" (*Transactions of Academician Pavlov's Physiological Laboratories*, Vol. I, Book 1, Leningrad, 1924, p. 119.) p. 108

[30] I. P. Pavlov's article "Internal Inhibition and Sleep Are Essentially the Same Physicochemical Process" was translated from his lecture under the same title (Lecture 15) published in the "Lectures on the Work of the Cerebral Hemispheres" (I. P. Pavlov, *Complete Works*, 2nd ed., Moscow and Leningrad, 1951, Vol. IV, pp. 263-78). The lecture published in the present edition is a somewhat altered version of I. P. Pavlov's article "Internal Inhibition of Conditioned Reflexes and Sleep Are the Same Process" written by Pavlov in 1922 for a book to have been published in

honour of A. P. Karpinsky, then President of the U.S.S.R. Academy of Sciences. The book was not published and the article was printed in the journal *Scandinavishes Archiv für Physiologie* (Bd. LXIV, 1923) and simultaneously in the book *Twenty Years of Experience* (I. P. Pavlov, *Complete Works*, 2nd ed., Vol. III, Book 1, Moscow and Leningrad, 1951, pp. 373-90).

The principal propositions and content of the lecture and those of the article *Twenty Years of Experience* essentially coincide; the present edition contains the lecture published three years later (1926) than the article. Pavlov somewhat supplemented and revised the lecture.

Pavlov's basic proposition that "internal inhibition and sleep are essentially the same process" was first formulated by him somewhat earlier in the report made to the Society of Finnish Physicians in Helsingfors, April 1922. The report was entitled "Normal Activity and General Constitution of the Cerebral Hemispheres" (I. P. Pavlov, *Complete Works*, 2nd ed., Vol. III, Book 1, Moscow and Leningrad, 1951, p. 365).

In the lecture published in the present edition the foregoing proposition was given thorough experimental substantiation.

All-round experimental substantiation was also given in the lecture to Pavlov's propositions on the "transition of inhibition to sleep and vice versa", on "replacement of inhibition with sleep" and on "summation of sleep and inhibition". The lecture clearly reveals Pavlov's dialectical interpretation of inhibition as "partial" sleep, as irradiated inhibition, and formulates the idea of the protective significance of inhibition and sleep. Of great interest is the fact that Pavlov considered this work one of his most important works on sleep (see I. P. Pavlov's article "The Problem of Sleep" in the present edition, p. 393). p. 109

[31] I. P. Pavlov's work "Transitional Phases Between the Animal's Waking and Complete Sleep (Hypnotic Phases)" was translated from the text of the lecture under the same title (Lecture 16) published in the "Lectures on the Work of the Cerebral Hemispheres" (I. P. Pavlov, *Complete Works*, 2nd ed., Vol. IV, Moscow and Leningrad, 1951, pp. 176-87).

Using extensive experimental material the lecture sets forth the basic regularities observed in the transitional states from waking to sleep, regularities concerning the spread and depth of the processes of inhibition in the cerebral cortex, and data on different extent and intensity of sleep. The experimental data on this question contained in the lecture give an insight into Pavlov's teaching on hypnosis and hypnotic phases. p. 126

[32] See the detailed description of L. N. Voskresensky's experiments in the article "Some Facts about the Physiology of Sleep" written by I. P. Pavlov jointly with L. N. Voskresensky (present edition, p. 53, see also Note 13). p. 127

[33] Here Pavlov cites B. N. Bierman's experiments described in his monograph "Experimental Sleep" (Gosizdat, 1925).

Pavlov approved of B. N. Bierman's monograph "Experimental Sleep". In the preface to the monograph he wrote: "Dr. B. N. Bierman's present experimental work brings us much closer to the final solution of the problem of the physiological mechanism of hypnosis. Another two or three details and the physiologist will have at his disposal the whole mechanism which has long been an enigma, has been shrouded in mystery" (I. P. Pavlov, *Complete Works*, 2nd ed., Moscow and Leningrad, 1951, Vol. IV, p. 428).

The most important conclusions drawn by B. N. Bierman from his experimental studies are his postulates that "hypnosis differs from sleep in its limited spread of the inhibitory process", that hypnosis is "sleep with partial waking" and owes its existence to a "sentry point" in the cortex. p. 128

34 Here Pavlov refers to I. P. Razenkov's experiments described in his work "Changes in the Stimulatory Process of the Cerebral Cortex of the Dog Under Difficult Conditions of Work" (*Russian Physiological Journal*, 1926, Vol. IX, Book 5-6). In this work Razenkov for the first time elucidated the main phasic states (hypnotic phases) in the cerebral hemispheres and gave their physiological characteristics. p. 132

35 Although Pavlov disagreed with certain postulates in N. Y. Vvedensky's teaching on the physiological essence of inhibition, he highly appraised his research in this question. Pavlov recognised that the various phases (discovered by Vvedensky) in the process of transition of the peripheral nerve fibre from excitation to inhibition under the influence of strong stimuli may also take place in the vital activity of the nerve cells of the cerebral hemispheres.

Pavlov very definitely expressed his point of view on this question as far back as 1923 in his work "Latest Achievements in the Objective Study of Higher Nervous Activity of Animals". He wrote: "In studying these deviations in the direction of predominance of inhibition, weakening of the process of excitation, we have convinced ourselves that one of the discoveries of our outstanding, now deceased, physiologist N. Y. Vvedensky is absolutely correct. Vvedensky has contributed a great deal to nervous physiology; he has had the good fortune of finding important facts, but has been for some reason insufficiently appreciated by the foreign press. Among other things, he is the author of the book *Excitation, Inhibition and Narcosis* in which he establishes changes in the nerve fibre under the influence of strong stimuli and distinguishes several phases. It has now developed that these peculiar phases are completely reproduced in the nerve cells when you greatly intensify the struggle between the processes of excitation and inhibition. I have no doubts that after this coincidence Vvedensky's works will finally be estimated at their true worth" (I. P. Pavlov, *Complete Works*, 2nd ed., Vol. III, Book 2, Moscow and Leningrad, 1951, p. 28). p. 133

36 The article "Different Types of Nervous System. Pathological States of the Cerebral Hemispheres as a Result of Functional

Influences Exerted on Them" was translated from the text of the lecture under the same title (Lecture 17) published in the "Lectures on the Work of the Cerebral Hemispheres" (I. P. Pavlov, *Complete Works*, 2nd ed., Vol. IV, Moscow and Leningrad, 1951, pp. 299-316). This article already distinguishes four types: two "extreme" (excitable and inhibitory) and two "intermediate", balanced types. However, this classification of types was subsequently modified, since it did not completely correspond to the classification of temperaments proposed by Hippocrates by which Pavlov guided himself. The same lecture contains data on functional pathological states ("experimental neuroses") produced by overstrain of the processes of excitation, inhibition, and their mobility. p. 147

[37] The article "Pathological States of the Cerebral Hemispheres as a Result of Functional Influences Exerted on Them" was translated from the text of the lecture under the same title (Lecture 18) published in the "Lectures on the Work of the Cerebral Hemispheres" (I. P. Pavlov, *Complete Works*, 2nd ed., Vol. IV, Moscow and Leningrad, 1951, pp. 317-35).

This lecture, a continuation of the preceding one, further elucidates the derangements of higher nervous activity ("experimental neuroses") produced by difficult tasks imposed on experimental animals and overstraining the basic nervous processes in the brain and the mobility of these processes. p. 167

[38] The article "Application to Man of Experimental Data Obtained on Animals" was translated from the text of the lecture under the same title (Lecture 23) published in the "Lectures on the Work of the Cerebral Hemispheres" (I. P. Pavlov, *Complete Works*, 2nd ed., Vol. IV, Moscow and Leningrad, 1951, pp. 414-33). In this last lecture Pavlov elucidates in detail the important and fundamental question of the justification of applying to man the experimental data obtained on animals. While recognising the possibility of such application, Pavlov calls for the greatest possible discretion considering the fact that it is precisely the higher nervous activity that "sharply distinguishes man from animals". This lecture for the first time raises the question of the peculiarities of man's higher nervous activity, the role of the word, speech, as a new physiological stimulus inherent only in man. In examining questions of hypnosis and suggestion Pavlov determines the peculiarities of these phenomena in man. Thus, Pavlov essentially for the first time expresses in this lecture his ideas on the second signalling system without as yet using this term. Concerning the teaching on neuroses, however, Pavlov still ascribes hysteria to neuroses in animals and does not consider it along with psychasthenia a specially human neurosis, as he did later. p. 187

[39] The work "Physiological Teaching on Types of Nervous System or Temperaments" was translated from the text of the article under the same title published in the second edition of I. P. Pavlov's *Complete Works* (Vol. III, Book 2, Moscow and Leningrad,

1951, pp. 77-88). This article constitutes Pavlov's report to the meeting of the Pirogov Russian Surgical Society dedicated to N. I. Pirogov's memory on December 6, 1927. In classifying the types of nervous system in dogs Pavlov divides the "intermediate" balanced type, according to the character of mobility of its nervous processes, into two types—the "lively" and the "inert". Thus he distinguishes four types which correspond to the four temperaments established by Hippocrates. The "excitable" type formerly recognised by Pavlov as corresponding to Hippocrates' sanguine temperament in this work corresponds to Hippocrates' choleric temperament. p. 208

[40] Nikolai Ivanovich Pirogov (1813-1881), great Russian surgeon and anatomist whose works laid the groundwork for the anatomo-experimental trend in practical surgery. Of great interest to neuropathologists and psychiatrists in his works on battlefield surgery is the teaching on the closed craniocerebral trauma, shellshock, in which he emphasised that the latter affected the entire organism. p. 208

[41] Leonid Vasilyevich Blumenau (1862-1931), outstanding Russian neuropathologist, known for his scientific contributions to the anatomy and physiology of the brain. Blumenau was one of the first clinical neuropathologists to use Pavlov's teaching in explaining the pathogenesis of functional diseases of the nervous system, hysteria in particular. Here Pavlov refers to Blumenau's work *Hysteria and Its Pathogenesis*, Leningrad, 1926. p. 218

[42] Only part of the article "Some Problems of the Physiology of the Cerebral Hemispheres" is published in the present edition. Only the fourth part of the article devoted to classification of types of nervous system was translated (I. P. Pavlov, *Complete Works*, 2nd ed., Vol. III, Book 2, Moscow and Leningrad, 1951, pp. 101-05). The article as a whole constitutes the Croon Lecture delivered by Pavlov to the London Royal Society, May 10, 1928. Specialists in the different branches of natural science are annually invited from all over the world to deliver a lecture for the Croon Prize. This work was published in English in the *Proceedings of the Royal Society*, Section B. Biological Sciences, Series B., Vol. 103, No. B. 721, 1928, pp. 106-10. p. 220

[43] The article "An Attempt of a Physiologist to Digress into the Domain of Psychiatry" was first published in the anniversary volume in honour of E. Gley and I. F. Heymans in the journal *Archives Internationales de Pharmacodynamie et Therapie* in 1930. It was also published under the same title in the booklet *Physiology and Pathology of Higher Nervous Activity* (Gosmedizdat, Leningrad and Moscow, 1930, pp. 37-45) and under the title of "Excursion of a Physiologist into the Field of Psychiatry" in the newspaper *Izvestia* (*Izvestia of the Central Executive Committee of the U.S.S.R.*, No. 122 [3969] May 5, 1930).

The article was translated from the text published in the second edition of I. P. Pavlov's *Complete Works* (Vol. III, Book 2, Moscow and Leningrad, 1951, pp. 126-32) and develops Pavlov's ideas in regard to his physiological interpretation of schizophrenia set forth in his article "Psychiatry as an Auxiliary to the Physiology of the Cerebral Hemispheres" (see p. 60 of the present edition and Note 15).

In this article Pavlov thoroughly analyses a group of symptoms observed in schizophrenic patients: negativism, stereotypy, echolalia and echopraxia, muscular rigidity, phenomena of hebephrenic silliness, and catatonic excitement. Pointing out that such symptoms also appear in healthy people during hypnosis Pavlov postulates more definitely the conclusion already planned in his work "Psychiatry as an Auxiliary to the Physiology of the Cerebral Hemispheres" that the "schizophrenic symptoms are an expression of a chronic hypnotic state" and that "in certain variations schizophrenia is really chronic hypnosis". According to Pavlov, this inhibition (hypnosis) is based on a "weak nervous system, special weakness of the cortical cells (hereditary and acquired) which easily become exhausted since normal stimuli are also too strong for such weakened cells. The exhaustion of the nerve cells is an impulse to the emergence of inhibition in them. But as long as the inhibitory process is effective the cortical cell is not deeply affected". Pavlov thus formulates his teaching on the healing and protective role of inhibition in schizophrenic patients. This teaching proved to be a deep theoretical substantiation of the formerly empiric treatment of schizophrenic patients with prolonged, artificially induced sleep. It also determined Pavlov's line in questions of organising psychiatric aid; Pavlov's statements on these questions are also of considerable interest.

Pavlov demands humane treatment of mental patients and consideration of the fact that some patients regard their very commitment to the hospital as a "violation of human rights". "Consequently," I. P. Pavlov writes, "it is necessary as quickly and as timely as possible to place such mentally diseased in the position of patients suffering from other illnesses which do not offend human dignity so manifestly" (present edition, p. 31).   p. 225

[44] Pavlov's article (written jointly with M. K. Petrova) "Physiology of the Hypnotic State of the Dog" was translated from the text published in the second edition of I. P. Pavlov's *Complete Works* (Vol. III, Book 2, Moscow and Leningrad, 1951, pp. 133-46). This work was first published in 1932 (*Transactions of Academician Pavlov's Laboratories*, Vol. IV, 1932). In 1934 this article was published in English under the title of "A Contribution to the Physiology of the Hypnotic State in Dogs. Character and Personality", (Vol. 2, No. 3, 1934, pp. 189-200). In the *Twenty Years of Experience* it was published only in the sixth edition in 1938. The work offers a deep physiological analysis of hypnosis in animals. Some hypnotic phenomena are interpreted on the basis of experimental data in the light of localisation and motion of hypnotic inhibition, phenomena of reciprocal induction and interactions of the cortex and subcortex.

The physiological analysis of hypnotic inhibition and negativism in the experimental dogs contained in this work is also of considerable importance in explaining a number of phenomena observed in the psychiatric clinic, the psychopathological symptoms in patients with the catatonic form of schizophrenia in particular. p. 232

[45] See the lecture on the "Transitional Phases Between the Animal's Waking and Complete Sleep (Hypnotic Phases)" published in the present edition (p. 126) and Note 16. p. 232

[46] See the article "Some Facts About the Physiology of Sleep" written by I. P. Pavlov jointly with L. N. Voskresensky (p. 53 in the present edition). The article contains a detailed description of the experiments with production of the hypnotic state in dogs, determining dissociation of the motor and secretory components in the conditioned food reflex. p. 237

[47] Here Pavlov confines himself merely to a general mention of the "broad representation" of the "internal world of the organism" in the cerebral cortex, a mention which serves as the basis for understanding the physiological mechanisms of verbal suggestion during hypnosis in man, as well as the possibility of influencing the vegetative processes in the organism, the activity of its internal organs, by means of such suggestion and autosuggestion. In the studies of Academician K. M. Bykov (1886-1959), Pavlov's closest pupil, as well as those of Bykov's collaborators the question of the relationships between the cortex and internal organs was very fruitfully and extensively elaborated.

On the basis of numerous experiments K. M. Bykov and his collaborators have established bilateral connections between the cortex and the internal organs; on the one hand, it is a regulating influence of the cortex on the activity of the internal organs by means of a trigger and co-ordinating mechanisms, and, on the other hand, it is the all-round "information" of the cortex on the state of the internal organs by numerous signals conveyed from the latter to the cortex and the formation of interoceptive conditioned reflexes (see K. M. Bykov, *Selected Works*, Vol. II, "The Cerebral Cortex and the Internal Organs", Moscow, 1954.)

In his work "The Problem of Sleep" published in the present edition (p. 393) Pavlov examines in greater detail the questions of the physiological mechanism of influencing the tissue processes, metabolism and activity of the internal organs by suggestion and autosuggestion. In this work he also explains at great length the "imaginary, autosuggested pregnancy" in hysteriacs.

Pavlov's statements in the "Lectures on the Work of the Cerebral Hemispheres" are very important for elucidating the physiological mechanism of verbal suggestion during hypnosis in the light of his teaching on the second signalling system and its interaction with the first signalling system. Pavlov's following statement is particularly important:

"Of the hypnotic phenomena in man so-called *suggestion* justly attracts special attention. How should it be understood physiologically? Of course, for man the word is as real a conditioned stimulus as all the other stimuli which man has in common with animals, but at the same time it is also more all-inclusive than any others and in this respect cannot in any way be either quantitatively or qualitatively compared with the conditioned stimuli of animals. Owing to the entire preceding life of the adult human being, the word is connected with all the external and internal stimuli reaching the cerebral hemispheres, signals them all, replaces them all, and can therefore evoke all the actions, reactions of the organism, which those stimuli condition. Thus, suggestion is man's most simplified and most typical conditioned reflex (present edition, p. 202). p. 240

[48] Reference is made to Pavlov's article "Brief Outline of Higher Nervous Activity" written in 1932 (I. P. Pavlov, *Complete Works*, 2nd ed., Vol. III, Book 2, Moscow and Leningrad, 1951, pp. 106-26). This article was also published in English in the American compilation *Proceedings and Papers* (New Jersey, the Psychol. Rev. Comp., Princeton, 1930, pp. 331-33). The article describes the successive spread of hypnotic inhibition in the motor area of the cortex in a certain dog during the act of eating. In this article Pavlov also dwells on the importance of "supermaximal stimuli" in the emergence of transmarginal inhibition and formation of phasic states in the cerebral cortex. p. 244

[49] Reference is made to V. V. Rikman's work "Discovery of Traces of Stimulation of the Centres of the Defensive Reaction as an Analogue of Traumatic Neurosis" *(Transactions of Academician Pavlov's Physiological Laboratories*, Vol. IV, p. 10, Leningrad, 1932). p. 245

[50] The article "On Neuroses in Man and Animals" was translated from the text published in the second edition of I. P. Pavlov's *Complete Works* (Vol. III, Book 2, Moscow and Leningrad, 1951, pp. 147-50). It is a review of the article "The Somatic Basis of the Neurosis" by the well-known Viennese psychiatrist Schilder who later lived in the U.S.A. The article was published in the American *Journal of Nervous and Mental Diseases*, 70, 502, November 1929. The review was published by Pavlov in the *Journal of the American Medical Association*, 1932, Vol. 99, No. 12, pp. 1012-1013 and in *The Bulletin of the Battle Greek Sanitarium and Hospital Clinic*, 1932. In the review Pavlov criticises Schilder for denying the importance physiological studies of neuroses in animals have for understanding neuroses in man. Schilder held that clinical observations of the "mental mechanism" should help to understand the data of experimental studies of higher nervous activity in animals. Pavlov's very interesting statements in this article concerning the methods of studying neuroses in man also deserve attention. p. 247

[51] The article "Experimental Neuroses" was translated from the text published in the second edition of I. P. Pavlov's *Complete Works* (Vol. III, Book 2, Moscow and Leningrad, 1951, pp. 189-94). The

article constitutes Pavlov's report to the First International Neurological Congress in Bern, delivered in German, September 3, 1931. This article was also published in the journals Deutsche Zeitschrift für Nervenheilkunde, 1932 Bd. 124, SS. 137-139; Ugeskr Laeg. 1932, Bd. 94, SS. 1135-1136. Of great importance in this article is Pavlov's exclusion of hysteria from the neuroses in animals. In his subsequent works he began to ascribe hysteria to specifically human neuroses. Pavlov's proposal to divide neurasthenia into two forms—hypersthenia (in the strong excitable type) and hyposthenia (in the weak inhibitory type)—also deserves attention. p. 251

[52] The article "Essay on the Physiological Concept of the Symptomatology of Hysteria" was translated from the text published in the second edition of I. P. Pavlov's *Complete Works* (Vol. III, Book 2, Moscow and Leningrad, 1951, pp. 195-218). This work was also published as a separate booklet under the same title by the U.S.S.R. Academy of Sciences (1932) and in French in the journal *L'Encéphale*, t. XXVIII, No. 4, 1933. In *L'Encéphale* it was published in an abridged form with notes of the translator W. Drabowitch. This entire issue of the journal was devoted to the clinical aspects and pathogenesis of hysteria treated from the most diverse points of view. It also contained an article contributed by G.Marinesko and M. Nicolesko on hysterical amnesia, elucidating the pathogenesis of this disease on the basis of the teaching on conditioned reflexes. The same article contains references to a number of formerly published works of G. Marinesko, O. Sager and A. Kreindler on hysteria in the light of Pavlov's conceptions. (*Revue neurologique*, 1930, June 3-11, 1932.)

The translator points out that Pavlov apparently did not know these works of G. Marinesko et al., in which the authors arrived at a conclusion closely corresponding to the inferences made in Pavlov's work, but they did not adequately consider the role of the weakness of the cortex in the development of hysteria.

Pavlov attached great importance to the article "Essay on the Physiological Concept of the Symptomatology of Hysteria" and regarded it as a "test of the extent to which the teaching on conditioned reflexes is justified in claiming to serve as a physiological substantiation of mental phenomena".

In this article Pavlov makes a deep physiological analysis of all the most characteristic symptoms of hysteria, the acute hysterical reactions, as well as the hysterical traits of the personality. It should be noted that in this article Pavlov offers a physiological explanation of hysterical nosophilia, the so-called "escape into disease" of the hysteriacs not infrequently superficially interpreted as manifestation of simulation. According to Pavlov, this presumably deliberate behaviour of hysteriacs is determined by conditioned reflexes and is a case of fatal physiological relations". In his concluding lecture in the "Lectures on the Work of the Cerebral Hemispheres" (see Note 38) Pavlov only outlined his conception of the first and second signalling systems, whereas in the present article he gives, for the first time, a broad definition of these two cortical signalling systems and describes the physiological peculiarities of each. In direct connection with the teaching of the signalling systems Pavlov offers, as a supplement to the classification of the types of nervous system in animals, a classification of specifically human types, depending on the interrelations between the first and second signalling systems. Using figurative expressions Pavlov divides people into "artists" and "thinkers" with an "intermediate" type between them. He establishes that the artistic type with its characteristic relatively weak first and relatively strong second signalling system is predisposed to hysteria. p. 255

[53] See Note 9. p. 261

[54] For the works of V. S. Galkin, A. D. Speransky's pupil, and the division of sleep into "passive" and "active" see the article "The Problem of Sleep" (present edition, p. 393 and Note 74). p. 261

[55] Rikman's experiments to which Pavlov refers were not published. p. 262

[56] The opinion that hysterical symptoms emerge only as a result of suggestion was expressed by the outstanding French neuropathologist Joseph Babinski (1857-1932) in 1907. It served as the subject of very heated discussions at many international congresses of neuropathologists and psychiatrists (see Babinski's work "Hysteriapithiatisme et troubles nerveux d'ordre reflexe en neurologie de guerre", P. 1917 (jointly with J. Froment). p. 274

[57] Reference is made to Bernheim's work "On Hypnotic Suggestion and Its Employment in the Treatment of Diseases". Odessa, 1887-88. p. 274

[58] Subsequently Pavlov relinquished the point of view that the second signalling system must be connected with the development of the frontal parts of the brain and generally doubted the legitimacy of localising the signalling systems anatomically. p. 276

[59] The article "Physiology of Higher Nervous Activity" was translated from the text published in the second edition of I. P. Pavlov's *Complete Works* (Vol. III, Book 2, Moscow and Leningrad, 1951, pp. 219-34). It is Pavlov's report to the Fourteenth International Physiological Congress in Rome, September 2, 1932.

This article was also published in the journal *Priroda (Nature)*, 1932, No. 11-12, pp. 1139-56, and in the *Latest Reports on Physiology and Pathology of Higher Nervous Activity*, Book 1, Leningrad, 1939, pp. 5-25. p. 282

[60] G. V. Volborth, one of Pavlov's pupils, organiser (1921) and for many years head of the Laboratory of Conditioned Reflexes at the Ukrainian Neuropsychiatric Institute in Kharkov. Of his scientific works the studies in efficiency and fatigue are of the greatest interest. p. 288

[61] See Note 9. p. 289

⁶² See the article "The Problem of Sleep" in the present edition (p. 393) and Note 74. p. 290
⁶³ Pavlov's theory of systematism in the work of the cerebral cortex and on dynamic patterns formed towards the beginning of the 1930's. Pavlov treated this question in great detail in his report to the Tenth International Psychological Congress in Copenhagen, August 24, 1932. See the article "Dynamic Stereotypy of the Higher Part of the Brain (*Complete Works*, 2nd ed., Vol. III, Book 2, Moscow and Leningrad, 1951, pp. 240-44). p. 293
⁶⁴ See "Essay on the Physiological Concept of the Symptomatology of Hysteria" (present edition, p. 255). p. 296
⁶⁵ In Pavlov's new statement on the second signalling system quoted in the article, Pavlov's indication of the importance of the second signalling system as the physiological basis of *abstract*, specially human, higher thinking and the definition of science as the "instrument of man's higher orientation in the surrounding world and within himself" merit attention. As in the preceding statement on the second signalling system (see present edition, p. 255 and Note 52) Pavlov still adheres to the point of view, subsequently relinquished by him, that the second signalling system is anatomically connected with the frontal parts of the brain (see Note 58).
p. 296
⁶⁶ The article "Example of an Experimentally Produced Neurosis and Its Cure in a Weak Type of Nervous System" was translated from the text published in the second edition of I. P. Pavlov's *Complete Works* (Vol. III, Book 2, Moscow and Leningrad, 1951, pp. 235-39).

The article contains the report made by Pavlov to the Sixth Scandinavian Neurological Congress in Copenhagen, August 25, 1932. It was published in the *Latest Reports on Physiology and Pathology of Higher Nervous Activity*, Book 1, Leningrad, U.S.S.R. Academy of Sciences, 1933, pp. 27-32.

The data on the treatment of neuroses with bromides and Pavlov's emphasis of the effectiveness of such treatment, if a proper correlation of the doses of bromides with the types of nervous system is ensured, deserves special attention.

Considerable interest in the treatment of neuroses, with bromides in particular, was displayed in Pavlov's laboratories for many years. The first attempts at treating neuroses and the studies in experimental therapy were carried out simultaneously with the beginning of the research in experimental neuroses.

Pavlov's special attention to questions of pharmacotherapy of nervous and mental diseases was determined, on the one hand, by the fact that during a considerable period of his activity (1895-1900) Pavlov worked as a pharmacologist, and on the other hand, by the fact that with the aid of therapy he expected to acquire so important and decisive a criterion of truth as practice. Pavlov wrote: "The power of our knowledge over the nervous system will, of course, appear to much greater advantage if we learn not only to injure the nervous system but also to restore it at will." (Present edition, pp. 366-67.)

431

On the question of applying Pavlov's pharmacotherapeutic conceptions in the psychiatric clinic see L. L. Rokhlin's article "Principles of Pharmacotherapy of Disorders of Higher Nervous Activity in Mental Patients" (*Physiological Journal of the Ukrainian Academy of Sciences*, 1956, Vol. II, No. 4). p. 298

[67] The article "Feelings of Possession (*Les sentiments d'emprise*) and the Ultraparadoxical Phase" was translated from the text published in the second edition of I. P. Pavlov's *Complete Works* (Vol. III, Book 2, Moscow and Leningrad, 1951, pp. 245-50). It is Pavlov's open letter to the well-known French psychologist and psychiatrist Pierre Janet.

This article was published in French in the *Journal de Psychologie* edited jointly by Pierre Janet and George Dumas in 1933 (No. 9-10, pp. 849-54) and in Russian in the *Latest Reports on Physiology and Pathology of Higher Nervous Activity*" (Book 2, Leningrad, 1933, pp. 5-11).

The thing that deserves attention in this article is I. P. Pavlov's frank appeal for collaboration between clinical psychiatrists, psychologists and physiologists. Pavlov wrote: "It seems that we should give proper consideration to our reciprocal work and cooperate in our research, for, after all, we are investigating the activity of one and the same organ (the brain—*Editor*) concerning which there can hardly be any doubt now."

Prompted by this striving Pavlov used the data on the ultraparadoxical phase, elaborated by that time in his laboratories, for physiological interpretation of certain forms of delirium described by P. Janet in the last part of his article "Feelings in the Delusion of Persecution" ("Les sentiments dans le délire de persecution"). This article was published by P. Janet in the *Journal de Psychologie*, 1932, pp. 161 and 401. It should be noted that in the French literature the role of the theory of conditioned reflexes in the interpretation of the pathogenesis of neuroses and mental disorders had been elucidated in a number of works of French authors as early as the 1920's-1930's (see Tinel, "Les réflexes conditionnels et les neuroses," *L'Encéphale*, XXIII, 1928; Delmas, "Le rôle des réflexes conditionnels en psychiatrie", *L'Encéphale*, XXV, 1930, etc.).

Pavlov also considered a number of other psychopathological phenomena—active negativism, controlism, ambivalence—to be based on the physiological mechanism of the ultraparadoxical hypnotic phase. During this hypnotic phase the reciprocal induction is perverted and responses to stimuli are contrary to adequate reactions. The phase itself emerges as a result of the exhaustion or weakening of the corresponding cortical cells to which the particular positive stimulus is addressed. In a number of his works Pavlov developed the idea of common physiological mechanisms for various psychopathological phenomena.

Pavlov displayed a special interest in P. Janet and repeatedly mentioned him in his statements on the "Wednesdays". On the "Wednesday" February 15, 1933 (*Pavlovian Wednesdays* Vol. 1,

Moscow and Leningrad, 1949, p. 287) he commented on the aforementioned open letter he had addressed to Janet. On the "Wednesday" February 20, 1935 he analysed two pathological cases from Janet's book *Beginning of Intellect*. At the same time he characterised Janet in an interesting manner.

He said: "Pierre Janet is an exceptional person. He is not a physician but a psychologist and, at the same time, a famous neuropathologist. He is undoubtedly an unusual, outstanding person." Then he evaluated Janet as a scientist. He said: "I am waging a big war against Pierre Janet as a psychologist and I shall do my best to vanquish him. But as a neuropathologist he is interesting. He has collected a mass of extraordinarily interesting and important pathological facts. I believe that as a psychologist he will in the end be defeated precisely by us, physiologists of higher nervous activity" (*Pavlovian Wednesdays*, Vol. III, Moscow and Leningrad, 1949, p. 95). p. 303

[68] The article "Attempt at a Physiological Interpretation of Compulsive Neurosis and Paranoia" was translated from the text published in the second edition of I. P. Pavlov's *Complete Works* (Vol. III, Book 2, Moscow and Leningrad, 1951, pp. 251-66).

It was also published in the booklet *Latest Reports on Physiology and Pathology of Higher Nervous Activity* (2nd ed., Leningrad, 1933, pp. 13-34), then in English in *The Journal of Mental Science* (1934, Vol. 80, pp. 187-97) and in French in *L'Encéphale* (1935, 30, pp. 381-93). This work is very important because it interprets physiologically such widespread and important psychopathological phenomena as delirium and obsession. For this purpose Pavlov utilised the theory of isolated pathological points and pathological inertness he had elaborated by that time on the basis of experimentally produced pathology of higher nervous activity in animals. On the basis of the conception of clinicians (P. Janet, E. Kretschmer, R. Malet) who held that obsessive ideas and delirium were closely related and could pass into each other, Pavlov underpinned these elements of clinical similarity with a similarity of physiological mechanisms: "pathological inertness of the process of excitation in a definite, physiologically conceived, isolated, pathological point of the brain". However, two reservations must be made here. Firstly, acknowledging the similarity Pavlov also sees the difference and points out "the degree of phases of the pathological state and certain additional features". The critical attitude during obsessive states and the uncritical attitude as a characteristic and invariable feature of delirium are determined by the different extent and intensity of the negative induction around the pathologically inert excited point and from the physiological basis in each of these psychopathological phenomena. Secondly, Pavlov does not establish the afore-described physiological mechanism for all, but only for a certain form of delirium, namely, delirium of a paranoiac structure. It should be noted that, in addition to recognising the possibility of a common physiological mechanism for the emergence of different psychopathological

433

phenomena, Pavlov also assumed the existence of different physiological mechanisms for the same type of psychopathological phenomena. This opinion is clearly illustrated in the article by a description of an inversion-type delirium which is based on the physiological mechanism of the ultraparadoxical phase. It is also important that the different physiological mechanisms of the same psychopathological phenomenon may, according to Pavlov, "exist separately or side by side, or alternately". It should be noted that Pavlov did not reduce the physiological bases of delirium of different structures to the two aforesaid physiological mechanisms (pathological inertness and the ultraparadoxical phase). For the deep feeble-minded, incongruous, megalomanic delirium in patients with progressive paralysis he searched the physiological bases in the regulating role of the second signalling system. (*Pavlovian Wednesdays*, Vol. III, Moscow and Leningrad, 1949, p.140.) p. 309

[69] Pavlov appreciated E. Kretschmer for his talent and the physiological trend in some of his works. At the same time he disagreed with a number of Kretschmer's incorrect methodological principles: his disregard for the qualitative differences between the normal and the pathological, biologisation of social phenomena, and autogenetic constructions. Concerning Kretschmer's book *Bodily Structure and Character,* which Pavlov had recently read, he said on the "Wednesday" October 23, 1935 that the book "nonplussed" him, that Kretschmer made a mistake "by wanting to drive the entire human race inhabiting the earth into the framework of his two clinical types: schizophrenics and cyclothymics. Of course, this is a wild statement of the question; why should the types prevailing in diseases and finally getting into psychiatric hospitals be regarded as basic? Indeed, the majority of humanity has nothing at all to do with these hospitals. Another strange thing is that he does not distinguish between type and character and this is, of course, also a flagrant mistake.

"We now firmly believe that man has inborn qualities and, on the other hand, qualities acquired in the course of life. This means that, if we speak of inborn qualities, we imply the type of nervous system, whereas, if it is a question of character, we refer to a mixture of inborn tendencies and drives and those instilled in him by the impressions he had received during his lifetime. Herein lies his mistake. He has confused it and has not made a clear distinction between the inborn type and the characteristics man acquires during his lifetime" (*Pavlovian Wednesdays*, Vol. III, Moscow and Leningrad, 1949, pp. 244-45). p. 321

[70] The article "General Types of Animal and Human Higher Nervous Activity" was translated from the text published in the second edition of I. P. Pavlov's *Complete Works* (Vol. III, Book 2, Moscow and Leningrad, 1951, pp. 267-93). It was also published in the booklet *Latest Reports on Physiology and Pathology of Higher Nervous Activity* (3rd ed., Moscow, 1935, pp. 5-41).

This article most comprehensively sums up the many years of research in the types of higher nervous activity conducted in Pavlov's laboratories. Particularly important in it is Pavlov's conception of the types of higher nervous activity. The fact that he attached great importance to the conditions of life in forming the type of higher nervous activity deserves attention. Pavlov wrote: "Human and animal behaviour is determined not only by congenital properties of the nervous system, but also by the influences to which the organism is continuously subjected during its individual existence; in other words, it depends on constant education and training in the broadest sense of these words." (Present edition, p. 327.)

The article lists the main criteria for determining the types of higher nervous activity (strength, balance and mobility of the nervous processes), clearly describes various types and examines different methods of studying them. Of considerable interest to psychiatrists are Pavlov's statements concerning the classification of types of people proposed by E. Kretschmer. Pointing out that Kretschmer's cycloid character coincides with his strong, unbalanced, "unrestrained" type (choleric temperament, according to Hippocrates) and the schizoid with the weak type (melancholic temperament, according to Hippocrates) Pavlov notes the inadequacy of this classification. He disagrees with Kretschmer in that the latter, proceeding from the data of the psychiatric clinic, from disease to health, rather than the other way round, dogmatically and schematically divides all people into two types—the schizothymic and cyclothymic. p. 325

[71] The article "Experimental Pathology of the Higher Nervous Activity" was translated from the text published in the second edition of I. P. Pavlov's *Complete Works* (Vol. III, Book 2, Moscow and Leningrad, 1951, pp. 294-314).

It constitutes the lecture delivered by Pavlov at the Institute for Advanced Medical Training in Leningrad, May 10, 1934. This article was also published as a separate booklet in Russian, German, English and French (Leningrad, Biomedgiz, 1935), in the book *Modern Problems of Theoretical Medicine* (Vol. I, Moscow and Leningrad, 1936, pp. 46-61) and the journal *Clinique* (1936, pp. 159-64).

Of interest in this article which sums up the many years of research in experimental pathology of higher nervous activity are Pavlov's indications of the significance of this research for the psychiatric clinic. Pavlov writes: "To a considerable degree the pathological nervous states produced by us conform to the so-called psychogenic diseases in human beings." (Present edition, p. 364.)

The article offers, also for the first time, a pathophysiological substantiation of combined therapy (bromides + caffeine) of nervous and mental diseases; Pavlov sees this pathophysiological substantiation in the fact that bromides and caffeine are "so to speak, two levers in the form of pharmaceutical remedies, two communicators towards the two chief apparatus, i.e., towards the two processes of nervous activity; then by putting into action and correspondingly changing the strength now of one, now of the other lever, we have a chance of restoring the distributed processes to their former place, into their proper correlations." (Present edition, p. 373.) p. 355

[72] The article "The Conditioned Reflex" is an excerpt from the work under the same title published in the second edition of I. P. Pavlov's *Complete Works* (Vol. III, Book 2, Moscow and Leningrad, 1951, pp. 335-43).

Published in the Big Soviet Encyclopedia and the Big Medical Encyclopedia (BSE, Vol. 56, 1936 and BME, Vol. 33, 1936) this article contains an extremely concise exposition of Pavlov's entire teaching on higher nervous activity. Besides, it was published in the *U.S.S.R. Physiological Journal,* (Vol. XIX, Book 1, 1935, p. 261). The concluding part of the article translated in the present edition deals with the parts of the teaching on higher nervous activity which are directly connected with the nervous and psychiatric clinics. In the teaching on types Pavlov's new statement on the interrelations of the inborn and the acquired deserves attention.

Pavlov writes: "The final, available nervous activity of the animal is an alloy of the type traits and the changes conditioned by the external·environment—phenotype, character." (I. P. Pavlov, *Complete Works,* 2nd ed., Vol. III, Book 2, p. 334.)

The physiological analysis of man's emotional life given in this article is also of considerable interest. Pavlov connects man's emotional life in its positive or negative tone with the course (easy or difficult) of the basic nervous processes in the cerebral hemispheres. It should be noted that, as regards the physiology of feelings, Pavlov expressed himself quite fully also in his other work "Dynamic Patterns of the Higher Part of the Brain", where he connected the emergence of emotions with changes in the dynamic pattern of nervous activity.

"I believe", Pavlov wrote in this work, "that there are sufficient grounds for assuming that the above-described physiological processes in the cerebral hemispheres conform to what we use to designate subjectively as our *senses,* and in the form of their numerous nuances and variations due to different combinations and intensities. Among these are the senses of difficulty and facility gaiety, and fatigue, satisfaction and chagrin, joy, triumph, despair, etc. It seems to me that the painful senses which often accompany a change in the habitual mode of life, an interruption of customary work, loss of close relations or friends to say nothing of mental crisis and collapse of beliefs, are, to a considerable degree, physiologically caused precisely by the change, the disturbance of the old dynamic stereotype and the difficulty of elaborating a new one." (I. P. Pavlov, *Complete Works,* 2nd ed., Vol. III, Book 2, Moscow and Leningrad, 1951, pp. 243-44.)

In this article Pavlov very concisely and clearly sums up all his formerly expressed ideas regarding the physiological interpretation of the different, most important psychopathological phenomena and mental diseases. He offers one more definition of the second signalling system (present edition, p. 378).   p. 378

[73] The article "Types of Higher Nervous Activity, Their Relationship to Neuroses and Psychoses, and the Physiological Mechanism of Neurotic and Psychotic Symptoms" was translated from the text published in the second edition of I. P. Pavlov's *Complete Works* (Vol. III, Book 2, Moscow and Leningrad, 1951, pp. 344-49). It contains the report made by Pavlov to a special conference arranged during the Second International Neurological Congress in London, July 30, 1935. The report was published in abbreviated form in the journal *Revue neurologique*, Vol. 64, No. 4, October, 1935, p. 633.

The new and most complete characterisation of the second signalling system deserves the principal attention in this article. In connection with this characterisation Pavlov again sets forth his teaching on specifically human types and on specifically human neuroses. Pavlov's clinical and pathophysiological characterisation of the basic forms of neuroses—neurasthenia, hysteria and psychasthenia—in this article is particularly clear and expressive. Although in his earlier works Pavlov had already mentioned pathological lability of the basic nervous processes, in addition to pathological inertness, in this article the question of pathological lability is most fully elucidated.   p. 387

[74] The article "The Problem of Sleep" was translated from the text published in the second-edition of I. P. Pavlov's *Complete Works* (Vol. III, Book 2, Moscow and Leningrad, 1951, pp. 409-27). This article is a shorthand record of Pavlov's report to the Conference of Neuropathologists and Psychiatrists of Leningrad in December 1935. It was first published in the first edition of I. P. Pavlov's *Complete Works* (Leningrad, 1940, Vol. I, p. 410). In his recollections N. Krasnogorsky mentions that Pavlov told him two weeks before his death that he planned to write a book on sleep (see preface to N. I. Krasnogorsky's book *Development of the Physiological Activity of the Brain in Children*, Moscow, 1939).

"The Problem of Sleep" is Pavlov's last work on sleep in which he summed up all his preceding statements on this subject. Of considerable interest in this work is the direct indication of the importance Pavlov attached to physiological investigations of sleep, his own investigations in particular. New and important in this work is also the emphasis he laid on the cortical regulation of sleep and his classical formulation of the role of the cortex in the vital activity of the organism in general: "The higher part controls all the phenomena which develop in the organism" (present edition, p. 394).

Pavlov's report and his answers to the questions put to him cover the very broad problem of sleep and related phenomena. The report contains a number of important statements on the physiological mechanism of sleep, hypnosis and dreams, the physiological mechanism of verbal suggestion, conditions of sleep, so-called "passive" sleep, etc. Pavlov criticises in his report the so-called "theory of the subcortical centre of sleep" and at the same time exhaustively explains in the light of his teaching the facts which formed the basis of this theory. According to the report, Pavlov no longer supports the proposition that sleep is irradiation only of internal inhibition, but holds that the initial moment in the emergence of sleep may be the process of inhibition of a most diverse character in the cortex. This coincides with F. P. Maiorov's statement that in a conversation with him on the question of classifying inhibitions in 1935 Pavlov noted that "hypnotic inhibition may be of either one or the other origin, i. e., it may develop from either "conditioned" or "unconditioned" inhibition (F. P. Maiorov, *History of the Teaching on Conditioned Reflexes*, Moscow, 1954, p. 296).

NAME INDEX

Andreyev, L. A., 82
Arkhangelsky, V. M., 120
Anokhin, P. K., 140

Babinski, J. F.F., 274
Bernheim, H. M., 274
Bierman, B. N., 83, 128, 136
Bleuler, P.E., 320
Blumenau, L. V., 218
Bykov, K. M., 138

Charcot, Jean M., 199
Chechulin, S. I., 116, 123
Clérambault, G., 324

Deryabin, V. S., 165

Filaretov, I. I., 309, 350
Frolov, Y. P., 83, 121, 191
Fursikov, D. S., 83, 122, 123
Fyodorov, L. N., 177

Galkin, V. S., 261, 290, 400, 402, 405
Gantt, W. M., 132
Goltz, Friedrich Leopold, 283

Hess, Leo, 404, 407, 408
Hippocrates, 216, 252, 339, 352, 360
Hoche, A., 272, 280
Hunter, W., 297

Ivanov-Smolensky, A. G., 177

Kalmykov, M. P., 83
Kircher, A., 70

Janet, Pierre, 85, 93, 194, 227, 230, 265, 277, 303, 316, 323, 376, 381, 389, 390

Kleijn, A. de, 93, 127
Kraepelin, Emil, 231
Krasnogorsky, N. I., 38, 81, 120
Kreps, Y. M., 80
Kretschmer, Ernst, 280, 316, 321, 322, 323, 353, 381, 389, 391
Kupalov, P. S., 114, 132

Lebedinskaya, S. I., 141

Magnus, 84, 93, 127
Maiorov F. P., 329
Martynov, A. V., 255

Narbutovich, I. O., 225
Nikiforovsky, P. M., 165

Ostankov, P. A., 225

Pavlova, A. M., 53
Petrova, M. K., 51, 53, 58, 77, 80, 114, 158, 178, 195, 232, 252, 298, 311, 330, 332, 350, 372, 392, 397
Pirogov, N. I., 208
Podkopayev, N. A., 192, 357
Popov, N. A., 115
Prorokov, I. R., 83, 139, 196

Raymond, Fulgence, 277
Razenkov, I. P., 78, 81, 82, 120, 132

439

Rikman, V. V., 80, 131, 168, 178, 193, 262, 291
Rozental, I. S., 119, 121, 124, 129, 137, 330
Rozhansky, N. A., 37, 53, 59, 127

Schiff, Moritz, 62
Schilder, Paul, 247, 250
Sechenov, I. M., 44, 46
Shenger-Krestovnikova, N. R., 45, 76, 154
Sherrington, Sir Charles Scott, 62, 356
Shishlo, A. A., 80, 137
Snarsky, A. T., 22
Speransky, A. D., 80, 102, 108, 143, 180, 261, 290, 400, 402, 405
Stroganov, V. V., 83
Strümpell, Adolf, 44, 261, 289, 400
Szondi, L., 254

Tigerstedt, Robert, 72
Tolochinov, I. F., 20, 355

Valkov, A. V., 82
Vasilyev, P. N., 52
Vishnevsky, A. S., 185
Volborth, G. V., 198, 199, 245, 288, 356
Voskresensky, L. N., 53, 63, 127
Vvedensky, N. Y., 86, 133
Vyrzhikovsky, S. N., 329, 348

Wilson, Samuel, 400
Wolfson, S. G., 17

Yakovleva, V. V., 332, 334
Yerofeyeva, M. N., 75, 111, 153, 160
Yurman, M. N., 177

Zavadsky, I. V., 290
Zelyony, G. P., 119
Zimkin, N. V., 136
Zimkina, A. M., 177

SUBJECT INDEX

A

Action
—passionate, 267
—rational, 267
—toxic, 68
Aim of physiological investigation, 16
Ambivalence, 307
Analgesia, during hysteria, mechanism of, 272
Analyser
—motor, 199, 243
—skin, 177, 193
—sound, 176
Analysis, 262, 285
—higher, 223
Apathy during schizophrenia, 225
Artists, as a group of human beings, 275, 381
Association, 283, 286
Automatism
—mental, 324
—of hypnotised persons, 201
Auto-Suggestion, 268, 273, 394

B

Brain
—balancing centres of, 93
Bromides, 78, 96, 165, 166, 177, 214, 252, 295, 296, 301, 310, 313, 331, 345, 367, 370, 380, 381
—administration of, 252, 381
—their mixture with caffeine, 373, 374, 381

C

Caffeine, 82, 136, 342, 373
—mixture of bromide and, 373, 374, 381
Castration, 252, 313, 317, 363, 366
Catalepsy, 62, 66, 232, 390
—in hypnosis, 84, 199
—in schizophrenics, 228
Cataplexy, 390
Catatonia, 226, 228, 231, 315, 383, 391
Centres
—balancing of the brain, 93
—nervous, the struggle of, 257, 287
—of Magnus de Kleijn, 127
—of sleep, 404
—reflex, 239
Cerebral cortex
— — activity of, under various strong influences, 86
— — chronc pathological states of, 185
— — chronic weakness of, during hysteria, 267
— — coupling role of, 89
— — dissociations of, 260
— — functional delimitation of separate points of, 73

441

—— individual peculiarities of, certain elements of, 68
—— injury to certain parts of, 105
—— isolated inhibition of the motor region of, 63, 65, 68, 70, 199
—— isolated pathological points of, 314, 370, 371
—— low excitability of, 82
————— in aged persons, 85
—— mosaic nature of, 90, 113, 293
—— pathological states of, 178
—— representation of the external world in, 240
—— representation of the organism's internal world in, 240
—— signalling role of, 89
—— thrombosis and haemorrhage in, 66
—— tone of, 406, 412
———— during hypnosis, 268
Cerebral hemispheres, 394
—— activity of, 213
———— exclusion of, 63
————— of the motor region of, 63
—— active state of, 44
———— conditions for, 44, 46, 49-70
—— as the chief organ of higher nervous activity, 87
—— as the nervous organ of the voluntary movements, 62
—— destruction of, in progressive paralysis, 66
—— influence of, on the subcortex, 265
—— laws governing the activity of, 256
———— disturbance of, during nervous and mental diseases, 189
———— elimination of, without the suppression of the lower parts of the brain, 62
—— minimum of stimulations necessary for the active state of, 44
—— pathological activity of, 66-67, 74
—— pathological states of, 153
—— physiological work of, 97
—— plastic character of the activity of, 224
—— resting states of, 44
—— sleep inhibition in, 65
—— thrombosis and haemorrhage in, 66
Character, types of, 213
Chloral hydrate, 140
Circularity
— after castration, 363
— of the nervous activity, 385
Collision between the excitatory and inhibitory processes, 77, 79, 97, 157, 168, 177, 185, 213, 313
———————— as the cause of nervous and mental diseases, 190
Complex, dynamic, structural, 370
Conditioning, biological significance of, 264
Confusion of opposite ideas, 308
Connection(s), temporary, 209, 283, 286
—— conditioned, 257
— between psychology and physiology, 297
Constitution, 208
Contralism, mechanism of, 307
Contraposition, general notion of, 305
Cortical cells, the limit of functional capacity of, 259, 288
—— different phases in the activity of, 98
—— exhaustion of, 119-120
—— functional destructibility of, 98, 105, 151
—— inhibited state of, 105
—— in the excitable type, 221
—— in the inhibitory type, 221

— — pathological state of, 359
— — refractive state of, 50
— — transition of, from the normal state of excitation to that of complete inhibition, 134
— — unreceptiveness of, 50
Cyclothymics, 352-354, 385

D

Decerebration, 62
Delimitation, functional, of separate points of cerebral cortex, 73-74
— of excitation and inhibition in space, 74
Delusion, 323-324
— of persecution, 206, 323, 376, 381
Development of depression (inhibition), 39, 73
— — speed of, 39, 40
Difference
— between external and internal inhibition, 73
— between unconditioned and conditioned reflexes, 88
Differentiation, 77, 78, 95, 155, 245, 262, 285
Disease(s)
— nervous, significance of the type of nervous system, in, 379
— — and mental, their causes, 190
— — — differences between, 189
— of cortical cells in schizophrenia, 231
— psychogenic, 364
Disinhibition, 81, 287
Disorders, nervous functional, conditions of, 190
— of nervous activity in the dog, phases of, 79
Dissociation
— functional, 289
— of the cortex, 360

Distortion of the action of conditioned stimuli, 80
Distraction, senile, 270
Dreams, 203, 296, 410
Drives, 223, 284

E

Echolalia, 228
Echopraxia, 228
Education and training, dependence of behaviour on, 327, 329-340
Emaciation, its effect on cortical cells, 121
Emotions, 284
Equilibrium
— of nervous processes, 74, 97, 325, 326, 330, 331, 387
— — — conditions, disturbing, 379
— of the organism, external and internal, 16
Eudetism in children, 275
Excitation, 132
— conflict between inhibition and, 74
— explosion of, 192
— in hysteriacs, 191
— latent focus of, 257
— movement through the cerebral cortex, of the process of inhibition and, 90
— relation between inhibition and, 72, 73, 74, 214
Excitatory process
— — changes of, 360
— — changes in the mobility of, 360, 391
— — collision between the inhibitory and, 77, 79, 97, 157, 168, 177, 185, 213
— — concentration of, 257
— — decline of, in old age, 269
— — explosiveness of, 350, 386
— — in connection with dissimilation, 292
— — inertness of, 324, 337, 338, 350, 360, 386, 391, 392

443

— — irradiation of, 292
— — lability of, 386
— — method of ascertaining the strength of, 340
— — strong, 341, 342
— — weak, 341, 342
— — weakening of, 390
Exhaustion of the elements of the cortex, 68
Experiments, psychical, 18, 20
Experimentum mirabile of Kircher, 70
Explosiveness, 360, 391
— of the excitatory process, 350, 386

F

Fatigue, 410
Fear, physiological mechanism of, 205
Feelings of possession, 303, 376, 381, 386, 390
Frontal lobes, 276
— — as the organ of human mentality, 297
Functions
— of the organism, involuntary, 241
— — voluntary, 241
— speech, 296

G

Generalisation, the law of, 324
Glands
— salivary, 13
— — activity of, 14
— — psychical reaction of, 17
— thyroid, 82

H

Hallucinations, 319
Hebephrenia, 226, 231
Human beings,
— — artists, as a group of, 275, 381
— thinkers, as a group of, 275, 276, 381

Hunger, and its effect on conditioned reflexes, 99
Hypersthenia in dogs, 254
Hypnotising
— hysteriacs, 199
— man, 198
Hypnosis, 32, 146, 199, 202, 234, 236, 289, 398, 411, 412
— and the state of the musculature, 235, 399
— animal, 70, 93, 130, 178
— degree of, 233, 234
— different stages of, 260
— human, 226
— loss of voluntary movements during, 199
— lowered positive tone in the cortex during, 268
— physiology of, 232, 239, 241
— verbal method of, 408
Hypnotics, 140
Hypnotism, 70, 198
Hypothalamus
— changes in, 404, 405
Hysteria, 191, 218, 255, 262, 264, 296, 365, 381
— affective, passionate action, 267
— analgesia, 272
— as a result of a weak nervous system, 265
— attacks of excitement, 192
— auto-suggestibility in, 268
— cortical inhibition in, 193
— cortical weakness, 218, 266
— destruction of general nervous equilibrium, 390
— disturbance of psychical synthesis in, 277
— emotivity, 267, 273, 390
— excitement, 191
— fantasticism, 274, 296, 390
— in dogs, 214, 254
— in the form of complete sleep, 266
— in the form of deep hypnosis, 266
— paralysis, 272
— perseveration, 314
— physiological phenomena, 278

444

— possibility of cure, 279
— refuge in illness, as a symptom of, 272, 279
— split ego, 277
— stereotypy, 314
— suggestibility, 218, 268
— symptoms of, 272
— synthesis of personality, the destruction of, 390
— twilight states, 274, 296
— type of nervous system in, 389
— weakness of the second signalling system, 390
Hysteriacs
— attacks of excitement in, 191

I

Illusions
— of people, 195
— visual, in dogs, 194
Impulses
— stimulating, 261
Induction, 125, 245, 257
— negative, 257, 287, 292, 324
— — in hysteriacs, 278
— positive, 192, 261, 290, 344, 345
— reciprocal, 83, 90, 256, 286, 287, 290, 307
Inertness, pathological, 313, 314, 317, 338, 360
— — as a result of catatonic attack, 315
— — basis for, 318
— — causes of, 318
— — chronic, 317
— — concentration of, 318
— — in compulsive neurosis, 315
— — in paranoia, 315
— — of nervous processes, in old age, 349
— — of the process of excitation, 314, 324, 337, 350, 359, 386, 391
Inhibition, 105, 394
— active, 258, 288, 331, 402

— as a law of induction, 257
— complete, 173, 174
— concentrated, 122
— concentration of, 40, 261
— conditioned, 37, 287
— — of the second order, 245
— conflict between excitation and, 73-74
— consecutive, 138, 344
— — cortical, 258, 331
— cortical localised, 199, 243
— difference between internal and external, 73
— diffuse, intensity of, 131
— equilibrium between excitation and, 74
— external, 72, 139, 201, 257, 287
— identity of sleep and, 123
— — in catatonic state, 383
— — in hysteriacs, 193-194
— — in schizophrenia, 230
— internal, 59, 62, 139, 288, 331
— irradiation of, 73
— kinds of, 258, 259, 260
— motion of, 90, 123, 259, 400
— of the activity of the cerebral hemispheres, 127
— of the motor region of the cerebral cortex, 63, 65, 66, 67, 70, 93
— partial, 200
— passive, 257, 287, 321
— relation between excitation and, 72, 73, 74, 80, 214, 268
— repetition of, 124, 125
— replacement of, with sleep, 121
— sleep, 64, 65
— speed of spread of, 38, 39, 40
— transmarginal, 259, 288, 350
— unconditioned, 257, 287
— weakness of, 344, 345
— which protects reactive cells of the organism, 226
Inhibitor
— conditioned, 36
— general, of conditioned reflex, 33, 34, 35

445

Inhibition
— limitation of the process of, 114
Inhibitory process, 105, 113, 114, 392
— — fundamental laws of, 286
— — in connection with assimilation, 292
— — inertness of, 338, 392
— — lability of, 392
— — overstrain of, 302
— — spreading of, 73, 90
— — weakening of, 82, 83, 391
Instinct(s), 87, 223, 273, 284
Inversion, 322, 382, 386, 390
Investigation
— objective, 29
— physiological, the aim of, 16
Irradiation, 40, 256, 286
— of excitation, 292
— of inhibition, 395
Isolated cortical points, pathological state of, 384
Iteration, 314, 385

L

Lability
— of the nervous processes, 348
— pathological, of the excitatory processes, 386
Law,
— governing the activity of cerebral hemispheres, 256, 285
— of concentration of the processes of excitation and inhibition, 256
— of coupling, 88, 97
— of induction see Induction
— of irradiation of the processes of excitation and inhibition, 256, 292
— of maximum, 291, 306
— of summation, 291
Lethargy, 266
Living being

— — general characteristic of, 208
— — its ability of adaptation, 209
— — specific activity of, 208

M

Mentality, higher, specially human, 297
Movements
— abortive, 234
— stereotypic, during schizophrenia, 225
— volitional, 292
— voluntary, 292

N

Narcolepsy, 390
Negativism, 233
— negative, 233, 234, 244
— phases of, 233, 244
— physiological mechanism of, 243, 307
— — positive, 233, 234, 244
Nervous activity,
— — basic processes of, 357
— — central, 386
— — circularity in, 385
— — higher, 188, 240, 285
— — — and stereotypic nervous activity, 239
— — — pathological state of, 361
— — — physiology of, 256, 262, 282
— — lower, 285
— — normal, 379
— — — disturbance of, 74
— — stereotypic, 239
Nervous processes
— — basic properties of, 357
— — concentration of, 65, 262
— — during hysteria, 278
— — equilibrium of, 325, 326, 339, 387

446

— — lability of, 348
— — mobility of, 325, 326, 332, 339, 345, 349, 387
— — — changes in, 350
— — — decline of, in old age, 349
— — methods causing their pathology, 358
— — strength of, 325, 326, 330, 339, 387
Nervous system
— — adaptation of, 213
— — central, 223
— — functional changes in, 94
— its plasticity, 224, 327
— — plasticity of, 327
— — state of, under hypnosis, 204
— — — chronic pathological, 154
— — test of adaptation of, 213
— — — of strength, 213
— — weakened, 194
Neurasthenia, 191, 217, 381
— as a pathological form inherent in the feeble-general and intermediate human type, 389
— forms of, 381
— in dogs, 214, 254
Neuroses, 214, 221, 247, 249
— compulsive, 309, 315, 319, 320, 385, 386
— experimental, 72, 165-166, 249, 251, 298, 316
— — after castration, 363
— human, 94, 365, 389
— of types of nervous system, significance in, 249, 251, 380, 389
— traumatic, 381
— treatment of, 195-197, 214, 252, 295, 298, 369, 380
— with predominance of excitation, 214
— — — of inhibition, 214

O

Objectification of an internal cerebral process, 372
Old age,
— — diminishing reactivity of the brain in, 201
Organism and its environment, 32, 37, 62, 89, 209, 210, 262, 276, 285
— its external and internal equilibrium, 16
Overstrain
— of the excitatory process, 311, 313, 318
— of the inhibitory process, 302

P

Pain
— cortical, 372
— mental, 372
Paralysis
— functional, 272
— progressive, 66
Paranoia, 309, 315, 316, 319, 321, 375, 385, 386, 391
— of types of nervous system, significance in, 320
Paranoia, pathological inertness in, 315, 320
Pattern(s), dynamic, 293
— of higher nervous activity, 142
Pavlov's advice concerning the treatment of the mentally ill, 231
Perseveration, 314, 385
Phases
— equalisation, 83, 91, 97, 134, 136, 172, 174, 181, 260, 289, 305, 359
— hypnotic, 93, 104, 126, 198, 226
— intermediate, between wakefulness and sleep, 90, 91, 93, 103, 126, 198, 226
— in the activity of the cells of the cerebral cortex, 98
— narcotic, 141, 202

447

— of complete inhibition, 83, 173, 174
— of pathological inertness, 321
— of sleep, 64, 145
— paradoxical, 83, 91, 92, 93, 94, 97, 106, 133, 136, 137, 138, 172, 174, 203, 243, 260, 272, 289, 305, 313, 359, 384
— — during hysteria, 278
— ultra-paradoxical, 138, 164, 183, 260, 289, 303, 305, 307, 313, 323, 359, 386
— — during delusion, 323, 376
Phobias, 107, 206
— of depth, 392
Physiology
— connection between psychology and, 297
— of hypnosis, 239
— of the higher nervous activity, 256, 262, 282
Points,
— isolated, pathological, of the cerebral cortex, 314, 370, 371, 384
— — — — — during hysteria, 278
— — — — — during compulsive neurosis, 375
— — — — — during paranoia, 375
— on duty (or on guard), 84, 410
Pregnancy, phantom, 240, 273, 394
Psychasthenia, 365, 390
— mechanisms of, 391
— weakness of the first signalling system during, 390
Psychology, its connection with physiology, 297
Psychopathology, experimental, 28
Psychoses, 189, 381
— endogenous, 218
— hysterical, 278
— manic-depressive, 353, 385, 389
Puerilism, hysterical, 278

R

Reaction(s), motor, 24
— — food, 235
— of the cerebral hemispheres to conditioned stimuli, 143
— psychical, 17
— secretory, 24
Reactivity of the brain, diminution of, in old age, 201
Reflexes, 12, 84, 206
— active, 32
— auto-curative, 236, 245
— conditioned, 20, 26, 46, 63, 72, 88, 94, 188, 210, 255, 257, 283, 356, 378
— difference between unconditioned and conditioned, 88
— disappearance of, 47
— equilibrating, 62, 66
— food, 87, 94, 210, 223, 241
— idea of, 87
— imitative, during hypnosis,
— inborn, 209, 210
— inhibitory, 179, 288
— initial inhibitory, 288
— interrelation between secretory and motor, 55, 56, 57
— investigating, 115, 118, 161, 179
— mechanism of, 88
— of caution, 179, 330
— of time, 310
— orienting, 292
— panic, 330
— passive, 32
— passive-defensive, 178, 198, 204
— self-protecting, 70
— signalling, 210
— sleep, 31-34
— social, 108
— spinal, 66
— study of, 210
— summation, 257, 286
— temporary, 209
— tonic, 62
— trace, 35
— unconditioned, 20, 26, 87, 210, 223, 284
— — centres of, 223

— variable, 209
Reflex, conditioned
— — biological significance of, 88
— — conditions for the formation of, 284
— — delayed, 290
— — effect of hunger on, 99
— — external phases of, 290-291
— — food, 75-77
— — formation of, 46, 89
— — inhibitory, 89, 94
— — inhibitors of, 33
— — method of, 99, 226, 255
— — negative, 89, 167, 188, 211, 362
— — place of origin of, 256
— — positive, 89, 167, 188, 211, 362
— — — formation of, in dogs, 220
— — reinforcement of, 47
— — step-by-step decline of, 140
— — theory of, 256
— — thermal, 49, 112
— — to sound, 64, 112
Relations
— between different kinds of inhibition, 259
— between the conscious and the unconscious, 206
— between excitation and inhibition, 72, 73, 74, 80, 268
— disturbances in, 214
— "psychic", 209

S

Schizophrenia, 218, 225, 383, 389
— apathy, 225
— as a chronic hypnosis, 230
— catatonic form of, 314, 383
— exhaustion of the nervous system, 230
— functional disease of cortical cells in, 231

— perseveration in, 314
— protective role of inhibition in, 230
— stereotypy in, 314
— symptoms of, 227, 228, 229, 230
— torpor in, 225
— weakness of cortical cells during, 230
Schizothymics, 352-53
Senses
— categories of, 294
— negative, 294
— positive, 294
Separate cortical elements, individual peculiarities of, 68
Signals
— first, of reality, 296
— of the second order, 388
— second set of, 296
Signalling system
— — first, 276, 296, 378, 310
— — in hysteria, 390
— — in psychastheniacs, 390
— — second, 276, 296, 378, 388, 310
Sleep, 31, 34, 44, 47, 48, 51, 52, 53, 93, 124, 226, 260, 289, 412
— accompanied by partial wakefulness, 84
— active, 260, 402
— after extirpation of the cerebral hemispheres, 403, 405
Sleep
— alternation between waking and, 125
— alternation of activity and, 125
— as a result of diminished sum of stimulations, 44, 45, 46
— as a result of inhibition of the investigating reflex, 116
— as an inhibitory process, 59, 90, 109, 110, 397, 400, 402
— centre of, 261, 404, 407, 408
— chemical causes of, 32
— continuous, 194, 230

449

— development of, in acoustic conditioned reflexes, 112
— — in thermal conditioned reflexes, 112
— deep, 56
— deep and chronic, 290
— effect of short, strong stimuli on, 130
— effect of weak, long-continued general stimulation on, 130
— encephalitic, 404
— hypnotic, 48
— identity with inhibition, 123
— influence of surroundings on, 37, 38, 48, 54, 56, 57, 58, 63, 119
— intensity of, 131
— interchange of wakefulness and, 412
— normal, 93, 289
— occurrence of fits during, 411
— overcoming, 51
— partial, 112
— passive, 260, 402
— phases of, 63, 64, 113
— transitional, between waking state and, 90, 91, 103, 126, 198, 226
— reflex, 408
— replacement of inhibition with, 121
— significance of continued or repeated stimulation for, 124
— significance of the duration of conditioned stimulation for, 112
— standing, 93, 194
— struggle against, 112
— with points on guard, 84
Sleepiness, 32, 122
So-called psychical phenomena, psychological explanation of, 255
Speech, 277, 296
State
— cataleptic, 61, 62, 66, 93, 127, 130
— waking, 44

— — internal inhibition as the most important factor of, 113
Stereotype, dynamic, 293, 294
Stereotypy, 314, 385, 391
Stimulation, 35
— mechanical, of the skin, 35, 49
— reflex, 32
— thermal, 31, 34, 49
Stimulus(i)
— absolute energy of, 91
— conditioned, isolated, 105, 110
— conditioned, 135, 142
— — distortion of the action of, 80
— — negative and positive, 113
— effect of the sum of, 22
— external, which act as direct inhibitors of the cortical cells, 178
— inhibitory, 288
— mechanical, of the skin, 49, 120
— negative, 113, 137
— positive, 113, 137
— strong, the action of, 178, 182, 185
— — as the cause of nervous and mental diseases in man, 190
— variety of, and their influence on the onset of sleep, 51
— weak, 178, 188
Stupor, 66, 71
Subcortex,
— influence of the state of cerebral hemispheres on, 266
— predominance of, during hysteria, 278
Suggestion, 48, 202, 203, 268
— hypnotic, 84, 268, 394
Sum of the stimuli, 22
Summation, the law of, 291
Symptoms, pathological, their causes, 67
— schizophrenic, 228, 229, 230
Synthesis, 206, 262, 284, 285
— higher, 223

T

Temperament(s), 208, 216, 222, 294, 339, 352, 387, 388
— choleric, 216, 217, 218, 222, 263, 339, 388
— classification of, 107, 216, 222
— dependence of, on the property of the cerebral hemispheres, 223
— melancholic, 107, 216, 218, 222, 388
— normal, 216
— pathological, 216
— phlegmatic, 216, 217, 222, 263, 294, 340, 354, 360, 388
— sanguine, 107, 216, 217, 222, 263, 294, 340, 354, 388
Thinking, concrete, elementary, 285
Thrombosis and haemorrhage in the cerebral hemispheres, 66
Timidity, 107, 205
Tone
— latent, 286
— of the cerebral cortex, 406
— — — in hypnosis, 268
Torpor in schizophrenia, 225
Transitional states, from excitation to inhibition, 79, 83, 134
Type(s) of nervous system, 41, 49-50, 96, 100, 106, 147, 148, 151, 152, 157, 164, 173, 174, 208, 213, 214, 216, 217, 218, 220, 221, 222-224, 251, 252, 262, 281, 293-295, 298, 330, 351, 352, 379, 387, 389

— — — and hysteria, 389-390
— — — and neurasthenia, 389-390
— — — and psychasthenia, 389-390
— — — as subjects of neuroses, 263, 295
— — — classification of, 252
— — — — according to Kretschmer, 353
— — — human, 216-217, 275, 276, 352, 381, 388, 389,
— — — main, 220, 252, 352, 388
— — — perfect, 332, 334
— — — effect of castration on, 252
Type of higher nervous activity, 142
— — — — definition of, 327
— — — — part played by, in the genesis of nervous and mental diseases, 387

U

Urethan, 62, 140

W

Wakefulness
— interchange of sleep and, 412
— partial, 84, 188
Word, significance of, for man, 202, 378, 388

451